Men'sHealth®

BETTER BODY BLUEPRINT

Men'sHealth®

BETTER BODY BLUEPRINT

The Start-Right, Stick-to-It Strength Training Plan

MICHAEL MEJIA, CSCS

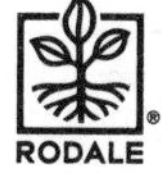

RODALE

Notice

The information in this book is meant to supplement, not replace, proper exercise training. All forms of exercise pose some inherent risks. The editors and publisher advise readers to take full responsibility for their safety and know their limits. Before practicing the exercises in this book, be sure that your equipment is well maintained, and do not take risks beyond your level of experience, aptitude, training, and fitness. The exercise and dietary programs in this book are not intended as a substitute for any exercise routine or dietary regimen that may have been prescribed by your doctor. As with all exercise and dietary programs, you should get your doctor's approval before beginning.

Mention of specific companies, organizations, or authorities in this book does not imply endorsement by the author or publisher, nor does mention of specific companies, organizations, or authorities imply that they endorse this book, its author, or the publisher.

Internet addresses and telephone numbers given in this book were accurate at the time it went to press.

Page 28: PowerBlock©, *courtesy of PowerBlock©*
Page 29: adjustable exercise bench and power cage equipment; page 32, adjustable cable station, stationary bike, elliptical machine; page 33, Smith Machine equipment; page 36, leg extension equipment and machine row equipment, *courtesy of Body-Solid Inc.*
Page 29: squat rack; page 33, hip abduction equipment; page 36, lat pulldown and pec deck equipment equipment; *courtesy of Life Fitness*
Page 30: ProSpot P-500 equipment, *courtesy of ProSpotFitness©P-500*
Page 31: Versa Climber equipment, *courtesy of Versa Climber*
All other photos, *courtesy of Mitch Mandel/Rodale Inc.*
Illustrations © by Karen Kuchar

Printed in the United States of America
Rodale Inc. makes every effort to use acid-free ♾, recycled paper ♻.

Book design by Anthony Serge

Library of Congress Cataloging-in-Publication Data

Mejia, Michael.
Men's health better body blueprint : the start-right, stick-to-it strength training plan / Michael Mejia.
p. cm.
Includes index.
ISBN-13 978–1–59486–331–8 hardcover
ISBN-10 1–59486–331–8 hardcover
1. Exercise for men. 2. Physical fitness for men. 3. Bodybuilding. I. Men's health (Magazine) II. Title.
GV482.5.M45 2006
613.7'0449—dc22 2006002097

Distributed to the trade by Holtzbrinck Publishers

2 4 6 8 10 9 7 5 3 1 hardcover

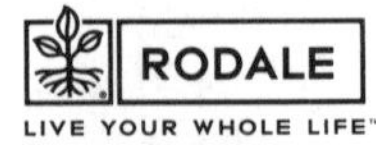

We inspire and enable people to improve their lives and the world around them

For more of our products visit **rodalestore.com** or call 800-848-4735

They say that behind every successful man is a good woman. Well, I'm lucky enough to have four women who stand beside me through everything I do. This book is therefore dedicated to them, without whom I would be completely lost.

To my mother, Catherine, who's served as my mentor, confidante, and assistant editor ever since I first started writing back in grade school. From my earliest years, you instilled in me the fervent belief that I could accomplish anything I set my mind to. Without your love, guidance, and undying support, I would never have turned into the man I am today.

To my wife, Michelle, whose tireless work ethic allowed me to pursue my dream of becoming a writer. You've supported me in every career decision I've ever made—whether you agreed with it or not. And on those occasions when things didn't work out, you simply worked harder so that our family wouldn't feel the hit. My love and appreciation for you and all that you do go beyond the scope of mere words.

And finally, to my daughters, Nicole and Brianna, without whom life simply wouldn't be worth living. You're the inspiration for everything that I do and every ambition I strive to fulfill. Together you've shown me the true meaning of life, as well as the importance of treasuring the things that matter most. I love you both more than you could possibly comprehend.

CONTENTS

INTRODUCTION

I know what you're thinking: "*Big* book." As if this whole fitness thing isn't confusing enough, the last thing you need is an encyclopedia-size reference guide just to drop a few pounds and fill out your shirtsleeves. After all, who's got time to sift through a tome like this? And even if you had the time, wouldn't it be better spent pumping and sweating your way to that chiseled physique you've dreamt about for so long? Wouldn't poring over this much information prior to even getting started basically amount to overkill?

I suppose that's an argument one could make. Seeing as how improving your fitness level and transforming your body into a visual specimen are both physical endeavors, the initial lack of physicality in this instance might seem a bit unsettling. You probably are chomping at the bit to get started and can't wait to get those first few workouts under your belt. Trust me when I tell you there'll be plenty of time for that soon enough. For right now, you need to learn how to go about things the right way. Maybe then you'll be able to avoid making some of the ridiculous—not to mention potentially dangerous—mistakes to which so many beginners fall victim. Mistakes that I myself made when I was first starting out and that I recount for you in painstaking detail in Chapter 1.

Not that I'm suggesting that you should read this entire book before ever engaging in a workout. But how are you supposed to have any clue about how to get started if you don't even know what type of beginner you are? Yes, believe it or not, there are different types. Chapter 2 will help you identify exactly which classification you fall into and help you lay out the appropriate training strategy. This first, seemingly insignificant step can go a long way toward determining whether or not you'll ultimately be successful in achieving the results you're looking for.

There's more to it than just classifying yourself as a particular kind of beginner. Once all the self-realization is complete, in Chapter 5 I'll ask you to put yourself through a pretty demanding set of tests to help identify your specific areas of weakness. Armed with the results from these tests, you can then proceed in a much more productive manner by custom-designing your own workout program. (Don't worry, I'll walk you through it every step of the way.) After that, there's a sort of break-in phase I call Basic Training, followed by a muscle-building phase, and then even a strength phase. Oh, and just in case you're interested in things like burning fat, improving your cardiovascular fitness, and becoming more flexible, I've addressed each of those critical fitness components at length throughout the entire book.

Before I go on, it might help to give you a little insight into my stance on this whole "getting in shape" thing. With more than 20 years of experience in the fitness industry, working with hundreds of people, I've developed some rather strong opinions on the subject. Perhaps none stronger than the idea that the better informed you are, the faster you're likely to progress. And isn't that really what it's all about—progression? Whether you're looking to get bigger, stronger, leaner, or more resistant to injury, the basic tenet is to improve yourself in some fashion. Otherwise, what's the point?

As you may have guessed from that last sentence, I'm not a big fan of training just for the sake of training. Don't get me wrong, I'm all for workouts being enjoyable—so long as they have some kind of purpose. You have to have some tangible goal to work toward, or else you'll just be spinning your wheels. It doesn't have to be grandiose; something as simple as dropping 5 pounds in a given time frame or being able to do 10 perfect pushups is fine. (We'll get into goal setting in much greater detail in Chapter 3.) Just simply going into a gym and indiscriminately pushing yourself is not the way to go.

Once you've established one or more goals, the next step is making sure you know the proper way to train in order to reach them. Not everyone has the money to plunk down for a personal trainer. Assuming you're one of the overwhelming majority who doesn't, you're going to have to turn to other sources to garner your fitness and nutritional information. Unfortunately, many of those "other sources" can be downright frightening in terms of the information they dole out.

All of which brings me to my reason for writing this book. Call it anger, call it frustration, call it a sense of duty if you want. I was just sick and tired of people who were starting out being given half-baked advice. It didn't matter whether those suggestions came from a know-it-all friend at work; the biggest, buffest guy at the gym; or the latest issue of *Muscle Monthly* magazine. Beginners were the red-headed stepchildren of the fitness industry, relegated to garnering what little knowledge they could from some of the most unreliable sources imaginable.

Until now. What I've done here is put together a comprehensive guide for beginners of all types. It doesn't matter if you've never picked up a dumbbell or you've tried and failed numerous times in the past to make fitness a regular part of your lifestyle. Nor does it matter how old you are. The information in the pages that follow takes into account the various changes your body goes through as you age and provides training advice and workout programs that are suitable to your current physical abilities.

Although it contains a multitude of different programs, this is not meant to be a book you occasionally consult when you need a new workout. It's meant to educate you about the proper way to get started. It will teach you things like what a realistic 1-month weight loss really is and how much you can expect to increase your bench press over the course of 2 months. Maybe along the way you'd also like to know whether it's better to use free weights or machines. Or whether exercises like squats and deadlifts are really as dangerous as you've heard. No matter what your question, you'll find the answer here.

Once you have finished the book and gone through all the programs specific to your individual needs, you'll have a decided edge over other beginners: You'll no longer be one of them. That's right, when you've read through all of the information, identified what type of beginner you are, put yourself through the self-assessment, and gone through the training programs in the sequential manner in which they're arranged, you will honestly be able to say that you are no longer a newbie. It may not seem like much, but take it from someone who knows, it's a level a lot of people never get to. Remember, there's no shame in being a beginner; the sad part is never progressing beyond that point.

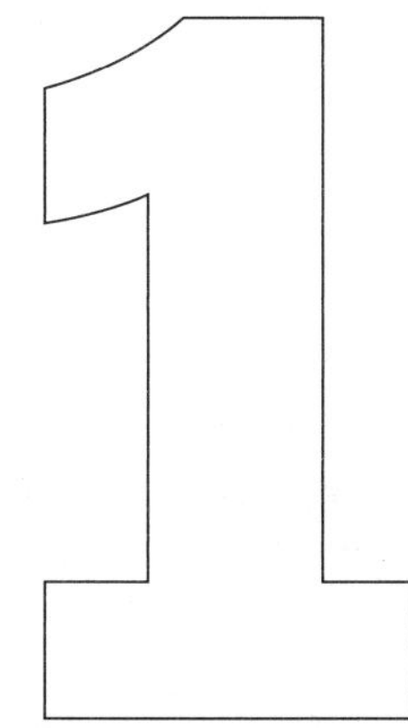

WE'RE ALL BEGINNERS AT SOME POINT

THE KEY IS LEARNING HOW TO PROGRESS BEYOND THAT POINT

I've got a bit of a confession to make. Now, I realize this might sound strange coming from someone in my position, but I didn't always know my way around a weight room. I mean, it's not as if I came out of the womb knowing how to design an effective training program, or able to demonstrate the proper form for a squat. There was once a time when, like you, I felt awkward and unsure of myself upon entering a gym. In fact, it didn't even have to be an actual "gym"; I used to feel self-conscious just working out in my buddy's basement back when I was a teenager. I guess what I'm trying to say is that despite having co-written several books and countless articles about fitness, not to mention having conducted thousands of training sessions with my clients over the years, I too was once a beginner.

Uh-oh, there it is: the "B" word. The one thing no self-respecting male will ever cop to being. You can call a man a lot of things—a liar, a cheat, a perfect candidate for a visit from the Queer Eye guys—but don't ever call him a beginner, particularly when it comes to working out. There's just something in the average guy's genetic code that makes it impossible for him to admit that he doesn't know what to do around the heavy iron.

Think I'm exaggerating? Go up to any guy who isn't—or at least looks as if he isn't—currently lifting weights and ask him why he's not. Assuming you don't just get punched square in the face, you're bound to hear excuses like "Who's got the time?" or "I just can't stand that whole gym atmosphere" or the ever-popular " I hurt myself lifting weights years ago and never got back into it."

About the only thing you *won't* hear is an honest admission of ignorance on the subject. And when you stop and think about it, why would you? After all, most of us have had at least some exposure to weight training by the time we hit 16, so there's some level of perceived familiarity there. Besides which, this stuff isn't exactly rocket science. Put weights on barbell. Pick bar up. Put bar down. Easy, right?

What if I told you there was more to it than that—a *lot* more? And what if I also told you that you don't know as much as you think you do, because most of what you've heard and read is dead wrong?

Okay, perhaps that was a bit strong. Suffice it to say that the bulk of diet and exercise information that's currently available is of little use to most beginners. It is often contradictory and places too much emphasis on reaching arbitrary goals, such as exercising at a specific heart rate or doing a particular number of strength-training sets and repetitions, rather than addressing your specific needs as an individual. These are factors that I'll discuss in detail shortly. For now, though, just realize that there's no shame in admitting you're not sure how to go about getting started. Even the best of us initially have trouble making sense of all of this.

BEEN THERE, DONE THAT

RECOUNTING SOME EARLY MISSTEPS

Trust me; I know what you're going through. When I first started training I thought it was going to be a piece of cake. I was convinced that the mere act of picking up a dumbbell was going to send my young, testosterone-laden body into a veritable muscle-building frenzy. Unfortunately, as I soon came to learn, it was a bit more complicated than that. Much of the complication stemmed from the fact that there is a whole lot more to this training thing than what I had learned back in high school gym class. Apparently, bench presses and biceps curls aren't the only exercises known to man. Go figure, huh? So you can imagine my surprise when I was first exposed to all the cool-looking machines and intriguing free-weight exercises there were to learn. And although I eventually did learn them, I had some rather interesting experiences along the way.

I remember one time in particular when I positioned myself on a machine facing the wrong direction. You can just imagine the amusement of the other gym members as I struggled to figure out how I could possibly pull handles that were a good $2\frac{1}{2}$ feet behind me without ripping my shoulders out of their sockets. I doubt anyone was looking at me that day and thinking, "There's a future contributing editor to a major men's health magazine." Then of course there was the time when I sent weights flying all over the place because I loaded more weight on one side of the bar than on the other and forgot to use collars. Let me tell you, nothing screams geek like heavy metal plates crashing to the floor in one loud, attention-grabbing crescendo.

And keep in mind, those were just the events other people witnessed. I suffered a string of private indignities right in the comfort of my own home before I ever got anywhere near a gym. Like the time I nearly broke my jaw by clocking myself in the chin with the bar while trying to do shoulder presses. Or how about when I fell to the floor in a heap because I hadn't properly secured my makeshift pullup bar in the door frame. The downstairs neighbors really appreciated that one. And how could I possibly forget nearly decapitating myself by taking all the weight off of one side of a loaded barbell, causing it to go whizzing past my face as it fell to the floor on the other side of the bench. Talk about seeing your life pass before your eyes!

It wasn't all bad, though. Like I said, I eventually started to figure things out. I pretty much had to. Otherwise I would've left myself open to the constant meddling of gym floor instructors (personal trainers were just *starting* to come into vogue back then) and other gym members who were always looking to "help out the new guy." Don't get me wrong—a little occasional guidance was nice, especially if the person offering the advice actually knew what he or she was talking about. Unfortunately, though, it was more often a case of the blind leading the blind. If I had a dime for all the half-baked advice and misinformation I was given when I was starting out, I'd be a multimillionaire with bad hair, hosting my own reality show on a major network by now.

One of the more humorous tidbits of information I was once offered was that I should start out with a "good, solid program—like the ones they have in the muscle mags." Ah yes, the muscle mags. Those bastions of fitness knowledge where training advice is readily dispensed by drug-induced mutants wearing clown pants and combat boots. I mean really now, where else could you go for tips on making your arms the size of tree trunks, courtesy of a guy with skin the color and texture of a leather sofa? Oh sure, it's funny now, but given my desperate state at the time, I was actually dumb enough to try some of those routines. I'm not sure whether it was due to the lack of results, the debilitating soreness, or my refusal to treat my body like a chemical dumping ground, but I soon figured out those magazines had little to offer in the way of viable training information.

To be fair, the advice coming from the instructors at the local gym wasn't much better. Granted, it was less extreme; they weren't recommending 30-set chest routines for people who'd never picked up a weight before. But it was every bit as misguided in its own way. For instance, when I first signed up and received my initial gym "orientation," I was led through a poorly conceived workout that gave no consideration to my age or current level of fitness, let alone to any of my individual goals. Not surprisingly, it also turned out to be the exact same workout given to a heavyset woman in Day-Glo spandex pants and an elderly gentleman with a noticeable limp. Thus began my skepticism with the way that beginners are treated in the weight room.

And I haven't even touched on the can of worms that is "cardio" training. You think the advice circulating about lifting is confusing? Try getting two different people to give you the same answer about the best way to burn fat or improve cardiovascular function. I'm telling you, it's not gonna happen. There are just too many conflicting opinions out there about such things as how much cardio you should do, how often, whether you should do it fast or slow, before weight training or after, do high impact or low impact, do it first thing in the morning on an empty stomach or later in the day, an hour or so after eating. And the list goes on and on. The sad part is that these are the *same* questions that people were asking 20 years ago, when I was first starting out. Yep, we've sure got a handle on this whole fitness thing all right.

LAND OF CONFUSION

SEEKING OUT THE RIGHT INFORMATION

I guess the point I'm trying to make here is that with all the confusion and misinformation that abounds in the fitness industry, there's no shame in admitting that you need a little help. It's one thing to refuse to ask for directions or to try to assemble something without following the instructions; that's for you and your significant other to work out. But if you think you can walk into a gym or any other type of training environment and just wing it, think again. Forget about looking foolish—there's a pretty good chance you could end up getting seriously hurt. Ironic, isn't it, that something designed to improve your overall health and physical appearance could, if done improperly, be potentially detrimental to it?

That's exactly why it's so important for you to have the right information from the get-go. There's no need for you to waste weeks, months, or even years constantly starting and then stopping a workout program because you can't get the results you're looking for. Believe me, every guy with huge arms, a chiseled midsection, or seemingly endless endurance was once a beginner, just like you. The only difference between the two of you is that he was able to figure out what worked for him and stick with it long enough to reap the rewards of all his hard work. And therein lies the "secret" to what makes a successful training program: individualization and discipline. It's really as simple as that.

You might not like hearing this, but there isn't any can't-miss formula for getting in better physical condition. How could there be? We're all so different. Just because something works for one person doesn't mean it's going to work for everyone else who tries it. As I alluded to earlier, there are simply too many factors that come into play: age, current fitness level, previous training experience, body type, etc. Beginners need more than vague generalizations like "start out slow" or "stick with the basics." What do phrases like that mean? Should you move slowly when performing the actual workout? Or maybe it means you shouldn't do too many sets and reps. Well, if that's the case, how are you supposed to determine what constitutes "too many"? You're a beginner, remember? You have no frame of reference to draw from.

And what about this whole stick-with-the-basics mantra? To some, it might suggest that beginners should stick mainly with machines since they lack the coordination and stabilization to work with free weights. To others—like me, for instance—it might suggest a need for *first* working with bodyweight and free-weight exercises in order to help develop coordination and stabilizer strength. And then there are even those few who feel that beginners should stick with cardiovascular and flexibility training and introduce strength work only later on, once they've improved their level of conditioning. In my best Chandler Bing voice, "That one couldn't *be* more off-base."

Now mind you, we're just talking about beginners in general here. Throw in the fact that there are different types of beginners, and the waters start to get even muddier. A guy who's never trained before will have to go about things much differently than a former athlete who used to work out religiously back in college. Just as an older guy with a sedentary job would be better off adopting a different approach than a teenager who's getting his first exposure to training. Each one of these guys is going to have different needs than the others.

The bottom line is there is no one set way to go about doing things. It's not as easy as pulling some generic workout out of a magazine or off a Web site or walking into a gym and having someone hand you a workout card and say, "Here, do this." Well, maybe it is if you have the financial means to hire a personal trainer to plan your workouts for you. When you're forced to go it alone, though, count on putting in a fair amount of work—not just in the gym but outside of it as well. That's because in order to be successful, your best strategy is to become as educated as you can about the way your body responds to physical conditioning. It takes patience, discipline, and intense desire to seek out the best information available to you. That's where this book comes in.

A GREAT PROGRAM . . . PERIOD!

DISCOVERING THE BENEFITS OF PERIODIZATION

Think of getting fit as a three-step process. Your first step, as is always the case, is to admit that you have a problem.

Okay, so you're a beginner. The good news is you don't have to be one for long. The second step is to seek out the appropriate information necessary to help you reach your goals. Easy enough—you've already bought this book, or you're at least considering buying it as you sit there, latte in hand, giving yourself this little free preview.

The third is to put the information contained within these pages to good use by taking the time to truly understand and appreciate the way *your* body works and not just looking at the book as a bunch of different programs to try out. Because that's certainly not the way it's intended to work.

This book is set up rather differently than other beginner's books for a variety of reasons. First off, as I mentioned earlier, there are many different types of beginners. It therefore makes absolutely no sense to prescribe generic workouts that fail to take into account people's individual differences. Don't get me wrong; there's only so much individualization you can include in any book. Suffice it to say that the programs contained in this one won't be full of the run-of-the-mill workouts you often see recommended to people who are just getting started. The next chapter will help you classify exactly what type of beginner you are and show you how to select workouts that are appropriate for your current skill level.

The other thing that makes this book so different is that it teaches you how to properly schedule your workouts so you can avoid training plateaus and ensure continued progress. One of the main reasons most people fail in their attempts to stick to a training program is that, after a while, their bodies completely adapt to what they're doing. A little adaptation is desirable—it's what causes your body to become stronger or leaner or more flexible as a result of the training stimulus. It's just that when the workout no longer poses a challenge, you have to alter it in some way in order to keep making gains. Coaches and trainers refer to this as periodization, a fancy term that means systematically changing the main focus of your training for brief periods in order to avoid the kind of training plateaus that doom other people's progress. So for instance, you might train to increase muscle mass for 1 month, to increase strength the next, and perhaps to build endurance the next.

With periodization, you don't neglect the other aspects of fitness in pursuit of a single goal; you simply give that goal priority for a brief period and strive to maintain everything else in the meantime. During an intensive muscle-building phase, for instance, you're still going to include cardiovascular exercise, just probably not to the same extent that you normally would. Then, just before your body starts to get the hang of that, you switch to a different goal for the next few weeks. Training this way, especially if the phases are sequenced in the appropriate manner, can lead to improvements above and beyond what you could expect with the more mainstream fitness approach beginners often favor.

That's why the programs contained in this book are arranged in the sequential manner in which they are, where each one builds on the one before it. It's a format that I've used successfully countless times and one that I'm hopeful more people will begin to adopt. I realize that some of you might be somewhat reluctant to embrace it. There are legions of guys who just want a workout that keeps them "in shape" and incorporates all aspects of fitness—particularly fat loss. They're not interested in training to increase muscle size or strength to any significant degree. If you're one of them, relax. I'm not looking to make bodybuilders out of anyone. What I am trying to do is show you that there's a right way and a wrong way to go after your goal.

Say you need to lose as much as 50 pounds. Shouldn't you concentrate exclusively on fat loss? Is it really a good idea for you to devote specific periods to becoming stronger or putting on more muscle mass? Absolutely! In fact, as long as you go about it the way I've outlined for you in the pages ahead, such an approach will actually accelerate your progress. Increased strength makes it easier to build muscle, and the more muscle you have on your frame, the easier it is to burn body fat. Seems somewhat counterintuitive, I'll admit, but it's a much more effective way to lose weight than spending hours on a treadmill and doing light, high-repetition strength training.

So you see, this approach really will work for just about everyone. Remember, this book isn't designed to show you how to train for the rest of your life. Its primary goal is to get you started in the right direction for the first 6 to 12 months so that you can make a regular commitment to keeping healthy and fit. In the process, it'll provide you with a good, working knowledge of the various aspects of fitness and how they interact to produce dramatic changes in the way you look and feel. In short, it's designed to give you the basic foundation you need to lose the beginner tag and gain a real appreciation for the way *your body* works.

So do us both a favor and, at the very least, read the next chapter to identify what type of beginner you are and how you should best proceed. While you're at it, you might also want to consider putting yourself through the self-assessment and corrective phases in Chapters 5 and 6 before you get started. At least this way you'll stand a better chance of not getting hurt and get a little better idea of what you're getting yourself into. Who knows, you also might become intrigued enough to abandon your hasty approach and do the programs in the intended order.

A warning for those of you in the "I just want to stay in shape" category: Don't just stick with the same program indefinitely. Once you've gone through the self-assessment and corrective phases, there's a "basic training" workout that equally incorporates all aspects of training. It's designed to be more or less an extension of the corrective phase, preparing you for the more intensive training to follow. It would be a mistake to stick with this type of workout exclusively, as your body will quickly adapt to it and your progress will soon cease. So try as best you can to do all of the phases in their intended order.

KNOWLEDGE IS POWER

APPLYING WHAT YOU LEARN

Look, we all have to start somewhere. I'm sure Michael Jordan didn't start dunking the first time he touched a basketball, nor did Tiger Woods likely sink the first putt he ever tried. Okay, maybe they did, but those guys are in a different stratosphere anyway. The point is, there are plenty of mere mortals, myself included, who weren't initially adept in their particular fields yet went on to achieve big things. So you're just starting out—so what? There's no shame in being a beginner. The only shame is in never progressing out of the beginner stage because you lack the knowledge and discipline to see things through.

You're being given a tremendous opportunity here, the kind that most beginners never seem to get. In the pages ahead you're going to be taught how to detect and subsequently eliminate your specific weaknesses, improve your overall level of physical conditioning, and increase your strength and muscularity far beyond what you ever imagined possible using a "beginner" approach. If you use this book appropriately, there's no reason you can't drop up to 40 pounds in as few as 3 to 4 months, or go from bench-pressing as much as a prepubescent girl to benching the combined body weight of multiple prepubescent girls. I've provided you with all of the information you need to reach your goals; the rest is up to you.

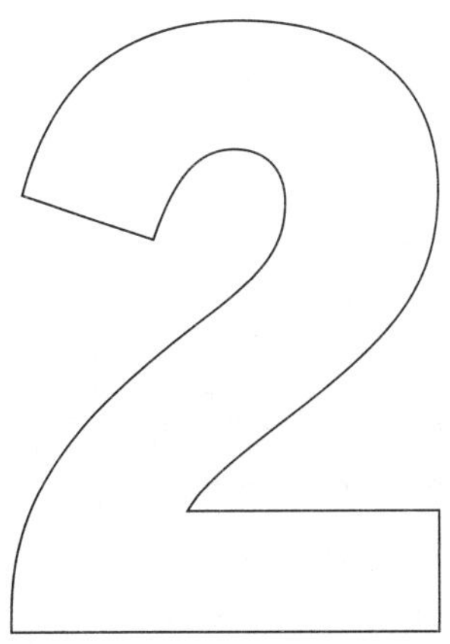

HAVING AN IDENTITY CRISIS?

IDENTIFYING WHAT TYPE OF BEGINNER YOU ARE IS HALF THE BATTLE

Now that you've come to grips with the fact that you are indeed a beginner, the next step must be to get started with the actual training program, right? Not so fast. Before you proceed, there's one more stop on your little voyage of self-discovery. To really get a handle on what you need to do to get your body in good working order, you're going to have to establish what *type* of beginner you are. It's not enough to say that you've "never really trained before" or that you've "taken an extended layoff from working out." If you're really serious about making a committed effort to keeping fit, you're going to need to be a lot more specific than that.

Remember my first workout, which I recounted for you in Chapter 1? You know, the one that was apparently so well designed it was applicable to people of all ages, genders, and physical abilities. Well, you probably won't be shocked to learn that I didn't get very much out of it. And, even though I was a complete novice at the time, I remember questioning the reasoning behind making everyone who came into the gym do the same exact thing. One day I finally worked up the nerve to question one of the instructors on this practice. He quickly shot back, "You're all beginners; you've gotta start somewhere." Agreed, just why all from the *same* place? This certainly doesn't address any of the aforementioned weaknesses that we all have to a certain degree.

Here's an example of one of the drawbacks of a one-size-fits-all beginner program. It's not uncommon to find some type of squat or leg press in a beginner's workout. These exercises are known as bilateral lifts, meaning that two limbs work together at the same time. If one limb is stronger than the other (as is almost always the case, due to such things as improved coordination of the dominant side or insufficient flexibility), the strength imbalance will never be corrected. Over time, this imbalance can manifest itself as an injury to a knee, hip, or even the lower back—most likely on the dominant side as it continues to pick up more and more of the stress as the weights increase over the course of the program.

Another important consideration for beginners is the amount of time they should spend on improving flexibility. Arguably one of the most important aspects of overall health and well-being, the ability to move freely and easily is often treated as an afterthought in many training programs. Adding resistance to an exercise too quickly, or attempting to burn more body fat by continually engaging in repetitive motions like cycling and stepping, can actually decrease movement efficiency as muscles become shortened. This problem is magnified for older individuals, whose muscles have already lost some of their elasticity due to the aging process. Yet most people are so busy trying to burn fat or build muscle that they devalue the importance of basic movement efficiency. This holds particularly true for beginners, who are almost always motivated to start exercising for aesthetic, rather than performance related, reasons.

Look, I realize that vanity is part of the deal here. But in our quest for that perfect physique, we shouldn't sacrifice the ability to move freely.

I could go on listing the numerous factors that ultimately determine your success or failure when beginning an exercise program. What I'd rather do instead is describe for you the several types of beginners and help you identify which group you fit into. This information, coupled with your results from the self-assessment in Chapter 5, will give you a definitive course of action for reaching your fitness goals. It will also go a long way toward helping you understand why different people need to work out in different ways. So, without further ado, let's meet the featured players.

THE NEW GUY

COMING TO GRIPS WITH THE FACT THAT YOU'RE A "NEWBIE"

First up, you've got what I like to call your total newbie. In gym lingo, the term *newbie* is used to describe someone who has absolutely no formal training experience whatsoever. These poor souls couldn't tell you the difference between a bench press and a situp. You belong in this category if you feel intimidated in a gym setting, if you work out in a jogging suit with a matching headband, or if you wear black socks with sneakers. Walking around the gym with a heavy leather weight-lifting belt cinched around your waist will also earn you entrance into this club.

I prefer to subdivide newbies by age since people come to realize the benefits of regular exercise at different points in their lives. Some start exercising when they're teenagers, while others wait until the signs of middle age become apparent.

There are even those rare few (actually a growing number over the past several years) who start exercising as senior citizens. Technically speaking, all of these people can be considered newbies, but does that mean they should all start a fitness program the same way?

Obviously, the answer is no. You simply can't expect a previously sedentary, middle-aged man or a recent retiree who's never picked up a weight in his life to do the same program as a college freshman. Forget that the kid doesn't have any experience either; the laws of aging dictate that he'll be able to handle more work and recover much more rapidly than the other two. There are a whole host of physical differences between an 18-year-old and a 45-year-old, and even more between an 18-year-old and a 70-year-old. That's why I propose different training guidelines based on age. However, since it would be impractical to address individuals of every age, I've chosen age 35 as the cutoff point, with those of you 35 and under following one set of guidelines and those of you over age 35 following another. I chose this number not for any scientific reasons but because it seems to represent a consensus among guys as to where physical abilities start to noticeably decline.

Being in the older group myself, I'm not happy about this cutoff. But whether we like it or not doesn't matter. What does matter is that following age-appropriate guidelines not only can make you less susceptible to injury but also can help you progress at a much faster rate than someone who chooses to ignore the influence of Father Time. Take flexibility, for instance. I just mentioned how, because of reduced muscle elasticity, we older individuals need to devote more attention to improving our range of motion than younger people do. This doesn't mean we should just throw in a few extra stretches at the end of our workout. It means we need to make flexibility a priority, even going so far as to put it ahead of strength training and perhaps even ahead of cardio work.

Don't get me wrong: Strength and cardiovascular health are both extremely important as you grow older. But the ability to move freely and efficiently must come first and foremost. Who cares whether you can leg-press a Hyundai if you can't bend forward to pick up a coin off the ground without fear of injuring yourself?

Another advantage the younger crowd has going for them is a superior ability to recover from intense training. We older guys need to allow for more recuperation between workouts (much the same way we need longer to recover from a night out with the boys than we did in our twenties). Our muscle fibers take longer to repair, our energy stores take longer to replenish, and our immune system function stays depressed for a longer period of time. So although we may be able to train as often as younger guys, we can't train as intensely and expect to recover at the same rate.

Last but not least, one other area where guys north of 35 come up short relates to nervous system function. As we age, the nervous system loses some of its ability to effectively recruit muscle fibers to contract, so it takes a little longer to become proficient at certain exercises. Where a 25-year-old might need to stick with a program for only 3 to 4 weeks before seeing results, a 55-year-old might need as many as 8 weeks. (Not that this is irreversible—even men well into their seventies and eighties have demonstrated improved muscle fiber recruitment as a result of regular resistance training.)

There are also a few general guidelines that apply to beginners of all types. One is the need to target any existing strength and flexibility imbalances (you'll learn to identify these in Chapter 5) before performing more complex movements like squats and various types of presses. Or, in the words of famed trainer and lecturer Paul Chek, "Isolate before you integrate." Seeing as how a chain is only as strong as its weakest link, doing so will leave you much less susceptible to injury. The other universal newbie rule is to stick with total-body workouts. Your arms, chest, back, or shoulders do not warrant their own separate training days. Total-body workouts, which require you to activate large amounts of muscle mass, are the preferred way to build size or strength or to just keep fit.

GLORY DAZE

WHEN YOU'RE NOT THE MAN YOU USED TO BE

Another group of beginners who warrant specific mention because of the unique problems they pose are the ex-jocks. These are the guys who played one or more sports back in high school and college but haven't done a thing since. Once they realized that they weren't going to be the next Derek Jeter or Kobe Bryant, they hung up their jockstraps and dove headlong into building their careers and families. So much so, in fact, that they lost most of the physical abilities that had made them good athletes in the first place. Just don't tell *them* that.

C'mon, admit it. If you fall into this category you're not going to let a little thing like the fact that you haven't done anything strenuous in more than a decade (or two) prevent you from tearing up the weight room the way you did back in the day. You probably think you could still light up the track the way you did 25 pounds ago; it would just take you a little longer to warm up now.

Well, I hate to be the one to break this to you, Captain Delusional, but your glory days are long gone. Try to jump right in and work out with the same fervor you did back when you were the big man on campus, and you'll be in for a world of hurt. Although the spirit may be willing, you'll quickly discover that your body is not.

As if your ego weren't enough of a potential liability, there's something else you need to be aware of before starting your new program. If you played sports at any sort of reasonably high level, it's a safe bet you probably accumulated a few battle scars along the way. Whether you have chronic back pain, a bad shoulder, a bum knee, or a trick elbow, you're likely going to need to modify certain exercises to make them more joint friendly. It's a

TRAINING GUIDELINES: KNOWING THE OVER/UNDER

Training Variable	Age 35 and Under	Over Age 35
Frequency		
Lifting	Moderate–high (2–4 days/week)	Moderate (2–3 days/week)
Cardio	Moderate–high (2–4 days/week)	Moderate (2–3 days/week)
Volume (number of sets and exercises)		
	Moderate–high (16–18 sets and 4–6 exercises)	Low–moderate (9–14 sets and 3–5 exercises)
Intensity		
Lifting: amount of weight	Moderate–High	Moderate
Cardio: Borg Rating of Perceived Exertion (See "Perception Is Reality" on p. 269.)	RPE: 14–18	RPE: 12–16
How Long You Should Stick with a Particular Workout	Low–moderate (3–4 weeks)	High (4–6 weeks)
Need to Modify Workouts Due to Orthopedic Problems or Other Preexisting Conditions	Low	High
Cardio Emphasis	Low (not a priority)	High (priority)
Flexibility Emphasis	Moderate (2–3 days/week)	High (3–5 days/week)

well-documented fact that ex-athletes have more joint-related problems than nonathletes. Don't sweat it; in the chapters that follow I'm going to teach you all kinds of neat little tricks for making otherwise painful exercises more manageable *and* effective.

You do have one positive going for you. Remember what I said about the central nervous system and how as you get older it takes longer for your body to recruit and use muscle groups in specific patterns? Well, the fact that you've trained previously gives you a big advantage over someone who hasn't. This is thanks to a little thing called muscle memory. You know, the old "It's like riding a bike" phenomenon. Once your muscles get reacquainted with some of the lifts you'll be doing, you'll soon notice that your strength levels will increase at a much more rapid rate than will those of a complete novice.

You just have to make sure that that old competitive fire doesn't allow your ego to start writing checks your body can't cash. The rate at which your strength levels return will be directly proportional to how far removed you are from your playing days. A guy who's been inactive for only 5 years or so will have a much easier time than one who hung up his letterman's sweater 30 years ago.

This is another reason why, just as I did with newbies, I like to divide ex-jocks into age groups, once again using 35 as the cutoff. Younger guys will follow one set of guidelines and older guys another, based on their particular needs.

SEASON'S FLEETINGS

SPORADIC EXERCISE HABITS JUST DON'T CUT IT

Last but not least comes a group of people who really can't be considered true beginners but who definitely deserve a mention. They're what I like to call the seasonal crowd, because their sole motivation to start exercising is some semiannual event like New Year's, spring break, or the start of bathing suit season. You may also occasionally notice some in the gym in the fall, making a last-ditch effort to look good for the holidays. Sadly, seasonals seldom stick with it for more than a few weeks at a time, and as a result, they never get the results they're looking for. They do too much, too soon, and end up burning themselves out before their bodies ever have a chance to adapt to the training.

If you fall into this category, you've got a completely different set of concerns than the first two groups. Unlike them, you've at least had some recent workout experience; obviously, it just didn't go very well, or you would have stuck with it longer. So for you, the issue isn't so much enhancing mobility or working around previous injuries (though you'll do the self-assessment and corrective phases just the same). Your major focus has to be finding a form of exercise that you enjoy, so you'll keep doing it, and setting realistic, short-term goals that you can reach. Oh sure, there'll be some other guidelines to make sure you don't hurt yourself and are progressing in the proper manner. But by and large, I'm convinced that your problem is more mental than physical, born out of a rapid transition from overzealousness to disinterest.

Trust me on this one; I've seen it enough times to know what I'm talking about. I've spent more than my share of time in gyms and fitness centers over the years, so I can spot one of these folks a mile away. They usually skulk in as if they're afraid to spark a "Where ya been?" type of comment from one of the other members. Last thing they want is to be chided about their shoddy gym attendance. Soon afterward, they're attacking the weights with reckless abandon, doing routines that make even the most seasoned gym rats raise their

WHO-O-O-OO ARE YOU?

Newbie, 35 and under: You're what an artist might refer to as a blank canvas. There's no previous training experience to cloud your thinking, so you should be open-minded and should respond well to just about anything you try. Just try not to start out too aggressively. This means following the programs as they're written and refraining from adding more sets and exercises along the way. Perhaps more than any other type of beginner, young newbies probably have the worst retention rates because they usually assume that their youth gives them the ability to push their bodies harder and faster than they're ready for. Avoid this mistake by adopting a well-rounded approach and not diving headlong into fat loss or muscle building right way.

Newbie, over age 35: Where ya been, pal? Never had the inclination to do any form of structured training before this? Oh well, better late than never. For you, flexibility will be one of the major focuses of the program. Expect to become really familiar with the various stretches and mobility sequences featured in Chapter 7. You'll also pay heavy attention to cardiovascular conditioning as well as strength building, both of which are key areas of concern for men as they grow older. As tempting as it may be, you're going to have to avoid the bench-press-and-biceps-curl-driven approach favored by the younger crowd.

Ex-jock, 35 and under: All right, tough guy. Remember, it's been several years since you single-handedly won the homecoming game. So what say you proceed with at least some level of caution? Improving flexibility will be key so you can regain some of the mobility you've lost while sitting behind that cushy desk. You'll probably find you can make pretty rapid gains in size and strength once you get into the teeth of the training program. Just remember that although you're still young, now is as good a time as any to start giving your heart the attention it deserves. So don't skimp on the cardio work in pursuit of getting buff again.

Ex-jock, over age 35: You may be a real shark in the business world, but your long stretch of inactivity has demoted you back to guppy status once you set foot in a gym. Restoring lost mobility is going to be a real priority, as is reeducating your body to the whole training process. Be patient and don't look to progress too quickly. Remember, just because you *can* lift something

eyebrows in disbelief. And cardio? Please—it's as if they think they can purge the sins of the entire holiday season with one endless ascent on the stairclimber. Most of these chronic re-starters end up becoming victims of their own good intentions.

So the question is, how do we get people in this category to (1) formulate the right plan for getting started and (2) learn that this whole fitness thing isn't something they should just discard once they reach some transient aesthetic goal like being able to fit into a bathing suit? In my view, it's as simple as providing them with the right information from the get-go. Because once they start feeling and seeing the results they can achieve with a better-balanced approach, there's no way they're going to want to stop exercising. By providing them with the right foundation for success, we'll effectively kill two birds with one stone by changing exercise from a chore into a habit. It's said that familiarity breeds contempt. Well, in the fitness industry, positive results breed adherence.

Proper planning is going to be a big part of the equation here. So much so, in fact, that I've devoted an entire chap-

doesn't necessarily mean it's a good idea to. Besides, you'll likely find that you'll need to modify the way you perform certain lifts, to compensate for those nagging little injuries you're always complaining about. There will be some holdover from your previous training experience, but it won't be anywhere near as much as you're expecting. Strive to improve your range of motion, allow your nervous system to reprogram itself by stressing form over weight, and gradually increase the intensity and frequency of your cardiovascular training.

Seasonal, 35 and under: Obviously, what you've been doing up to this point hasn't worked. If it had, you would've made exercise a habit long ago and you would have no need for this book. So your objective is to follow to a tee the progression laid out in these pages. I've never seen this type of approach fail, and since your approach has, well, you do the math. The biggest challenge for you is going to be finding exercises you enjoy and ways to make the things you dislike about exercise more enjoyable. Say you hate to stretch because you find it completely boring. Well, the flexibility workouts in this book were designed to be anything but. Or maybe you never seem to be able to gain muscle because you can't devote endless hours to being in the gym. The muscle-building workouts featured in Chapter 8 will enable you to build plenty of muscle in just a couple of brief, intense workouts per week. Whatever your goals are, there'll be enough information in here to pique your interest and help you commit to exercising on a more regular basis.

Seasonal, over age 35: You, my friend, are a bit of an anomaly. Most guys your age gave up trying to look good at the beach years ago. Although at your age, it's probably more of a wanting-to-look-good-at-a-reunion type of thing. Whatever the case, you'll follow guidelines similar to those for the other beginners who are over 35: heavy flexibility and cardiovascular emphasis, with lots of attention to building strength. Your main objective will be to try to make it work this time, because bodies—especially older bodies—don't like being put through arbitrary periods of increased physical exertion. So more than anything else, work on making exercise a habit this time around.

ter to it immediately following this one. In addition, there are a few other things that those of you who favor the seasonal approach need to look out for if you ever want to get off your little exercise roller coaster. When you attack a workout program like a bunch of Huns raiding a buffet table, there's a pretty good chance your body's going to take exception. Whether this manifests itself as pain, injury, or dramatic changes to your metabolism depends on just how hard and fast you come out of the gate.

Take your tendons and ligaments, for instance. You probably don't give them much thought, but these connective tissues provide your joints with the stability they need to carry out everyday functions like climbing stairs or lifting heavy objects. However, due to their poor blood supply, they tend to adapt to training at a much slower rate than your muscles do. Seeing as how tendons attach muscles to bone, you can begin to see why developing one ahead of the other could potentially pose a problem. Add in the ligaments, which attach bone to bone and also get little in the way of blood supply, and you've suddenly got a situation where muscles are getting much stronger than their support structures.

This is why, once you've done all of the specific strengthening and stretching in the corrective workouts, you're going to switch over to much-higher-repetition training (12 to 15 reps per set) in order to increase bloodflow and bolster tendon and ligament strength. This will help you avoid the all-too-common joint pain that often sabotages people who start out too aggressively in an attempt to reach an unrealistic goal in a ridiculously short time frame. Short of going to a plastic surgeon, it's impossible to lose 20 pounds or shave 6 inches off your waist in a couple of weeks. Unfortunately, that's more than enough time to strain or sprain a ligament or to develop a nasty case of tendonitis as a result of pushing your body beyond its capabilities.

Need more convincing? Let's talk metabolism. Strenuous exercise boosts metabolic rate, plain and simple. The harder you exercise, the greater the increase in your metabolism. Work out hard for a couple of weeks to a couple of months, and you're going to give your metabolism a serious boost, which, in turn, is going to kick your appetite into high gear. The trouble begins when your exercise jones fades but your newfound appetite stays revved up for a few weeks. All of a sudden, you're 5 to 10 pounds heavier than when you started.

Now that you know the potential pitfalls of sporadic, unregulated exercise, the next step is to make sure that you never fall prey to them again. How do you do that? Well, for starters, you don't just pick up the first workout program you see and say, "Yeah, I'll do this." That's definitely not the way to use this book. Over the next few hundred pages, you'll be exposed to several different workout plans. Some focus on building muscle, while others are geared toward strength development, cardiovascular fitness, or fat loss. As effective as they are, skipping ahead to them at this point would be a huge mistake, making this book just another piece of worthless fitness paraphernalia you turn to in desperation a couple of times a year.

GETTING TO KNOW YOU

CLASSIFYING WHAT TYPE OF BEGINNER YOU ARE

By now, you must be saying to yourself, "What good is knowing what kind of beginner I am if I have no idea how to fix it?" After all, to this point I haven't really provided you with any hard and fast guidelines for getting started. There's a reason for that. Before you can eliminate a problem, you first have to identify it. Now that you've become familiar with some of the unique challenges specific to your situation, you have a better understanding of what it's going to take to overcome them. That's exactly why I painted with wide strokes here and didn't go into finite training recommendations for each type of beginner yet. There's plenty of time for that later on, when we get to the actual program design.

So if you're still confused as to how much weight to use, how many sets you should do or what the optimal intensity and duration of your cardio workouts should be, sit tight. We'll get to all of that in due time. For now, take solace in the fact that you already know more about your body—and what it's going to take to improve it—than most people in your shoes know. Now comes the fun part: learning how to apply that knowledge.

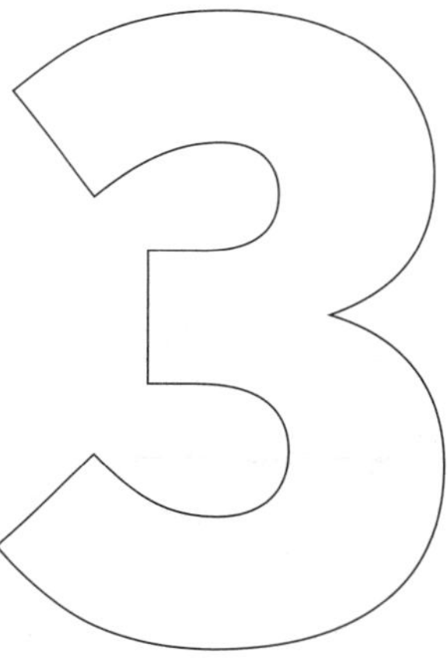

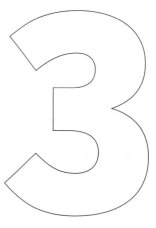

THE POWER OF PLANNING

YOU CAN'T GET WHERE YOU WANT TO GO ON DEDICATION ALONE

You've probably heard this a thousand times before, but it bears repeating: If you fail to plan, you're planning to fail. I know it's a cliché, but it's also an extremely accurate statement in most instances. There are very few things in life that you can enter into without any kind of forethought or preparation and expect to be successful. Sure, a couple of things come to mind—like, say, getting married or perhaps running for president. For the most part, though, you pretty much have to think things through before you act. Otherwise, you're practically ensuring that whatever you're attempting to do will be wrought with problems.

This is the case with exercise. If you approach your workouts irrationally, thinking that in a few short weeks you can undo the damage caused by years of inactivity, you can forget it. I've seen too many people go down that road only to end up injured or turned off to the whole idea of training altogether. It doesn't matter what your goals are—burning fat, improving cardiovascular fitness, getting stronger, or all of the above—there's a systematic way to go about making them happen. And it all starts with having enough patience to formulate the right plan.

So here's what I want you to do: Stop reading right now and go get a pen. You'll need to write down, by filling out the form on page 20, some of the things we're going to go over in this chapter. Those things include short- and long-term conditioning goals, a realistic training schedule that fits your lifestyle, and nutritional strategies that will help you reach your goals as quickly as possible. Don't worry if you have no idea how to determine these strategies; I'm about to walk you through it step-by-step. By the time we're done, you'll have a completely new appreciation of just what it takes to start an exercise program.

FITTING IN FITNESS

MAKING THE TIME TO EXERCISE

If all you had to do all day was work out, you'd probably be in phenomenal shape. Movie stars are a perfect example of this. When an actor is preparing for a role, he's not distracted by the everyday pressures that you and I have. You know, little things like worrying about making ends meet, a hellish commute, or running a thousand different errands. I'm not saying celebrities don't work hard on their bodies—take it easy, Brad. It's just that it's a little easier to focus on getting buff when you don't have to wonder how you're supposed to fit your workouts into your hectic schedule (not to mention when you have a personal trainer and a private chef).

Let's face it, you could have the best workout program bar none, but if you can't find the time to do it, what good is it? There's no sense committing to a 4-day-per-week workout schedule when you know full well you have only 2 days to exercise. So the aim of this section is to help you to set up a realistic training schedule based on your goals, needs, *and* available workout time. You might be pleasantly surprised to find out that it doesn't take as much of a time commitment as you assumed. At least initially, that is. If you have aspirations to take your physical development to great heights—like, say, *Men's Health* cover model material—you'll find that the time commitment increases exponentially. But that's a ways down the road yet anyway.

The first thing you need to do is figure out how many days per week you can set aside time to exercise. I suggest a minimum of 2 and a maximum of 5 scheduled training days per week (that includes both strength and cardio training), depending on what type of beginner you are. In my experience, older lifters of all types are usually best off opting for fewer training sessions per week. Younger lifters, so long as their schedules allow, do better with more frequent workouts. You should certainly feel free to experiment and see what works best for you. The best thing about this kind of moderate training frequency is that it helps establish exercise as a habit, without overwhelming you or leaving you tired and sore all the time.

Once you've figured out your training frequency, the next thing you have to decipher is how much time you have available to work out each training day. One of the biggest complaints I hear from beginners is how long it takes to work out. When you add up a warmup, stretching, strength work, cardio training, and then a cooldown with yet more stretching, it can sometimes take as long as 90 minutes to do a single training session. That can be a bit much for someone just getting started. Add in a potential commute to and from the gym, and maybe a shower, and now you're talking about a significant chunk of time. Which, by the way, is going to require waking up at the crack of dawn to train before work, risking getting fired by doing it on your lunch hour, or alienating your family by coming home late.

Thankfully, it doesn't have to be that way. Such marathon training sessions are a product of the generic approach to fitness and do little more than promote overtraining. The way the workouts in this book are designed, you'll spend, on average, between 15 and 25 minutes for strength workouts, 12 and 20 minutes for cardio, and all of 5 to 10 minutes on warmups and stretching. In my opinion, if you are a beginner and you are not completely finished with your workouts in under an hour—and sometimes in significantly less time—then you're doing something wrong. Here's why.

If you're able to commit to 4 or 5 training days per week, you're likely going to be dividing your strength and cardio workouts into separate workouts anyway. You want to make exercise a habit by making it a regular part of your day. Because you won't be training with as much volume (number of strength-training exercises and sets of exercises) as guys who aren't beginners, and because most of the cardio workouts in this book focus on intensity rather than duration, none of your workouts is going to take very long. You'll probably be done in 30 to 40 minutes, or less in some instances.

Even assuming that you can only make time to work out 2 or 3 times per week, and therefore need to combine strength training and cardio on the same days, your workouts will still be designed in such a way that each session will take under an hour. Consider the following two examples:

Newbie, Age 45

Goals: Increase strength and cardiovascular fitness and improve flexibility

Available workout days per week: 2

Available workout time: 50 to 60 minutes per session

Sample Workout: Monday and Thursday

Warmup: 5–7 minutes

Strength training: 20 minutes

Cardio: 10–15 minutes

Core training (working all of the muscles from the base of your chest to the top of your hips, on the front, back, and sides of your body): 5–7 minutes

Stretching: 5–7 minutes

Total time: 45–56 minutes

Ex-Jock, Age 30

Goals: Increase muscle mass, improve flexibility, and decrease body fat

Available workout days per week: 4

Available workout time: 45 minutes per session

Sample Workout: Monday and Friday

Warmup: 5–7 minutes

Strength training: 20–25 minutes

Stretching: 5–7 minutes

Total time: 30–39 minutes

Sample Workout: Tuesday and Sunday

Warmup: 5 minutes

Cardio: 15–20 minutes

Core training: 7–10 minutes

Stretching: 5 minutes

Total time: 32–40 minutes

As you can see, neither of these programs requires a tremendous initial time commitment. The older, less conditioned guy is looking at 2 hours per week max of total workout time, with some daily flexibility work sprinkled in for good measure. Whereas the younger guy is only being asked to make a 3-hour weekly commitment, despite the fact that he's exercising twice as many days. So if you're worried that a workout program is going to eat up all your free time, relax. Going about it this way will leave you plenty of time for family, friends, and anything else you want to do.

FIRST AND GOAL

HAVING SOMETHING TO SHOOT FOR

I'm going to be honest with you: I absolutely hate asking a new client what his goals are. Not because I don't care or don't want to know—I am, after all, a trainer, and as such I need to have some insight into exactly what it is this person is trying to accomplish. The reason I hate asking is because of the responses I get. Things like "To get back in shape." Or "I just want to lose and tone." The only enjoyment I get out of this process is when I look the client dead in the eye and ask, "Okay, what does that mean?" To which he usually responds, in a state of shocked confusion, "*You're* the trainer. Don't *you* know?"

No, I don't know. And the reason I don't is because those aren't really goals. They're nothing more than popular ambiguities that perpetuate the generic approach to fitness that still reigns supreme. Consider the phrase "get back in shape" for a moment. What does this really mean? What exactly is considered "in shape"? Is it possessing a high level of cardiovascular fitness? Being able to squat 1½ to 2 times your body weight? Or maybe it means having above-average flexibility? Being in shape means different things to different people, so it's pretty pointless to offer it up as a goal unless you have some way to quantify it.

And don't even get me started on the "lose and tone" comment. Lose what? Hopefully not weight, because weight includes fat, water, *and* muscle tissue. Losing the first one is fine, but losing too much of the latter two can adversely affect both your strength levels and metabolism. Sure, the numbers on the scale might temporarily look more palatable, but in addition to the decline in physical performance, you'll probably just end up gaining all the weight back anyway.

I'd much rather hear things like, "I want to be able to run 5 miles a day again." Now that's a goal! Or maybe, "I want to add 2 inches to my shoulders and lose 2 inches from my waist." That's another goal. I'd even take something as seemingly ambiguous as "I just want to be able to play with my kids." Not as finite a goal as the others, but there's enough there to go on to formulate a plan. Kids run around a lot, so improving cardiovascular fitness and flexibility would be key. There would also probably be some lifting and even a little wrestling involved. That means increasing total body strength would also be a priority.

Granted, none of these examples mentions a specific time frame, but we'll get to that soon enough. At least we've attached some tangible objectives to what before were nothing more than vague concepts.

DIVIDE AND CONQUER

TRYING NOT TO ACHIEVE ALL OF YOUR GOALS AT ONCE

As you can see, there's a lot more to goal setting than meets the eye. The first step is identifying specific results you want to achieve and can in some way quantify. The next is to put a time frame on how you can achieve them. I'm not talking about setting some unreasonable deadline. You could say you want to lose 25 pounds in a month or add 2 inches to your arms in 2 weeks. Obviously, though, short of a hunger strike or a visit to Jose Canseco's house, neither one is going to happen. Reasonable weight loss—assuming you want to lose mostly fat and not water and lean tissue, which would slow metabolism—is 1 to 2 pounds per week. Losing inches takes a little longer because when you lose 2 pounds that fat doesn't necessarily all come off your waist. Two inches per month is realistic. As far as adding muscle, if you add an inch or two to your arms over the course of 2 to 3 months, you're doing pretty well.

The key to reaching your goals is to break them down into manageable segments that when added up equal a more long-term objective. Say your long-term goal is to drop 30 pounds, lose 8 inches off your waist, and add 50 to 75 pounds to your bench press. Let's also assume that you want to do all of this within 6 months. Regardless of what type of beginner you are, that's a pretty daunting task. But what if you broke it into parts? Like, say, dropping 15 pounds, taking 4 inches off your waist, and increasing your bench by 25 to 35 pounds in 3 months. Sounds a lot better, right? And what if you took it even further by setting a 1-month goal of losing 5 pounds, slimming your waistline by 2 inches, and improving your bench press by 10 to 15 pounds? All of a sudden, this is looking extremely doable.

Okay, pick up that pen I asked you to get earlier and think about what you want to achieve by embarking on this program. Remember, try to be as specific as you can. Write your goals at the top of the next page. Next, underneath your goals you'll notice that I've listed the following time intervals in order: 2 weeks, 1 month, 3 months, 6 months, and 1 year. What this will do is provide you with a more manageable timetable and show you the proper way to progress to avoid overtraining and/or injury. (See "Sample Goal-Setting Worksheet" on page 21 examples.)

Now I know some of you are probably wondering exactly what you're supposed to accomplish in 2 weeks. And that's a fair question; 2 weeks really isn't a whole lot of time for training adaptations like reduced body fat or improved strength levels to occur. What you can do is begin to establish good habits by setting a small, extremely reachable goal in this time frame. It might be something as simple as getting in a specific number of strength and cardiovascular workouts per week or setting aside 10 to 15 minutes per day to stretch. Remember, at this point it's all about establishing good habits, and a goal of this type is just what you need to start off on the right foot.

From there, you simply break down your larger goal into more manageable segments, with the key being that you don't focus too far down the road. I know that most people who suddenly start exercising want to see immediate results. And to be honest, using the approach that's laid out for you in this book will allow you to progress rather quickly. Keeping in mind that not everyone responds to training the same way, you just might find that you start reaching some of your short-term goals ahead of schedule. I have, after all, been doing this for quite some time, and I've learned what works and what doesn't for most people. I just ask that you don't let your impatience to reach long-term goals sabotage your progress. Being down 10 pounds in a month, for instance, is extremely doable; being down 20 to 30 is going to take you a little longer.

That doesn't mean that you can't reap plenty of short-term benefits along the way. Among the more immediate changes you'll likely experience is marked improvement in your energy levels. Whether it's an increase in those often talked about endorphins or simply more blood and oxygen regularly being transported to your working muscles, you'll notice a pronounced bounce in your step just a couple of weeks into your new program. And the best part is, besides the improvement to your overall mood, more energy means you'll be able to push that much harder during your workouts, so it's really a self-sustaining process.

Need more? How does quickly ridding yourself of a few of those unwanted pounds sound? Transforming yourself from the King of the Couch Potatoes into a bona fide fitness fanatic is going to send your metabolism into overdrive to compensate for all the increased activity. Couple that with all of the sweating you'll be doing, and it's possible to lose as much as 5 pounds in your first week of training. Granted, much of this will be water weight, so that rate of weight loss won't continue. But at the very least the mental lift you'll get from seeing those numbers on the scale start shrinking could be just the kick start you need to lead to more long-term weight loss.

What about those of you who are looking to gain weight—that is, muscle mass? Surely you can't expect the same sort of short-term payoff, right? Well, yes and no. While it may take 6 to 10 weeks to start seeing

GOAL-SETTING WORKSHEET

Goals:	**3 Months:**
2 Weeks:	**6 Months:**
1 Month:	**1 Year:**

noticeable gains in muscle mass, it is possible to increase strength much more rapidly. Thanks to your central nervous system becoming more efficient at recruiting your muscle fibers to contract, you might find that the amount of weight you're lifting from one workout to the next increases substantially. Initially you may see gains of 10 to 15 percent, though as you progress that will slow down, getting closer to your genetic "ceiling." The more weight you can handle, the more muscle you'll ultimately be able to build (once you start providing your body with the proper amounts and types of nutrients it needs to get bigger—more on this in Chapter 8 on muscle building).

So while you might not necessarily experience eye-popping changes overnight, there will be enough things happening in the short term to keep you motivated enough to press on. And of course, the longer you stick with it, the more these incremental changes will start to add up to some really noticeable differences. It's a pretty simple formula: Start slowly and then watch your progress snowball into something truly amazing.

I've seen this approach work enough times to be completely confident in recommending it to you. Not just for the many clients I've helped through the years, but for myself as well. When I had to put on some more muscle mass for my previous book, *Scrawny to Brawny*, I figured I needed to gain a good 20 to 25 pounds in order to properly promote it. (As you might have guessed from the title, it's a how-to guide for skinny guys who want to bulk up.) Only trouble was, being a fully mature adult (at least physically, that is), it seemed pretty tough to put on that much weight, most of it in the form of muscle mass, especially in a 5-month time frame. But when I broke down the weight gain into monthly goals, I realized I had

Sample Goal-Setting Worksheet

Goals: Gain 15 to 20 pounds (mostly muscle); be able to do a set of 10 chinups (currently at 0); add 2 inches to thighs, chest, and shoulders and 1½ inches to arms.

2 Weeks: Establish good exercise habits by getting in two total-body strength and two cardio workouts per week. Work on flexibility every other day.

1 Month: Maintain same workout frequency. Shoot for a 2- to 3-pound weight gain. Be able to do a set of 5 to 6 controlled negative chinups. Introduce daily flexibility drills.

3 Months: Increase workout frequency (optional) to three total-body strength and three cardio workouts per week. Be up 6 to 8 pounds. Be able to do 2 to 4 consecutive unassisted chinups. Be ½ to 1 inch bigger in the thighs, chest, and shoulders and ¼ to ½ inch bigger in the arms.

6 Months: Maintain new workout frequency, but switch from total-body to alternating upper-/lower-body strength workouts. Increase intensity of cardio workouts. Be up 12 to 15 pounds. Be able to do a set of 6 to 8 chinups. Be 1 to 1½ inches bigger in the chest, shoulders, and thighs and 1 inch bigger in the arms.

1 Year: Realization of all goals and reassessment of physical abilities. Set new goals going forward.

to shoot for only 4 to 5 pounds per month. And when I realized that was only 1 to 1½ pounds per week, I was no longer worried about the prospect of doing it. Because when you break down those goals, they suddenly don't seem anywhere near as difficult.

NUTRITION 101

LAYING THE FOUNDATION FOR NUTRITIONAL SUCCESS

Planning your new fitness program wouldn't be complete without giving at least some thought to nutrition. You might initially see some results by starting your new exercise regimen without altering your current eating habits. But if you're serious about making major changes to the way your body looks and performs, sooner or later you're going to have to get your diet in order. So, seeing as how you're already making one life-altering change by committing to a regular exercise schedule, why not make it two for two and start learning the basics of a healthy diet right now? It'll only make things easier once we start getting a little more intricate with the nutritional guidelines as the program progresses.

To make sure you don't become too bogged down with all the information I'm throwing at you, I'm going to keep the recommendations in this chapter rather simple. The three main areas we're going to focus on are energy balance (calories in versus calories out), meal frequency (how many times per day you should eat), and hydration. These are the three areas where beginners need the most help. Before you start obsessing about things like the amount of proteins, carbs, and fats you're ingesting, or what type of supplements to take, you need to have these basics down pat. By simply developing a good working knowledge of these three factors and the impact they have on your body's ability to function at optimal levels, you'll be well on your way to reaching some of your short-term goals.

CALORIE COUNTING

DETERMINING YOUR DAILY ENERGY NEEDS

Energy balance, or the number of calories going into your body versus the number you expend throughout the day, is without question one of the trickiest aspects of nutrition. Oh sure, it seems simple enough—if you want to weigh less, just eat less. If it were really that simple, though, anyone who's ever gone on a diet and radically restricted their caloric intake would have the body of their dreams. Needless to say, this couldn't be farther from the truth. So, what gives?

What gives is that restricting the amount of energy you put into your body will work for only so long before your metabolism starts slowing down. Once that happens, your body starts learning to make do with less food. It begins more readily holding on to body fat because it's not getting enough of the right kinds of fats in your diet. As if that weren't bad enough, it's also pretty quick to eat into your existing muscle tissue if your daily protein intake isn't quite up to par. Before you know it, you start feeling tired and sluggish all of the time, you get sick more often because your body isn't receiving all of the nutrients it needs, and, oh yeah, you also don't end up burning any fat. Which, in case you forgot, is the main reason you're restricting calories in the first place.

Please don't misinterpret what I'm saying; you do need to create an energy deficit when you're trying to lose fat. The question is, how much of a deficit? Before you can answer that, you first need to know how much energy your body needs on a given day to function at optimal levels.

And don't think calorie counting is just for people who want to drop a few pounds. If you're serious about building muscle, you'd better not only know what your daily energy requirements are but also be prepared to exceed them by 300 to 500 calories per day.

There are a lot of different formulas for calculating daily energy requirements. Few, however, are as accurate as the Harris-Benedict formula, a method that uses such factors as your sex, age, and weight. The first step in the formula is to calculate your basal metabolic rate, or BMR. Your BMR is your resting metabolism, the rate at which your body burns calories just to keep you alive—to keep your lungs inflating, your heart pumping, your brain thinking, and so on. To do this, you need to know your weight in kilograms, which is equal to your weight in pounds divided by 2.2. You also need to know your height in centimeters, which is equal to your height in inches multiplied by 2.54. Then plug those numbers into the following formula.

$$66 + (13.7 \times \text{weight in kg}) + (5 \times \text{height in cm}) - (6.8 \times \text{age in years}) = \text{BMR}$$

Once you've calculated your BMR, the formula incorporates a daily activity multiplier to account for the calories you expend in the course of daily life.

Sedentary (little or no exercise, desk job): BMR × 1.2

Lightly active (light exercise or sports 1 to 3 days/week): BMR × 1.375

Moderately active (moderate exercise or sports 3 to 5 days/week): BMR × 1.55

Very active (hard exercise or sports 6 or 7 days/week): BMR × 1.725

Extremely active (hard daily exercise or sports and physical job): BMR × 1.9

You simply multiply your BMR by your activity multiplier to come up with your total daily energy requirement.

Activity multiplier × BMR = Total daily energy requirement

For example, let's say you're a 35-year-old, 6'1", 220-pound male. Using the Harris-Benedict formula, your numbers would look like this:

BMR = 66 + (13.7 × 91) + (5 × 185) – (6.8 × 35)

BMR = 66 + (1,247) + (925) – (238)

BMR = 2,000 calories

Next you need to factor in the energy you expend during your daily activities. Assuming you fall into the sedentary category, your numbers would change as follows:

BMR of 2,000 × Activity factor of 1.2 = 2,400 calories Total daily energy requirement

Once you know your total daily energy requirement, it's simply a matter of consuming anywhere from 15 to 20 percent fewer calories or from 5 to 20 percent more calories, depending on whether you're interested in losing or gaining weight, respectively.

THE ENERGY CRISIS

FUELING UP TO TRIM DOWN

Generally speaking, ingesting 15 to 20 percent less than your total daily energy requirement should lead to about a 1-pound weight reduction each week. Restricting calories in this manner will help ensure that most of the weight loss comes from stored body fat, as opposed to extremely low-calorie, starvation diets that leave you dehydrated and rob your body of precious muscle mass. So, the formula for our 35-year-old, 6'1", 220-pound-example guy to lose about a pound per week would be as follows.

2,400 – 15 to 20% (360 to 480) = 2,040 to 1,920 calories

It's possible that you'll come up with a number of calories that far exceeds what you've been taking in up to now. And despite that, it may seem that you still can't shed fat. The problem here is that you've slowed your metabolism to such an extent that your body has learned to get by on substantially fewer calories than it needs to function at optimal levels. You're not burning any fat because your body refuses to let go of it, not knowing when it's going to get the good, healthy fats it needs from your diet (mono- and polyunsaturated fats such as those found in olive oil, canola oil, flax oil, nuts, seeds, and avocados).

And you certainly won't build any muscle mass, regardless of how diligent you become about strength training. At best, all you can hope for is to retain what little muscle you do have. So, what do you do?

Even though you do need to increase your caloric intake to get your metabolism firing again, it would be a mistake to jump right up to the higher number of calories. An increase like that would be too much for your body to handle and you'd likely end up gaining body fat. Instead, every 2 weeks, increase your daily caloric intake by 200 to 250 calories. This way, it would take you 8 to 10 weeks to get up to the higher number. This will allow your metabolism to slowly adjust to the increased food intake. Together with the increased physical activity from your new workout program, this gradual increase in calories will help get your metabolism back on its feet again and enable you to finally start burning some of that unwanted fat.

I realize that the idea of eating more to lose weight may be counterintuitive. But think of your daily caloric intake as fuel for a jet engine. If you don't give that engine enough fuel, it's never going to transport you where you want to go. The same holds true for your metabolism. If you want it firing on all cylinders, you'd better start giving it everything it needs to get the job done.

Of course, not everyone who's trying to trim down has been eating too little. Some—dare I say most—guys reading this are currently eating way more food than they need to. For all of you guys, regular exercise combined with moderate caloric restriction is definitely the way to go.

THE NEED TO FEED

THE BASICS OF MUSCLE-BUILDING NUTRITION

There's more to working out than just burning fat, though. Despite being in the minority, there are, believe it or not, some people who actually want to *gain* weight. Mind you, we're talking muscle mass here.

If you fall into this category, being aware of and subsequently surpassing your daily energy needs is absolutely essential to adding the muscle you so desperately seek. Take it from someone who knows firsthand how difficult it can be to gain muscle mass. The amount of muscle you build over a given time frame has an awful lot to do with how much of a caloric surplus you consume. Some guys prefer to take the slow, steady route, where they gain just a couple of pounds of muscle each year and stay relatively lean while doing so. If you're one of them, your caloric consumption should be only somewhat slightly north of your daily energy requirements—say 5 to 10 percent higher.

Others—like me, for instance—prefer the more aggressive approach. This entails consuming 15 to 20 percent more than your daily caloric needs in order to bring about big gains in a relatively short period of time. How big? A gain of 15 to 20 pounds of muscle within a year's time is certainly possible. That is, of course, after you strip off any additional fat you accumulated along the way. And trust me, you will pick up a few extra pounds of fat when using this approach.

CHOW TIME

PLANNING YOUR MEALS

Once you've established how many daily calories you're going to eat, the next thing you have to do is figure out how to divvy up those calories into several meals throughout the course of the day. It's not as simple as eating three squares or, worse yet, two big meals per day. Whether your goal is to burn fat, build muscle, or just improve overall health and well-being, to get the most out of those calories you're going to have to spread them out throughout the day. Doing so will lead to better digestion and absorption of nutrients and will get your metabolism firing on all cylinders. You'll feel more energetic and attentive and much less prone to periods of lethargy throughout the day. And, because you'll be processing your food so much more efficiently, you'll see better and faster results from your training.

Planning your meals is not an exact science. You could eat three meals and three snacks, four or five smallish meals, whatever works for your schedule. Here's a sample meal breakdown for someone consuming approximately 3,000 calories per day:

7 a.m. (breakfast), 800 calories: 2 cups cooked oatmeal, 2 whole eggs plus 4 egg whites, 2 turkey sausage links, 1 banana, and 1 cup orange juice

10 a.m. (mid-morning snack), 400 calories: 1 cup plain yogurt and ¼ cup walnuts

1 p.m. (lunch), 600 calories: 6 ounces grilled chicken, 2 cups pasta salad, and 1 cup steamed vegetables

4 p.m. (mid-afternoon snack), 400 calories: 2 tablespoons peanut butter on 2 slices of whole grain bread

7 p.m. (dinner), 500 calories: 4 ounces grilled salmon and green salad with 1 tablespoon olive oil

9:30 p.m. (snack), 300 calories: 2 cups cottage cheese and 1 cup sliced fruit

WATER WORKS

GET IN THE KNOW ABOUT H_2O

Last but not least amongst our basic nutritional recommendations is the importance of proper hydration. Contrary to popular belief, dehydration doesn't take place only under conditions of extreme heat. It's no stretch to say that thousands of Americans walk around at least partially dehydrated on a daily basis. Because we're a society that relies so heavily on sugar-filled soft drinks and juices, many of us just don't get the correct amount of water our bodies need to function properly. Add in the diuretic effects of caffeinated beverages like soda and those $4 double lattes and the problem is only made worse.

Even a mild case of dehydration can lead to stress, lowered performance, increased fatigue, and longer recovery time between workouts. If dehydration gets worse, you could experience severe fatigue, joint pain, digestive disturbances, and weakened immune function.

Although it's difficult for the average person to have a good handle on his or her state of hydration, if you are prone to drinking caffeinated or high-sugar beverages, often feel fatigued, and have a tendency to get sick, chances are you need to start drinking more water. The liquid you ingest when drinking other beverages doesn't count. To improve the way your body feels, looks, and functions, you need to drink good old-fashioned H_2O.

How much water should you drink? While the long-established guideline of eight 8-ounce glasses per day is a good start and might represent a marked improvement, count on upping that amount significantly to account for your newly active lifestyle. Think more in the range of 1½ to 2 gallons, especially on workout days. You'll have to work up to that gradually, otherwise you'll wear out a path to the bathroom. Besides, as with any major physiological change, it's always best to go slowly to give your body time to adapt.

THE BEST LAID PLANS . . .

PATIENCE AND PERSEVERANCE ARE KEY

Okay, now you've got a definitive plan of action. You've armed yourself with the kind of information most people in your situation never seem to access. But just because you've figured out your daily energy requirements, clearly identified your short- and long-term goals, and committed yourself to a schedule for reaching those goals, that doesn't necessarily mean you're going to be successful. By deviating from the very plan you just worked so hard to create, you could still end up like countless other frustrated beginners. Don't give in to the temptations of quick results promised by "can't miss" workouts and seemingly too-good-to-be-true nutritional supplements.

Building the body you want takes time, hard work, and the right plan. That doesn't mean you won't see some quick, inspiring changes along the way. As I mentioned earlier, if you do things properly, there will be plenty of little short-term rewards like improved energy levels and a gradually shrinking waistline. Just know going in that dramatic, head-turning physical transformations aren't going to happen overnight. That's why I liken the process of becoming fit to a journey, rather than to a destination. As with any journey worth taking, you need to have a plan in place in order to get where you want to go.

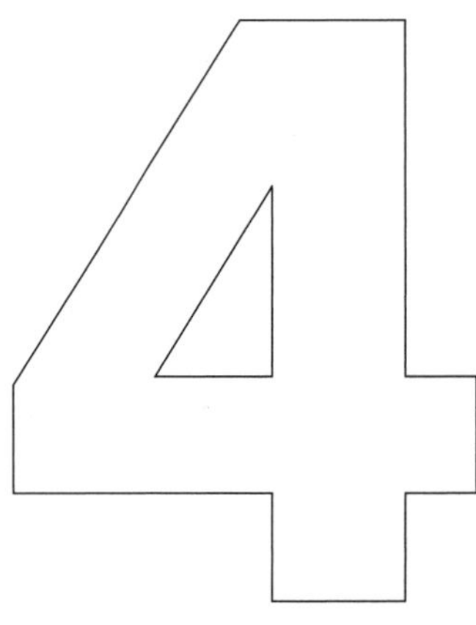

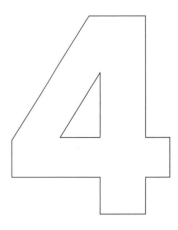

TOOLS OF THE TRADE

HERE'S THE EQUIPMENT YOU NEED FOR THE BODY YOU WANT

No matter how committed you are to starting and sticking with an exercise program, you'll never achieve the results you're looking for if you don't have the right equipment. This doesn't necessarily mean you have to commit to an expensive gym membership; too many people make that mistake every January as a knee-jerk response to their overindulgence during the holiday season. It just means you should know what your options are. To that end, here's an inventory of all the different types of equipment that are out there.

Jump rope: A good jump rope can cost you anywhere from $10 to $25. The only differences in the more expensive models are things like weighted handles and a more comfortable grip. In my opinion, the old-fashioned brown leather type you can get for 10 bucks is just fine.

Stationary bike: This can run from $300 up to several thousand dollars. Some of the best-selling brands are Schwinn, Fitness Quest, and Keys.

Treadmill: Expect to spend a bit more here. You can't get a decent treadmill for under $1,000. You can't go wrong with anything made by Precor or ProForm.

Rower: Only one choice here in my view: the Concept 2 rower. This is the granddaddy of them all and quite simply head and shoulders above the rest. The in-home models start at around $800.

Vertical climber: Like the treadmill, this can be rather expensive. If you have the money, though, it probably offers the best cardiovascular workout going. VersaClimber is the original (and most expensive).

Stairclimber: Any model put out by StairMaster is probably your best bet. Tunturi also has some decent in-home models. Expect to spend between $800 and $2,500.

Elliptical machine: Its increasing popularity has brought the prices down in recent years. A good model runs between $750 and $2,000. Schwinn, ProForm, and Reebok are among the best.

Medicine ball. Unlike the oversize leather ball held together by shoestrings that Sylvester Stallone used to heave around back in his Rocky days, today medicine balls come in a variety of shapes and sizes. The right size for you is dependent on a number of factors, including your initial fitness level, the types of exercises you'll be using it for, and your individual goals. With that in mind, the following recommendations should help you decide which ones are appropriate for you.

- 1 and 2 kilograms: Good for dynamic warmups and various core drills for all types of trainees, these can also be used for strength and power training in older and more deconditioned populations.

- 3 to 5 kilograms: Still useful for dynamic warmups and core training in more experienced exercisers, they're also a useful strength-building tool for beginning and intermediate trainees.

- 6 to 8 kilograms: Excellent tools for core training and power development in intermediate to advanced exercisers, these are good strength-training tools for beginners.

- 9 kilograms and up: These heaviest balls are best used by more advanced trainees, although beginners and intermediates can still use them for controlled strength exercises like squatting and overhead presses.

Dumbbells. In my opinion, an adjustable dumbbell system called PowerBlocks is quite simply the best piece of fitness equipment ever developed. PowerBlocks are easy to use, incredibly versatile, and sturdy as can be. They come in a variety of sizes and let you change weights with just the pull of a pin, going from 3 to 21 pounds, from 5 to 45 pounds, or from 5 to 125 pounds in no time at all. You'd probably be fine with the 5-to-45-pound set since it enables you to add onto it as you become stronger. It retails for around $250, with the additional stand priced at $120. The Pro Rexan set, which allows you to use weights ranging from 2½ pounds all the way up to 85 pounds, sells for about $600, and the stand goes for $130. Best of all, their unique design makes PowerBlocks a real space saver. Two PowerBlocks, plus the stand they're set on, take up only 3 square feet. True, they can be a serious investment, but with a 10-year guarantee and the amount of space and money they'll save you in the long run, they can't be beat. You can find out more at www.powerblock.com.

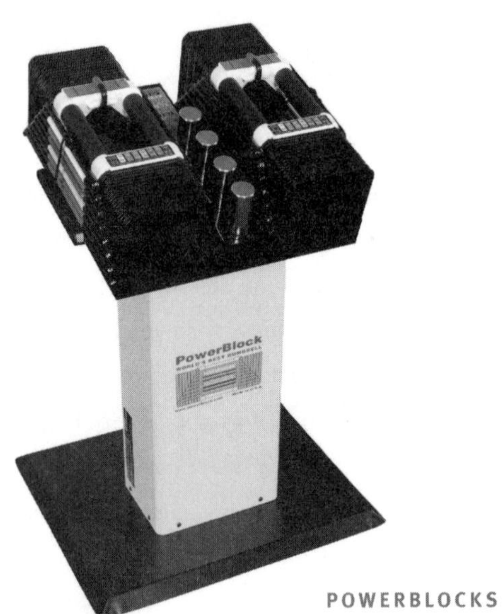

POWERBLOCKS

Barbell and weight sets. Your first option here is the standard barbell set. This retails for between $60 and $120 and comes with a 7-foot standard bar, 85 pounds of weight plates, two dumbbell handles, and two collars (clips used for holding the weights in place on the bar).

Then there's the 300-pound Olympic set with bar. This set consists of a 7-foot Olympic bar and 255 pounds of weight plates and collars for as low as $100. Or you can purchase the bar and weight separately as you get stronger. The bar can be purchased separately starting at $85 and the plates for as low as 50 cents per pound.

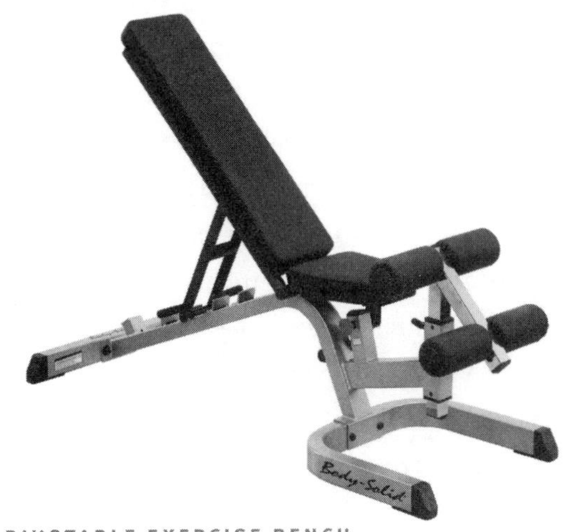

ADJUSTABLE EXERCISE BENCH

Adjustable bench. This is just a sturdy bench you can set to various angles (incline, decline, etc.) and use for a wide variety of exercises, including bench presses and dumbbell rows. A good one will set you back anywhere from $150 to $300.

Squat rack or power cage. These are just sturdy supports on which you can set the weights when doing heavy exercises like squats, bench presses, and overhead presses. Aside from giving you something to lift the weights off from, their biggest benefit is that they allow you to lift relatively heavy weights without the aid of a spotter. Simply set the supports near the bottom of your range of motion and, if you get in trouble, just set the weights down on top of them.

If you are going to work out at home and want to buy your own squat rack or power cage, Body-Solid is one manufacturer in particular that offers extremely durable pieces at reasonable prices. As far as power cages go,

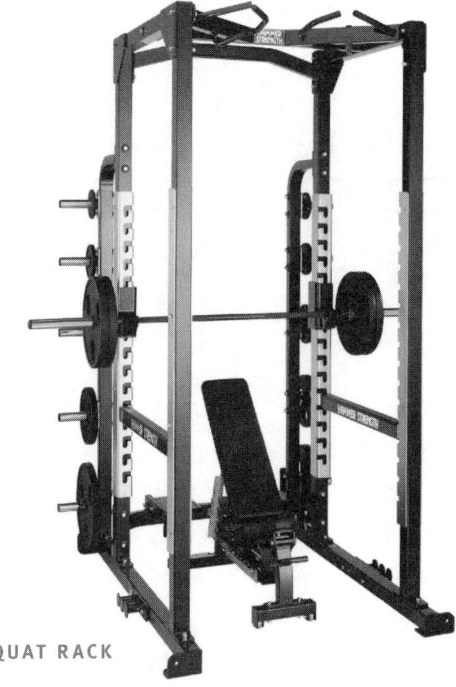

SQUAT RACK

Power Tec has one of the best. It sells for about $360, comes with an overhead chinning bar, and enables you to add on an optional dip station and/or lat pulldown/low row. Their squat rack is also first rate and sells for around $360.

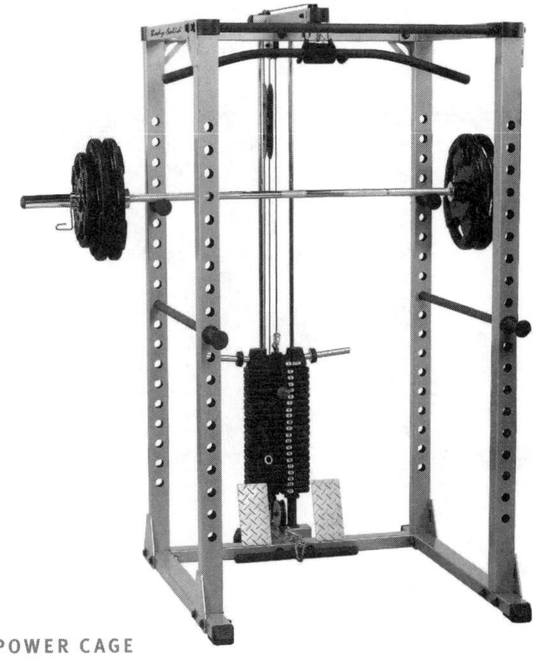

POWER CAGE

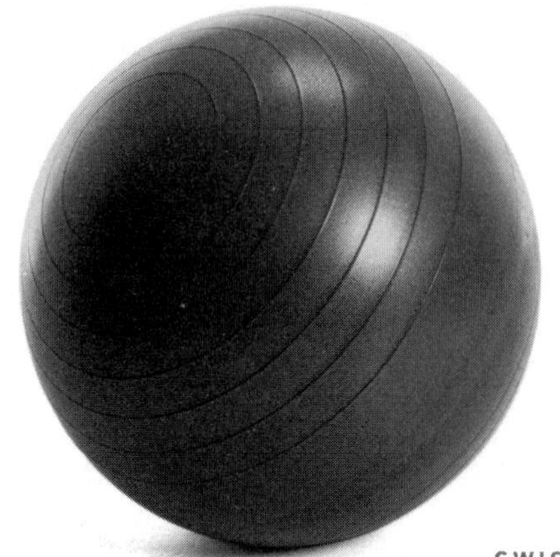

SWISS BALL

Stability balls and exercise mats. Balls run in the \$25-to-\$40 range, with mats being slightly more expensive. Neither is an absolute must have, but if you have the extra cash, they'll help add tons of variety and comfort to your workout. The balls, also known as Swiss balls, are brightly colored, thick-plastic orbs that come in a variety of sizes and allow you to do everything from challenging core exercises to flexibility drills. They can even double as benches to support you when performing various free-weight exercises. Make sure that you get the burst-resistant variety and that it's the proper size for you. Guys 5'7" and under will need the 55-centimeter ball; 5'8" to 6'2", the 65-centimeter; and 6'3" and taller the 75-centimeter size. For home use, you can purchase mats as well as balls at most sporting goods stores and through nationally recognized athletic equipment companies like Power Systems (www.power-systems.com) and Perform Better (www.performbetter.com).

Weight machines. These allow you to work out just about every muscle in your body, and they're a little less intimidating if you lack the strength, stability, or even confidence to jump right to free weights. Two of the best are the Bowflex Xtreme 2 and the ProSpot P-500. However, before you decide to lay out the money for one of these bad boys, I suggest you take some time to weigh all of the pros and cons of working out on machines.

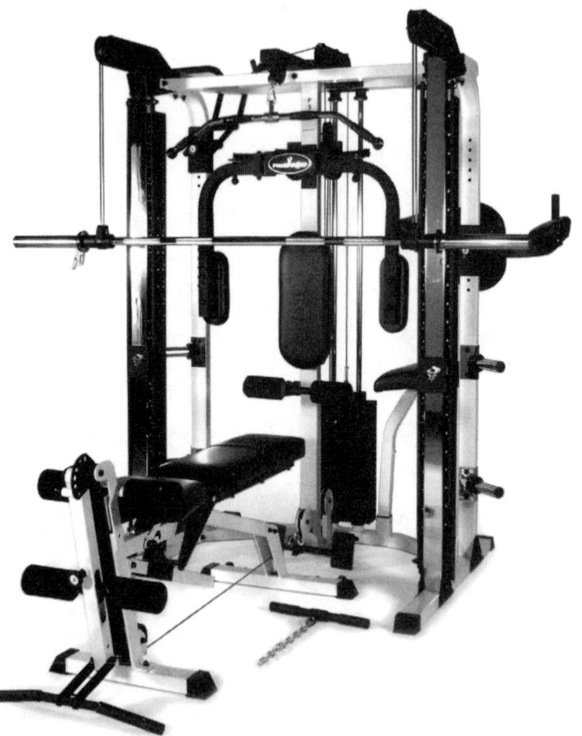

PROSPOT P-500

STRENGTHS AND WEAKNESSES

MACHINES HAVE THEM, JUST LIKE YOU DO

I'm not a big fan of machines. It's not that I think all of them are useless—quite the contrary. There are several types that can actually be quite beneficial if used properly. I like the FreeMotion line, developed by renowned conditioning specialist Juan Carlos Santana. Unlike most other machines, which lock you into a set path of motion, these adjustable, cable-based machines allow you to alter the range of motion to suit the way your body moves. In doing so, they place far less strain on joints and connective tissue and more accurately mimic the types of movements you'll do when you're outside the gym.

High-ticket items like these are most likely out of the

question if you train at home, though. There are numerous types of home gym machines on the market that claim to have tremendous versatility. While some are probably better than others, none gives you the versatility you can get from some free weights and a bench. As far as cardio goes, if you've got the money, a good treadmill or an elliptical machine can always come in handy. Then again, to get your heart rate going and burn a few extra calories you could also jump-rope, go for a run, or do a free-weight circuit.

The point I'm trying to make is that while weight and cardio machines may make exercise a little bit easier at times, you don't really *need* them to get a good workout. That said, if you like all the bells and whistles and know you'll adhere to a program better if it involves machines, then go for it. There are also some people who simply won't do cardio work unless they can zone out in front of a television while they're working out. If you fit into either category, by all means use those machines to your heart's content. I may be a purist, but I'm flexible enough to acknowledge that some exercise is better than none. If working on machines is the only way you'll commit to a program, be my guest.

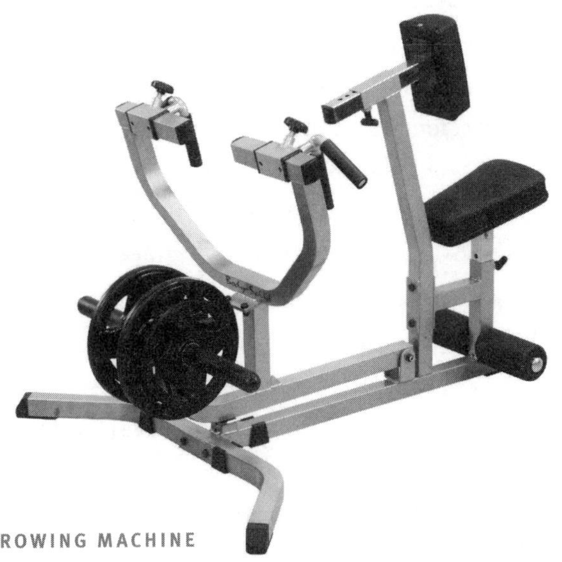

ROWING MACHINE

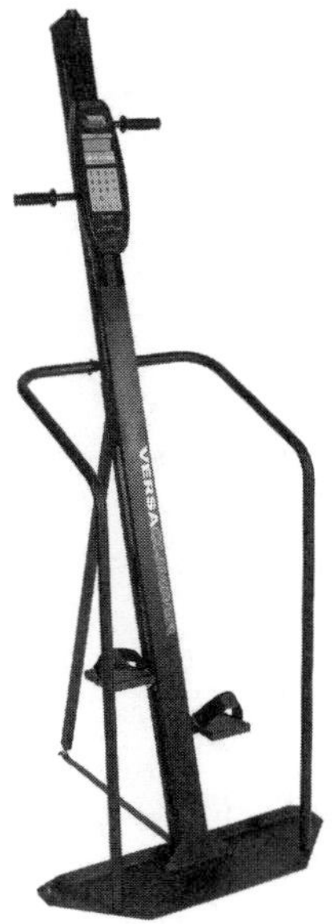

VERSACLIMBER

Just to be fair about it, I've decided to provide you with a list of machines that are well worth the effort.

Rowing machine. I'm referring mainly to resistance-type rowing machines that are used for upper-back strengthening. These include cable rows, machine rows, and even plate-loaded, free-weight rowing machines, although cardio rowers like the Concept 2 are also quite useful. The great thing about these exercisers is that they target the oft-overlooked upper back musculature that helps pull back, or retract, your shoulder blades. By helping to promote proper posture and more balanced development of the muscles that surround the shoulder joint, these machines offset the overemphasis on chest and front deltoid work typical of most workout programs. Definitely an underused resource, in my opinion.

VersaClimber. Like the Concept 2 rower, this is an apparatus that will give your heart a real workout. Its simulated climbing motion works so many muscles at the same time that you can't help but become more fit by using it on a regular basis. It combines upper- and lower-body movement through a large range of motion, for the ultimate cardiovascular, calorie-burning stimulus. And

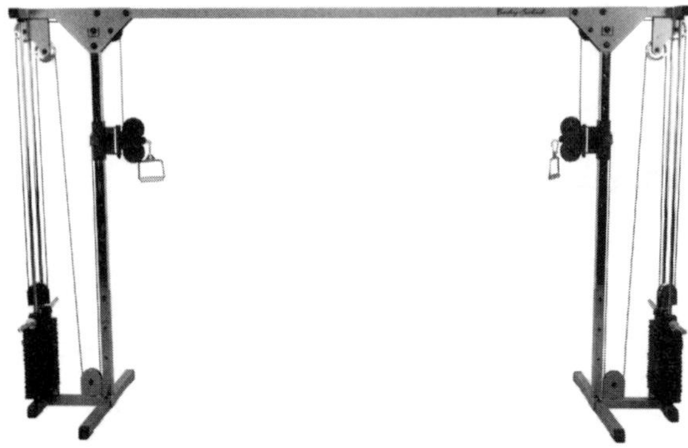

ADJUSTABLE CABLE STATION

the best part is, if you work out in a gym that has this machine, you'll almost never have to wait to use it, because most people just aren't willing to expend that much effort. A VersaClimber is also a lot cheaper and a lot smaller than a treadmill, making it a great choice for home use as well.

Adjustable cable station. The great thing about this is that it's so versatile. It allows you to do everything from rowing to lunging to core exercises. Best of all, since you're not locked into one set path of motion, a cable station allows you to make little alterations in the range of motion that give the exercises more of an individualized feel.

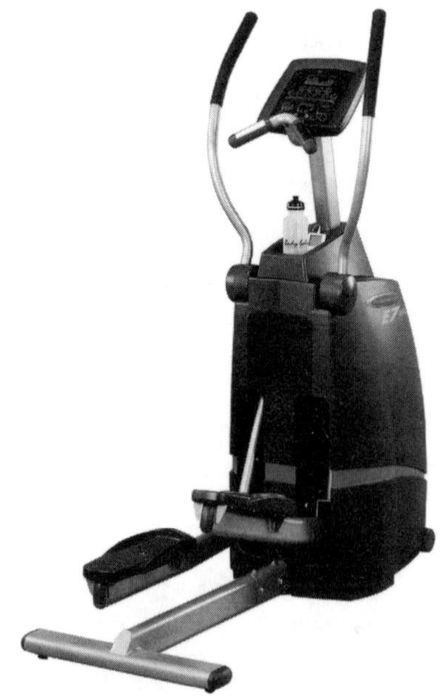

ELLIPTICAL MACHINE

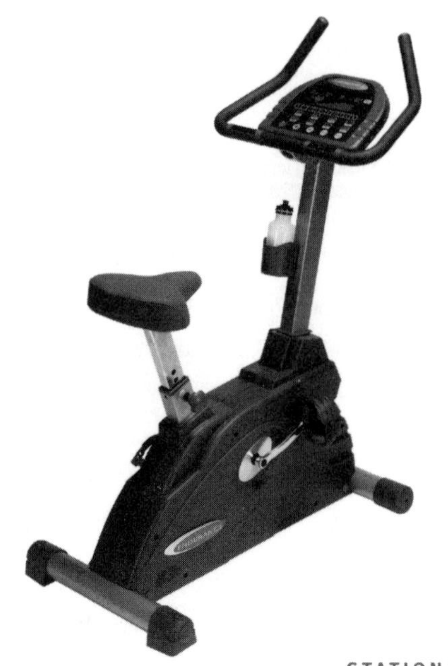

STATIONARY BIKE

Low-impact cardio machines (elliptical trainers, stationary bikes, and upper-body ergometers, or UBEs, which are basically stationary bikes for the upper body). Let's face it, not everyone is able to run. Although some may live for it, the constant pounding and jarring make it more of an exercise in futility for others. For older individuals or people who are significantly overweight, running, skipping rope, and high-impact aerobic classes are simply out of the question. If you fit into this category, low-impact forms of cardiovascular training, like elliptical trainers and stationary bikes, are a much better and safer way to go. They'll give you all of the same benefits without the unwanted orthopedic stress that often accompanies these activities.

Hip abduction/adduction machines. These enable you to do some targeted strengthening of muscles that play an important role in stabilizing the knee joint during movements like squatting and lunging. So despite their reputation as "chick machines," these have plenty of application for macho types as well.

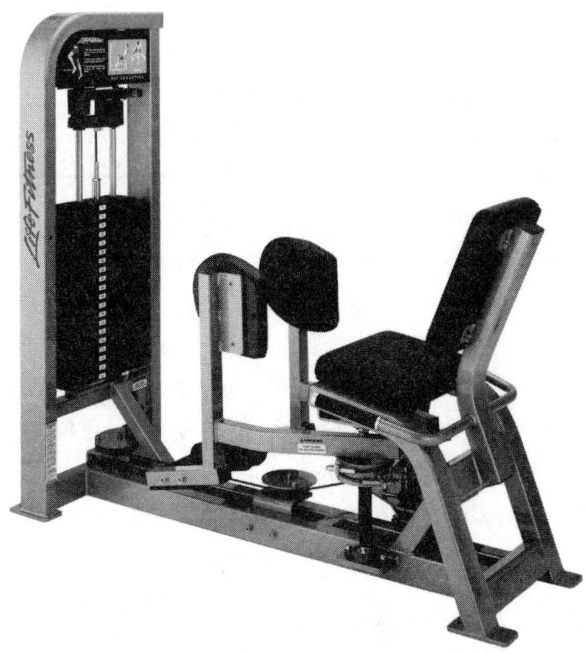

HIP ABDUCTION/ADDUCTION MACHINE

RAGE AGAINST THE MACHINES

ONES TO BE WARY OF

While I may accept and respect your decision to opt for machines over free weights, I'd be remiss if I didn't point out some of my least favorite machines and the potential dangers they pose, even when used correctly. If orthopedic surgeons were to come up with a most-wanted list à la the FBI, these are the machines that John Walsh would be warning you about every Saturday night.

Smith machine. A lot of people like this one because of the perceived level of safety it provides. Because the bar travels attached to two guiding cables and has safety hooks at several different levels, it's easy to just hang up the weight if you get into trouble. However, this safety feature is outweighed by the fact that the machine locks you into a linear movement pattern when performing exercises like squats, bench presses, shoulder presses, and rows. This is not the way your body was intended to move, and as a result, it places a lot of unnecessary strain on joints and connective tissue.

Pec deck. This is among the first strength-training machines to ever hit the market. Designed to target your chest, this little biomechanical nightmare combines horizontal abduction and external rotation of the shoulders. Yes, that's as bad as it sounds. It basically means holding your arms up at right angles as if you were the target of a stickup. This can be a tough enough position to get into without any additional load. Asking your shoulders to actually move a weight from this position is pretty much asking for trouble.

Leg extension machine. Sure, it seems innocuous enough: Just sit in a big ol' easy chair and kick your legs out in front of you. Trouble is, the position of the weight in relation to your knees places a tremendous amount of

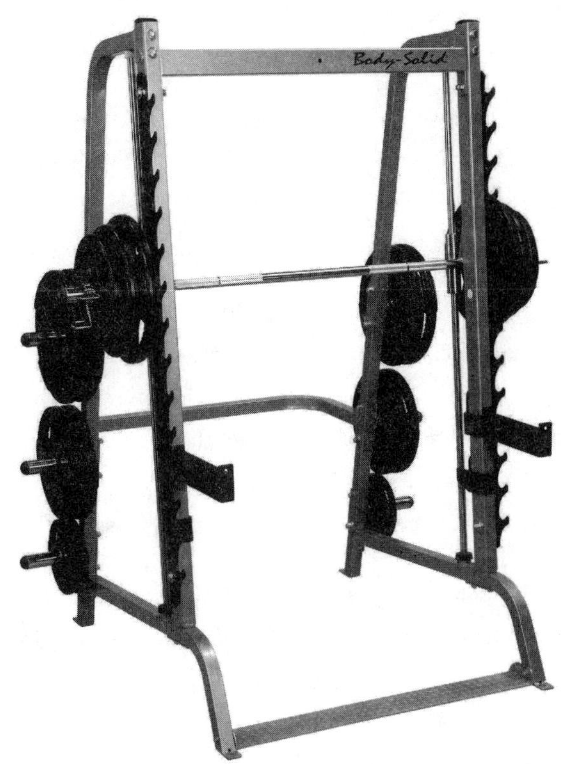

SMITH MACHINE

(continued on page 36)

Your guide to fitting in while you're working out

Believe it or not, there is a certain way one is supposed to conduct oneself when working out in a gym full of people. It's pretty easy for a newbie like you to screw up and do something that totally alienates you from the rest of the members. In addition to knowing and following the written rules like always showing your membership card upon entering and not working out in your street clothes, there are a whole slew of unwritten rules you need to know to peacefully coexist with those around you. Here's a list of the 10 biggies.

Always exercise good personal hygiene. Few things are more unpleasant than working out next to someone with killer BO. I understand that it's impractical to take a shower before you work out, especially if you train first thing in the morning, but a swipe of deodorant under each arm shouldn't be too much to ask. Nor is it unreasonable for your fellow members to expect you to show up with clean workout attire each time you train. Please make sure to wash your gym clothes after each use.

Clean up after yourself. Other people don't want to lie on a bench or use a treadmill soaked in your sweat. It doesn't take too much effort to throw an extra towel into your gym bag and wipe down the equipment once you're finished with it. Doing so will save you the embarrassment of being known as "that sweaty guy."

Put back any equipment you've finished using. You'd be amazed at how many people have trouble grasping this idea. Walk into many gyms and you'll likely see loaded barbells left unattended and dumbbells lying all over the floor. There are even some inconsiderate clods who load machines with tons of weight only to let someone (usually a much smaller and weaker someone) strip down the weight just so they can use the equipment. Needless to say, this behavior goes over about as well as a lead balloon with your fellow gymmates. Not to mention the fact that it can get your membership revoked if the management ever catches you. This is more than just inconvenient to those around you; it's potentially dangerous. It's easy to trip over a wayward dumbbell or drop a weight on your foot while unloading a machine. Rather than risk alienating everyone at your gym, just do the sensible thing and put your stuff away.

Don't monopolize the equipment. Most gyms post time limits for the cardio machines, especially during the busiest times of the day (the early a.m. and after-work hours). Going over your allotted time is a quick way to get on people's bad sides. It doesn't matter if you feel your training goals dictate that you "need" the equipment more than someone else (because you have more body fat to lose). The rules exist for a reason, so make sure you follow them.

Hogging equipment can also be a problem in the weight room. Using a given machine or other piece of equipment doesn't mean you have exclusive access to it until you've finished all of your sets. During rest intervals, it's customary to allow someone else to use the equipment until it's time for your next set. This is known as working in, and it works both ways: It's perfectly acceptable for you to approach someone and ask to share the equipment while they're resting between sets. When sharing a machine, you can do this with just about anyone since changing the weight is as simple as pulling out a pin. With free weights, however, it gets a bit more complicated. In this situation, you want to be sure that you and the other person are of similar strength levels. Nothing disrupts the flow of a workout more than having to load and unload large amounts of weight after each set.

Never talk to someone while they're doing a set. The reasoning here is pretty simple: Lifting weight is hard, and it takes a great deal of focus. The last thing someone needs when in the process of lifting a couple of hundred pounds is you distracting them by asking when they're going to be done with the equipment. If you see someone in the middle of a set, have the courtesy to wait for them to finish before speaking to them. You also might want to stand out of their line of sight. Even if you're not speaking to them, looming over someone while they're lifting can be every bit as annoying.

Respect other people's space. I don't know about you, but I can't stand being crowded. There's more than enough space in the average gym that you don't have to work out on top of other people. Besides being incredibly annoying, working out too close to a fellow member is also potentially dangerous. You could get hit with a weight, limb, or other moving object. So before you start to perform an exercise, make sure you have ample space around you to execute it properly without infringing on anyone else.

Don't block access to equipment you're not using. Unfortunately, this sort of thing happens all too frequently and is often done by even the most seasoned gym rats. Performing an exercise in such a way that it prevents another member from using a different piece of equipment is one of the most inconsiderate and dangerous things you can do. Whether it's performing dumbbell exercises too close to the rack so no one else can get the weights they need, or doing crunches right behind a treadmill so people have to step over you to use it (sadly, I've seen this happen), you're bound to get on someone's nerves.

Use the equipment for its intended purpose. This refers to performing exercises in inappropriate places—like, say, doing biceps curls in the squat rack or cranking out a set of stepups on the bench press. Certain pieces of equipment serve specific purposes. A squat rack, for instance, is made for . . . squats! Yes, it allows you to grasp a bar set just below waist level so you can do a set of curls without having to bend over and pick up the bar, but that's completely beside the point. You could do that same set of curls anywhere in the gym; someone who wants to squat can only do so in that rack. Break this rule and you run the risk of angering some of the biggest, strongest guys in the gym.

Keep the noise to a minimum. Yelling, screaming, and other types of histrionics really aren't necessary just to lift a weight. I know there are guys in every gym who do this, but trust me, you don't want to be one of them. It's obnoxious, and it really annoys the people around you. It doesn't make you any stronger, either. So if you think a primal scream or two will help you eke out that extra rep, you're sadly mistaken. For what it's worth, singing aloud to the tunes on your MP3 player while on the treadmill is almost as bad.

Keep all personal belongings in your locker. This includes things like your wallet, car keys, gym bag and, most important, your cell phone. Lugging your bag with you from station to station and leaving it on equipment you're not using is inconsiderate to other members. There's enough to worry about in a gym without having to be careful not to trip over, or inadvertently place a weight on top of, someone's personal effects. The locker rooms exist for a reason and are included in the price of your membership, so take full advantage of them. Besides, talking on a cell phone at the gym makes you look like a self-important dweeb.

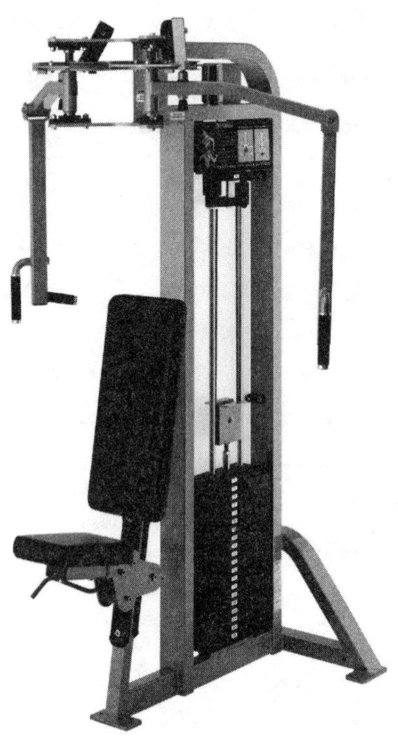

PEC DECK

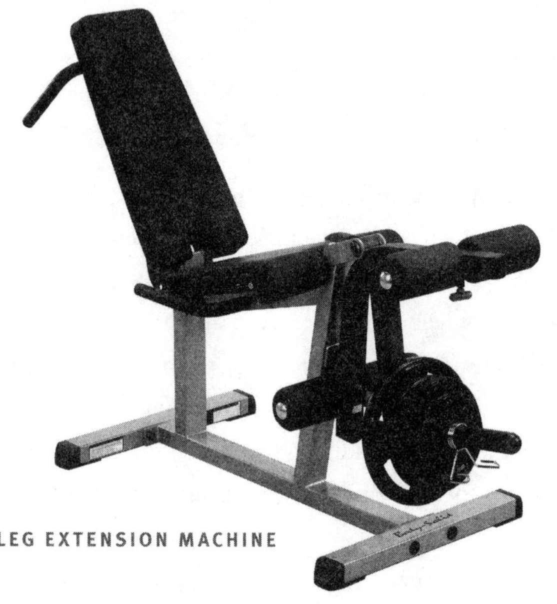

LEG EXTENSION MACHINE

shearing force on the joints (yep, that's bad)—a force that only gets compounded the higher you raise the leg. Never mind the fact that it's a practically worthless movement that has little if any carryover to everyday movements like squatting and lunging.

Ab machines. These are absolutely laughable. Most beginners lack the core strength to get their shoulder blades to leave the floor when they're attempting to perform a situp. The last thing they need is to make the movement harder by adding external resistance! I cringe whenever I see people on these various crunch machines, grabbing the handles and basically just jerking the weight up with their arms. Not that the unweighted ones are any better, mind you. In fact, they go to the opposite extreme, making the exercises too easy by giving you a biomechanical advantage to get the weight up. There are tons of other, more effective and functional ways to work your abs (this book is full of them). My advice: Take a pass.

Lat pulldown machine. The actual machine isn't the problem. If you lack the strength to do a pullup (that's going to have to change, by the way), using the lat pulldown is the next best thing. My issue is with using the machine to do a version of the lat pulldown exercise in which you pull the weight down behind your head to the base of your neck. Once again, it causes you to employ that dreaded combination of horizontal abduction and external rotation of the shoulders. Besides potentially straining the small muscles of the rotator cuff that are integral to stabilizing the shoulder joint, this movement also places tremendous stress on the anterior (front) aspect of the shoulders, leaving you open to potential subluxations, or dislocations, if you do the exercise often enough. Do yourself a favor: If you must do pulldowns, do them to the front.

The important thing to remember about all machines is that, while they're not completely useless, neither are they crucial to getting a good workout. With your own body weight and simple free weights, you can do enough to keep your body in good working order. Some of you

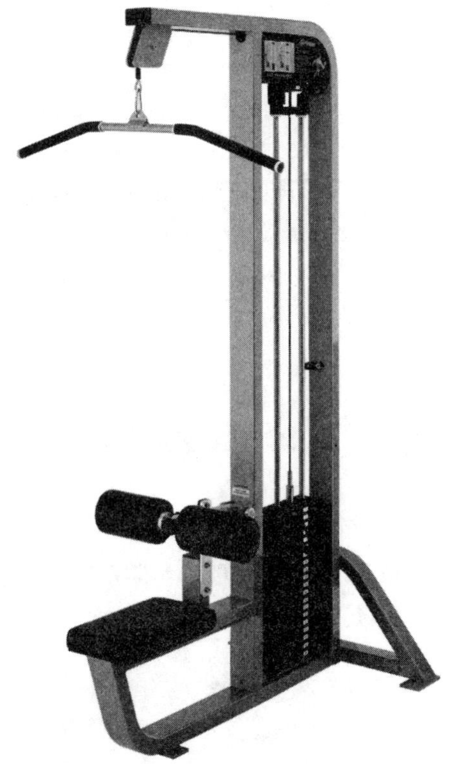

LAT PULLDOWN MACHINE

may find that the ease and comfort that machines offer make working out more appealing. If training with machines makes you feel like you're getting more out of your workouts, by all means, use them as much as you like. Just know that while some may be beneficial, there are those that may actually do you more harm than good.

THE RIGHT TOOLS FOR THE JOB

MATCHING YOUR GEAR TO YOUR GOALS

Now that you have an inventory of available exercise tools, let's take an in-depth look at exactly what you can accomplish with different types of equipment. Then you can examine your budget to see whether you'll be able to provide yourself with everything you need to achieve the goals you've set.

Goal: Improved cardiovascular function. You can get an excellent cardiovascular workout by simply stringing together several bodyweight calisthenic exercises. Assuming that doesn't do it for you, you might also need a good pair of running and/or hiking shoes and a jump rope. Or you might want to opt for a more high-tech approach like a treadmill, stationary bike, or rower. For a home gym, either the VersaClimber or a stairclimber is probably your best bet in terms of the amount of space they take up.

Goal: Improved flexibility. There's not much you're going to need here. As long as you've got ample space and a mat or comfortable floor to lie on, you're all set. Simply follow the exercise descriptions and pictures I'll provide in Chapters 6 and 7.

You may not realize that you can also increase flexibility with light dumbbells and barbells. Yes, I'm talking about the same free weights you see the meatheads at the local gym hurling around with reckless abandon. When used improperly, they can turn you into a muscle-bound, poorly proportioned mess with the flexibility of a stone. Ah, but if you use them the right way, the wonders you will find.

Increasing flexibility with free weights requires doing some fairly odd-looking exercises and using some pretty unconventional training methods. On the bright side, the end definitely justifies the means. See the flexibility workouts on page 104.

Goal: Increased size and strength. If you're interested in increasing strength or building muscle mass, bodyweight exercises like pushups, pullups, dips, and lunges will produce some improvements, at least in the beginning. As you progress, though, you'll probably need to introduce some form of external resistance—that is, weights—into your workouts. This is especially true if your main focus is to increase strength, although you will find a rather intense bodyweight strength workout in Chapter 9. At best, you're probably looking at 6 to 8 weeks before you need to start adding some additional weight to your exercises. As far as building muscle is concerned, it's possible to increase the size of your muscles using only your body weight and the proper nutritional approach. The physiques of competitive gymnasts and martial artists are a testament to this fact. Of course, much of this has to do with the countless hours of grueling training they put in each day, as well as the many advanced exercises they're able to perform. It's unlikely that a beginner like yourself could expect similar results.

So at the very least, a set of simple dumbbells will come in extremely handy. However, seeing as how you'll probably need a lot of different weights to do the various exercises in your program, a bunch of dumbbells could quickly get cumbersome if you work out at home. Enter the PowerBlock.

You'll also likely need a bench, preferably an adjustable one. Adding on from there, a barbell, some weight plates, and a support structure like a squat rack or power cage would also be helpful, especially if increasing strength is your primary goal.

If price is no object and you prefer machines to free weights, there are several good home workout machines on the market that offer a variety of options. Some of the best include the Bowflex Xtreme 2 and the ProSpot P-500. Finally, no gym is complete without Swiss, or stability, balls.

Goal: Fat loss. Perhaps more than any of the other goals, this offers the most diversity in terms of how you can approach it. You can opt to go with just your own body weight, low-tech cardio exercises like running or skipping rope, traditional machine-based cardio like treadmills and stationary bikes, or intensive weight training. The choice is really up to you.

The idea of weight training being an effective way to burn body fat or improve flexibility is probably a very intriguing concept to you. The average person assumes that free weights are best suited to people who want to get bigger and stronger. Walk into any gym, and I guarantee you'll find a lot more people pumping up with them than using them to become leaner.

LOCATION, LOCATION, LOCATION

SELECTING THE BEST PLACE TO WORK OUT

Now that you've got the lowdown on the types of equipment necessary to reach various goals, the next step is deciding whether to work out at home or in a commercial gym. You may have already made your decision based on financial or logistical reasons. If money and space are no object and you're still on the fence, perhaps I can help shed some light on which might be the best choice for your particular situation.

The truth is, there is no objective best place to work out. Some people get great results at home with modest equipment, while others prefer the diversity afforded by a health club. The key is making sure you know the pros and cons of each. The following information should prove quite helpful in pointing you in the right direction.

Home Sweet Home

The Benefits of Being a Homebody

There are an awful lot of advantages to training in the privacy of your own home. For starters, the commute is an absolute breeze. You'll rarely, if ever, experience any traffic tie-ups going from the bedroom to the basement. You also don't have to wait to use any of the equipment or worry about wiping other people's sweat off it before you do. Another nice perk is being able to shower barefoot once you've finished training, something I definitely don't advocate trying in a commercial health club.

If you ask me, it's pretty tough to beat training at home. The privacy and unobstructed access to equipment is a far cry from what often goes on in gyms. No one can tell you what to wear or what kind of music to play, and the place is never closed!

That said, working out at home is not completely without drawbacks. If you make the effort to go all the way to the gym, that's it, you're there. At home, you can get distracted by household chores, intrusive family members, and ill-timed phone calls. Still, as long as you're capable of tuning these things out and you have the financial wherewithal to get all of the equipment you need, training at home is a great way to go.

Join the Club

What to Look for When Joining a Gym

What if you don't have the money or space to covert your home into your own private fitness palace? Don't sweat it; you can get a great workout by opting for one of the increasing number of gyms that seem to keep popping up all over the place. As a matter of fact, unless you're in Bill Gates's tax bracket, it'd be tough—if not downright impossible—to fill your home with the diversity of equipment found in most gyms. Of course, along with all that fancy equipment comes a whole host of other things you need to be aware of when you decide to join a gym.

Some people just can't train unless they're in a gym atmosphere. Whether it's due to the perceived superiority of exercising with high-priced equipment or the social aspect of being around others with similar interests, they just seem to feed off it. I've even known guys who will drive all the way to the gym just to stretch because they "can't get into it" at home.

And you know what? That's fine. As long as you're doing something to improve your health and well-being, who cares where you do it? Just realize that not all gyms are created equal. There are a lot of things you need to consider before committing to something that could become a regular part of your life for months, if not years, to come. Don't just sign up at the first place where you see weights and a couple of treadmills. A number of factors—including some you probably haven't even thought of—could significantly impact your level of satisfaction with a potential new gym. Here are a few of the more pressing concerns.

Location: It doesn't matter how nice a gym is or how impressed you are with its equipment or amenities: If it's inconvenient to get to, your visits will be few and far between. Try to pick someplace that's close to your home or place of work. This will allow you to train either before or after work, or maybe even sneak in a workout on your lunch hour.

Price: Beware of gyms that look for huge financial commitments up front. These days, most gyms offer affordable monthly dues after an initial registration fee. Also look for gyms that allow you to pay as you go. The last thing you need is a monthly bill for a gym membership you have no intention of ever using again.

Staffing: Whether or not you opt to use a personal trainer is up to you. At the very least, your membership dues should provide you with an initial evaluation and orientation where you'll be shown how to use the equipment. There should also be at least one instructor working the gym floor at all times to assist members and answer any questions they may have. All of the instructors should possess some type of certification, preferably from a nationally recognized certification body like the National Strength and Conditioning Association

(NSCA), the National Academy of Sports Medicine (NASM), or the International Sport Sciences Association (ISSA). Quite often gym floor instructors are kids fresh out of college who haven't yet secured jobs in their chosen fields, so be sure to ask. The last thing you need is to have your heart rate manipulated by some kid who could just as easily be asking you if you want fries with your order.

Equipment: You now know that it doesn't take much, but be sure that whatever equipment the gym has is to your liking and appears to be well maintained. Ripped upholstery and rusted metal should serve as major red flags that member service may not be a priority. If the management doesn't care enough to keep the equipment looking nice, you can't help but wonder what kind of working order it's in.

Hours: Make sure the gym is open at the times when you're able to get there. If you work odd hours and can exercise only extremely early in the morning or late at night, you need to ensure that the gym can accommodate your schedule. Additionally, be on the lookout for discounted memberships for off-peak times. A lot of gyms offer cheaper memberships to people who can work out in the middle of the day, when gyms typically aren't as busy. And speaking of peak times, make sure to find out when those are. Nothing can ruin your workout faster than an overcrowded gym.

Cleanliness: Though it's not much of an issue to some people, if you ask me, a dirty, stinky gym can be a real turnoff. I don't expect the place to be spotless or to smell like potpourri, but it's pretty gross when people leave sweat angels on the benches and the locker room looks like it hasn't been cleaned since the Reagan administration. So don't be afraid to ask if the gym has a maintenance staff and how often the place is cleaned.

ALL GEARED UP

UNDERSTANDING THE IMPORTANCE OF HAVING THE RIGHT EQUIPMENT

Hopefully the information presented in this chapter has impressed upon you that determining exactly what constitutes the "right" equipment is half the battle. A lot of it has to do with how open-minded you are and how hard you're willing to work. If you're the type who refuses to embrace nontraditional conditioning concepts or who thinks that a bunch of high-tech exercise gadgets will basically do all of the work for you, you can pretty much forget about ever getting into the kind of condition you're looking for.

In the end, the best tool at your disposal isn't something you can buy in a sporting goods store or from one of those cheesy infomercials. No piece of equipment, regardless of how well it's designed, could ever take the place of a strong work ethic. There's a tremendous amount you can accomplish just using your own body, whether training at home with simple free weights or working out in a state-of-the-art gym. In the end, how you go about things is up to you. Just know that the only limitations you have are imagination and desire, because you can get a good workout just about anywhere if you put your mind to it.

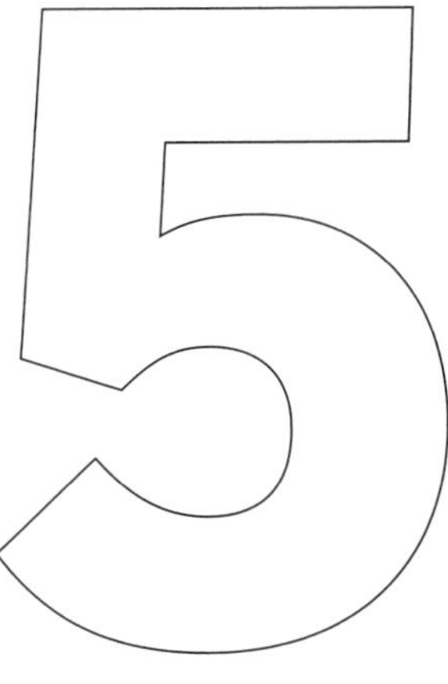

TAKE STOCK OF YOURSELF

PHASE 1: IT'S TIME TO SEE HOW YOU MEASURE UP

Get ready to be humbled. You're about to experience one of the most difficult and potentially frustrating parts of your new program: the part where you find out just what this body of yours can do. Yep, this could get ugly all right. The battery of tests you're about to put yourself through is designed to flesh out all those little imbalances and weaknesses I've been warning you about for the past few chapters. Some of the tests are difficult to do, will be extremely foreign even to those of you with some training experience, and may even require you to enlist the help of a friend or relative to record your results. In other words, you may find them to be somewhat inconvenient. Too bad. I want you to do them anyway.

Why put yourself through a testing protocol that may potentially make you feel worse instead of better? After all, low self-esteem is probably one of the reasons you want to start exercising in the first place. Won't poor results here just serve as confirmation of how much your physical abilities have eroded?

You can't look at it that way. The only way to avoid the pitfalls other people encounter when they're just starting out is to individualize your program as much as possible. And that starts with having an accurate assessment of where *your* strengths and weaknesses currently lie.

I know it's no fun to put yourself through a bunch of tests, especially when those tests are specifically intended to expose flaws in the way your body functions. The truth is, it's absolutely necessary if you're really serious about making any kind of sustained progress. Anybody can just arbitrarily start exercising, but rare is the individual who sets out to do it with the aim of restoring balance and structural integrity to his physique before focusing on aesthetic goals.

Call me an idealist, but I feel that the best way to help beginners make exercise a regular habit is to promote function over form. First get your body functioning properly and reduce your likelihood of injury, then improve its performance, and *then* worry about how it looks. I realize this is the exact opposite of the way most people go about things, but most people give up long before they've achieved their first objective of looking better, let alone the other two. With the system I'm proposing, because you'd be going about things the right way, you'd actually get visible results even sooner than expected, despite the fact that you'd focus more on structure and function.

How can that be? Simple. When you do things like restore lost range of motion to a muscle group that was previously restricted, or create more balance in the muscles that act around a particular joint, not only are you improving the way your body functions, but by increasing its performance potential, you're suddenly able to do more work. Freeing up your running stride, for instance, would lead to longer, more productive runs. Just as adding more balance to the muscles that comprise the rotator cuff (a small group of muscles that help stabilize the shoulder joint) would

KNOWING THE PERCENTAGES

The "skinny" on measuring body fat

You often hear about people using body fat percentage as a way to gauge their fitness progress. There are a variety of different techniques for assessing how much body fat a person is carrying on his or her frame. They range from the simple and relatively inexpensive to the complicated and often cost prohibitive. While some people go out of their way to have their body fat percentage tested on a regular basis, most of these methods—besides being costly and time consuming—are simply inaccurate. Here's a listing of some of the various techniques along with their proposed benefits and shortcomings.

Hydrostatic weighing. Long considered the gold standard of body fat measurement techniques, this involved procedure is based on Archimedes' principle, which states that the volume of an object is equal to the object's loss of weight in water (assuming the density of water is equal to 1). Skilled technicians are required to administer the test, and it is usually available only in a hospital or university setting. It's also rather time-consuming, often taking upward of a half hour to complete. Yet despite its lofty status as the king of body measurement techniques, it still has an error rate of approximately 2.5 percent—meaning that if it measures your body fat as 15 percent, your true percentage could actually be anywhere from 12.5 to 17.5 percent. It becomes an even less appealing option when you throw in the facts that it costs anywhere from $25 to $50 and can be pretty uncomfortable.

Skinfolds. This is a common test that is offered in most gyms and fitness centers. It involves an instructor using a pinching device called a *caliper* to measure the amount of fat you have stored underneath your skin at various locations on your body. Typically, 5 to 7 different sites are used, although some formulas allow for more. The sum of these skinfolds is then added up and plugged into a formula to give you your body fat percentage. The problem with this method, in addition to its 3 to 4 percent rate of error, is that the

allow you to train with more challenging loads. In either case, the end result will be a greater work output as a direct result of the functional improvements you'll have made.

The same cannot be said when you train for vanity first. A perfect example is the overemphasis most guys place on their "mirror muscles," aka the chest, lats, biceps, abdominals, and quadriceps. What this does is tend to promote imbalances between the muscles that act on the anterior (front) and posterior (rear) aspects of certain joints. Take the shoulder, for instance. Too much chest and lat work at the expense of more upper-back strengthening can contribute to an inward rotation of the upper arms, giving the shoulders a "slumped forward" look. Besides looking rather unattractive, this kind of internal rotation dominance, as it's known, can predispose the shoulder to numerous injuries. Things like shoulder impingements and rotator cuff tears are all too common in weight rooms because of the lack of balance that exists in the average trainee's program.

Similar problems also occur at the knee because of quadriceps (front thigh muscles) that get overworked in relation to the muscles that act on the posterior aspect of the joint, most notably the hamstrings. With all the emphasis on exercises like squats, lunges, and

reading is only as accurate as your technician is skilled. I can tell you from personal experience that taking body fat measurements is not easy and that it requires a significant amount of practice to become adept at it. So not only are you at the mercy of your technician's skill level, but to ensure the most accurate results you also have to make sure that you're measured by the same person each time.

Bioelectrical impedance. This method uses electrical current to measure body fat. Electrodes are placed on your wrist and ankle and a low current is passed through your body. The error rate for this test is 3 to 5 percent, and your results can be further impacted by any event that can alter your actual weight—things like eating a large meal, or losing a lot of sweat through exercise.

DEXA (dual energy x-ray absorptiometry). This highly involved procedure uses a whole-body scanner and two low-dose x-rays to read bone mass and soft tissue mass. Its accuracy is on a par with that of hydrostatic weighing, without all the discomfort. It will set you back about $100, though some insurance companies do cover it.

Circumferences and girths. With this method you simply use a tape measure to record the circumferences of several key points on your body and then plug your results into a formula to get your body fat percentage. This is highly inaccurate but not completely without merit. As with skinfolds, as long as you can get the same person to test you each time, circumferences can be valuable tools in assessing your progress. Forget about plugging your measurements into some silly formula—if your numbers consistently shrink, you'll know you're on the right track.

Ultimately, even an accurate body fat percentage is of questionable value, since most people wouldn't know what a healthy percentage is anyway. For the record, between 10 and 14 percent for men and 15 and 18 percent for women is considered optimal.

leg extensions, it's hard for the hamstrings to keep up. When the muscles on one side of a joint become significantly stronger than the muscles on the other side of that joint, sooner or later you're going to run into problems. Not that they necessarily have to be the same strength—most people's quadriceps are in fact about one-third stronger than their hamstrings. You just can't have too much of a disparity or else you stand a good chance of suffering an injury somewhere down the line.

Hopefully by now you're starting to gain an appreciation for just how important it is to assess your current physical standing before getting started. It's like they say, you have to know where you are in order to know where you're going. And where you are is right on the precipice of a whole new way of thinking when it comes to working out. If the information in this chapter teaches you nothing else, it should crystallize the fact that when it comes to exercise, every*body* is different. We all have certain strengths, as well as specific weaknesses, that need to be addressed. Unfortunately, simply following along with what most of the other people around you are doing in the gym isn't going to be of any great benefit to you. So get used to the idea of standing out and being an individual when it comes to your workouts. Who knows, if your progress is noticeable enough, you might become the guy at the gym whom everyone starts emulating.

Before you start the testing, let's record some relatively simple data. Enjoy this for now; things are going to get a lot tougher in a few minutes. The first thing you need to do is establish a starting weight for the program. Not that all of your success is going to be measured by how much weight you lose or gain (depending on what your goals are), but it's helpful to at least have a baseline value for comparison later on.

Starting weight: ____________

TEST DRIVEN

COMPILING THE DATA THAT WILL DRIVE YOUR NEW PROGRAM

The tests you're about to undergo are divided into a couple of different categories. In compiling them, I enlisted the help of biomechanics experts Eric Cressey and Mike Robertson, who wrote a brilliant series of articles entitled "Neanderthal No More: The Complete Guide to Fixing Your Caveman Posture" that was featured in *Testosterone* magazine (www.t-nation.com). I found the information in these articles to be so valuable that, with Eric and Mike's permission, I just had to share it with a larger audience. The articles were quite in-depth and at times a bit technical, so I've chosen to share with you what I deem to be the most important bits and pieces from the series.

As you go through the tests, be sure to check off the appropriate area on the score sheet provided on page 56. You'll need this to construct your own workouts in the corrective phase that follows this chapter. All you'll have to do is choose from a template of various exercises and stretches that correspond to the weaknesses and imbalances you've identified during the testing.

Well, what are you waiting for? Time to get to work!

Postural Assessment

I realize that for someone who's anxious to start a fitness program, good posture usually doesn't rank too high on the ol' priority list. After all, there's the gut that needs shrinking, the muscles that need pumping, and the heart that needs to start working more efficiently. Surely posture can be assigned a lower level of importance. The truth is, good posture isn't just a vanity thing. It allows you to breathe better, move more freely, and even metabolize your food more efficiently. Perhaps most important, proper posture can take unnecessary strain off joints and connective tissue, making you much less susceptible to injury. The following tests will give you a good handle on how you stack up.

Standing profile. For this test, all you need is a friend and a camera. Simply stand relaxed with your arms at your sides and have your buddy take a picture of your profile. Remember, I said "relaxed"—no sucking in that gut! Once you've got the photo in hand, the first thing I want you to focus on is your basic postural alignment. Starting at your feet, draw a line from the middle of your foot going upward toward your head. Ideally, that line should travel straight up through your knee, hip, acromion process (the bony prominence located where your shoulder blade meets your clavicle) and mastoid process (the bony prominence just below and behind your ear).

Not that your body should be perfectly straight; there are three distinct spinal curves that we all possess. The question is, do any or all of these curves deviate from the norm? For example, you can tell that you have an exaggerated curvature of the lower back, called *lordosis*, if the waistband of your underwear tilts down in front instead of running parallel to the floor. Cressey notes that an excessive lordotic curve and anterior tilting of the pelvis usually go hand-in-hand and can lead to injuries, overuse conditions, and faulty movement patterns.

Then there's the classic round-shouldered posture emblematic of an exaggerated kyphosis (or humpback). This can be either slight, where your arms are carried in front of your body instead of alongside it, or severe, where you can see your upper back when

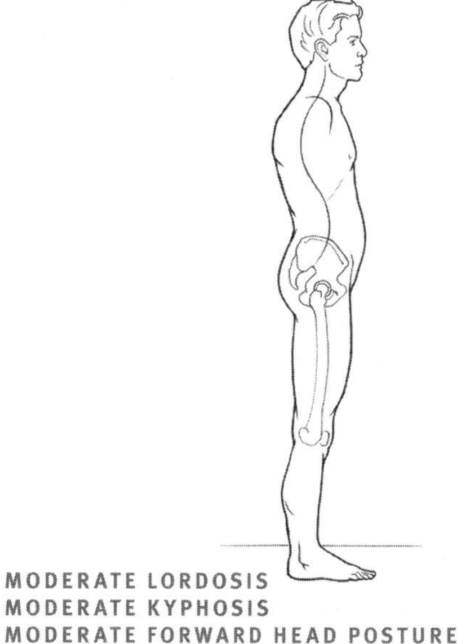

MODERATE LORDOSIS
MODERATE KYPHOSIS
MODERATE FORWARD HEAD POSTURE

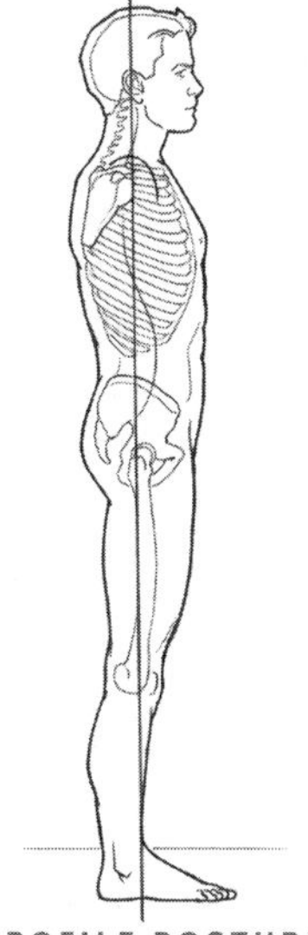

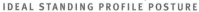

IDEAL STANDING PROFILE POSTURE

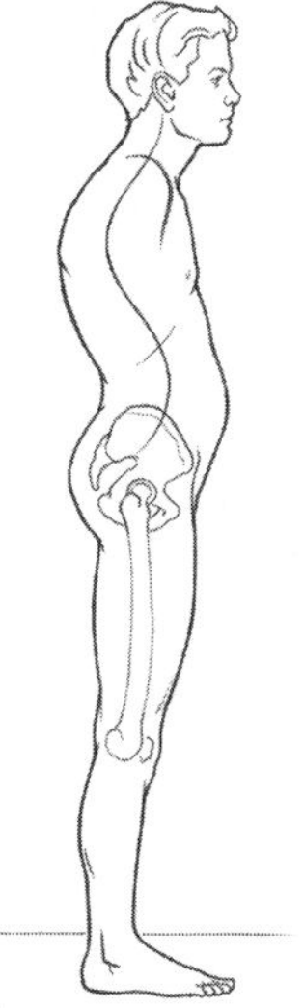

SEVERE LORDOSIS
SEVERE KYPHOSIS
SEVERE FORWARD HEAD POSTURE

standing in profile. Either way, it's something you're going to want to correct for both functional and aesthetic reasons.

Finally, there's the all-too-common forward head posture, where your head enters a room before the rest of your body. This one is pretty prevalent among people who sit in front of computers all day, and it can be a real pain in the neck.

Standing facing forward. Again stand relaxed with your arms at your sides and have your buddy take a picture, but this time from the front. We've already garnered a lot of information regarding your upper body by analyzing your profile picture, so we'll confine our analysis to the lower body for this one. Just as we did with the profile picture, I want you to once again focus on your feet. Can you draw a straight line from your feet up through your knees and hips? Or is there a visible collapsing of your feet (with your arches caving in toward the floor), external rotation of the feet (due to tightness in your hips), or "pinching in" of your knees? If you answered yes to the second question, you could be suffering from excessive pronation of the feet, internal rotation of your upper thighs, or both. Whatever the case, you'll be subjecting your knees to unnecessary strain once you start loading your lower body with exercises like squats and leg presses. So be sure to place a check in the appropriate column(s) so you can select the right exercises and stretches you need to correct the problem from the next chapter.

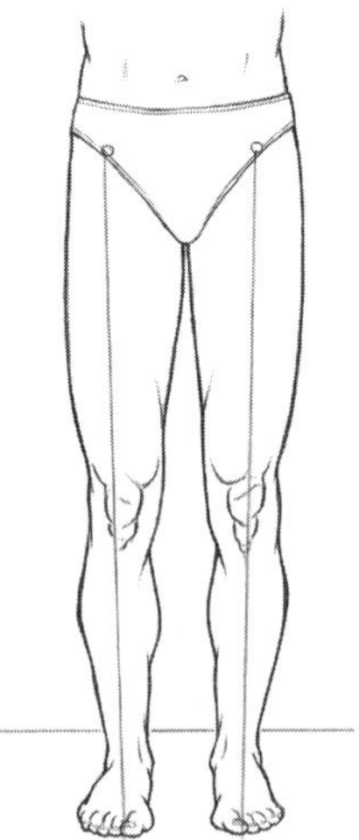

IDEAL LOWER-BODY ALIGNMENT

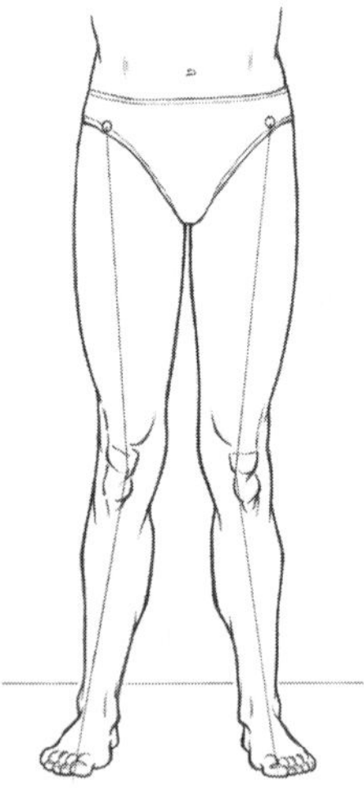

OVERPRONATION OF THE FEET
INTERNAL ROTATION OF THE UPPER THIGHS

Standing facing backward. One last time stand relaxed with your arms at your sides and have your buddy take a picture, but this time from the back. This is the easiest posture test of the lot. All you have to focus on this time is your shoulder blades. Ideally, the inner, lower borders of your shoulder blades should be down and back, somewhat close together. If you have excessive curvature of your upper back, however, they may wing out forward and to the sides. There's also a third possibility: shoulder blades that are somewhat elevated, indicative of an overactive upper trapezius and a weak, inhibited middle and lower trapezius.

Cressey and Robertson note that the latter two conditions can exist to varying degrees from one side to the other, meaning that you could have a left shoulder blade

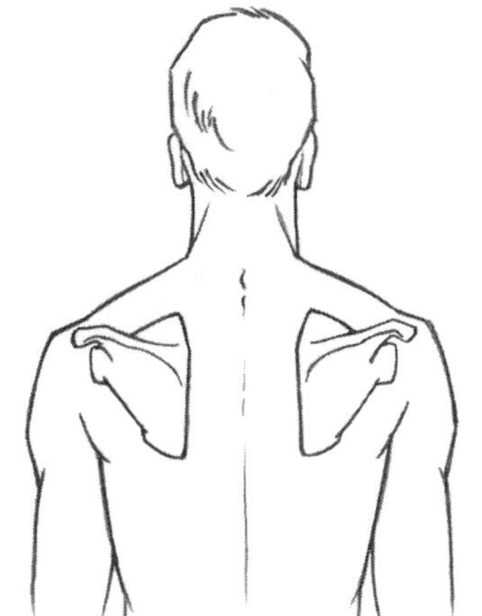

IDEAL SHOULDER BLADE POSITION

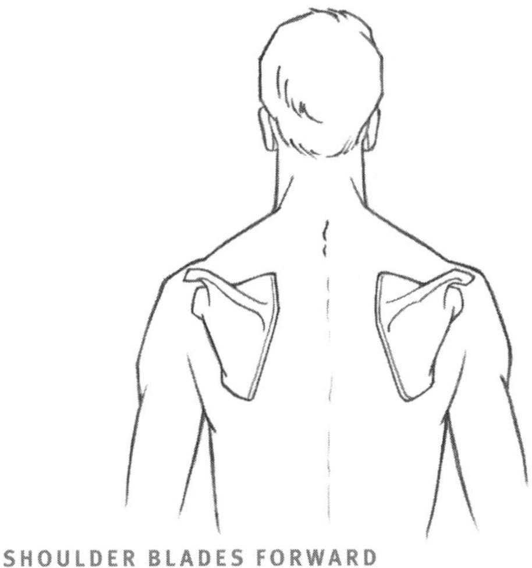

SHOULDER BLADES FORWARD AND OUT TO THE SIDES

SHOULDER BLADES ELEVATED

that wings out more than the right and/or a right one that rides up higher than the left. Not to worry, though; you'll learn exactly how to correct any of these conditions in the next chapter. For now, just be as diligent as you can in recording your results.

Flexibility Tests

Overhead squat. Besides being an excellent measure of total-body flexibility, this test will reveal a lot about your functional strength as well as how efficiently your nervous system coordinates the contraction of various muscle groups working simultaneously. I recommend having a friend take photos—or better yet, shoot videotape—of you performing this test from several angles.

To execute the test, grasp a broomstick with a wide, or "snatch," grip (typically about twice shoulder width) and stand with your feet spread approximately shoulder-width apart and *slightly* turned out (using a clock reference where straight ahead is equivalent to 12 o'clock, your right foot should be turned out no farther than 1 and your left no farther than 11 o'clock). Next, lift the broomstick over your head. Then, with

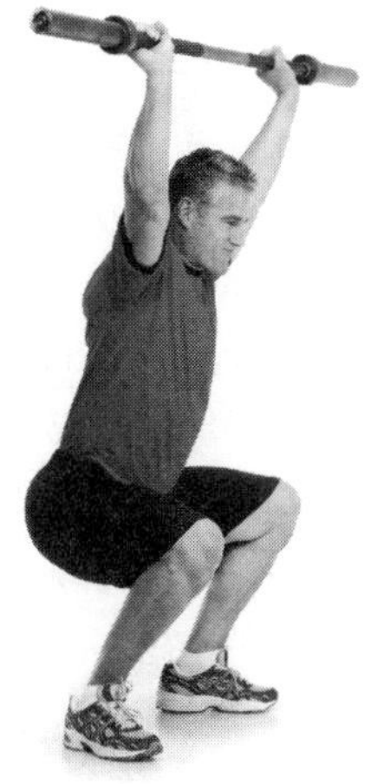

IDEAL OVERHEAD SQUAT

your arms completely straight, slowly squat down as far as you comfortably can. Upon reaching your lowest point, pause momentarily before standing back up to the starting position.

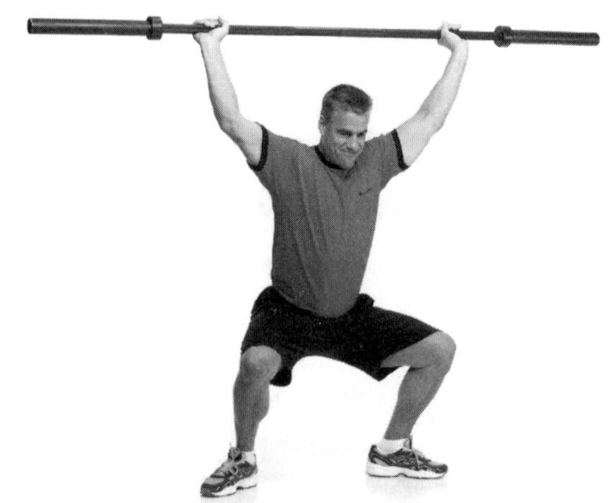

OVERHEAD SQUAT WITH FEET EXTERNALLY ROTATING

Depending on your flexibility and strength levels, there are several things you may have noticed. Cressey goes into great detail in the analysis of this test in his article "You Don't Know Squat" at *Rugged* magazine (www.ruggedmag.com), but I'll highlight a few key points. Feet that flatten out, or overpronate (with arches collapsing inward), as you descend could indicate tightness in the calves and/or weak glutes. If your feet turn out, or externally rotate, that could once again be indicative of tightness in the calves, hamstrings, or piriformis. Whereas, knees that pinch inward could be the result of tight adductors (inner thighs) and once again, weak glutes. Your butt excessively sticking out and your back excessively arching (lordosis) could mean tightness in the hip flexors, tensor fascia latae (TFL), spinal erectors, and lats. On the opposite side of the coin, a butt that tails underneath you and rounds would point to tight hamstrings. Finally, arms that drift forward instead of staying back and even with your ears point to tight pecs and lats as well as weakness in your lower trapezius and rhomboids.

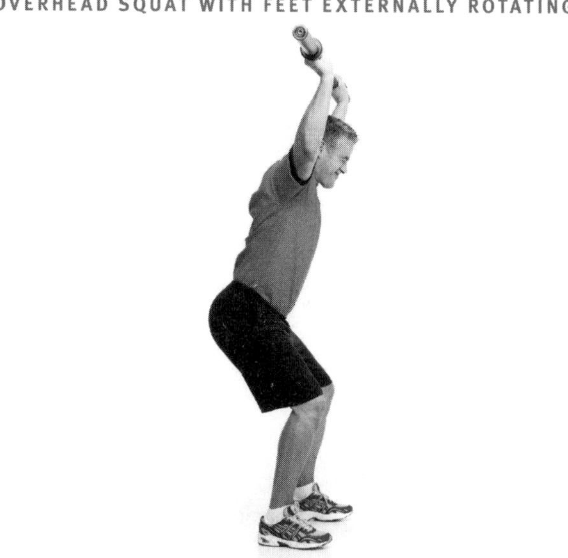

OVERHEAD SQUAT WITH EXCESSIVE BACK ARCH

If you aren't sure about where some of these affected muscles are, don't sweat it. Refer to the illustrations on pages 311 and 312 to become familiar with their locations. For now, all I want you to do is record where and how your form is deviating from the ideal example of an overhead squat in the photo on page 47. Once you've done that, it's just a matter of learning the appropriate exercises and stretches in the next chapter. And just in case you're still wondering why you need to bother doing this, consider that any deviations in your form are occurring when you're working with an unweighted broomstick. Can you imagine what would happen if you

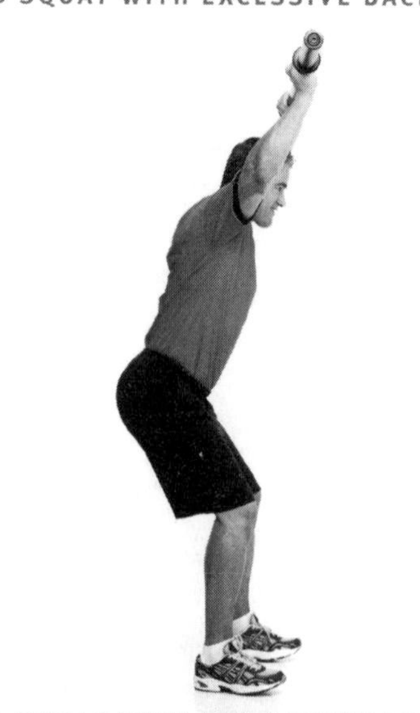

OVERHEAD SQUAT WITH ARMS DRIFTING FORWARD

attempted to squat a barbell loaded with dozens of pounds? Granted, you wouldn't be holding it up over your head, but trust me, it still wouldn't be pretty.

Lower-body rotational test. Like the overhead squat, this test requires both flexibility and strength. It's an excellent indicator of the rotational strength and range of motion of your core musculature. To begin, lie on your back and place both arms out to your sides, palms down and in line with your shoulders. Next, lift your legs so they're extended straight over your hips with the soles of your feet pointed toward the ceiling. (Lack of hamstring flexibility may make it difficult to keep your legs straight, so bending your knees *slightly* is permissible.) Now comes the hard part: Keeping your entire back pressed against the floor, slowly allow your legs to rotate over toward the floor to one side. As you do this, be sure to not let your back arch or your opposite shoulder blade come up off the floor. When you've gone as low as you can, pause for a second before using your core muscles to bring your legs back to the starting position, and then repeat to the other side. Be careful not to use any bouncing or momentum to bring your legs back up.

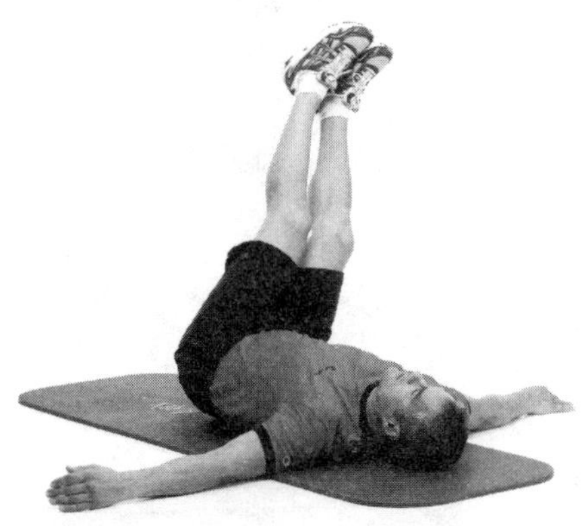

LOWER-BODY ROTATIONAL TEST WITH LIMITED ROTATIONAL ABILITY

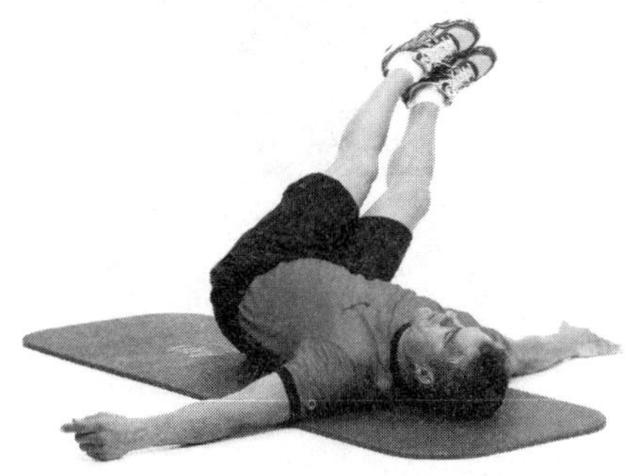

LOWER-BODY ROTATIONAL TEST WITH GOOD ROTATIONAL ABILITY

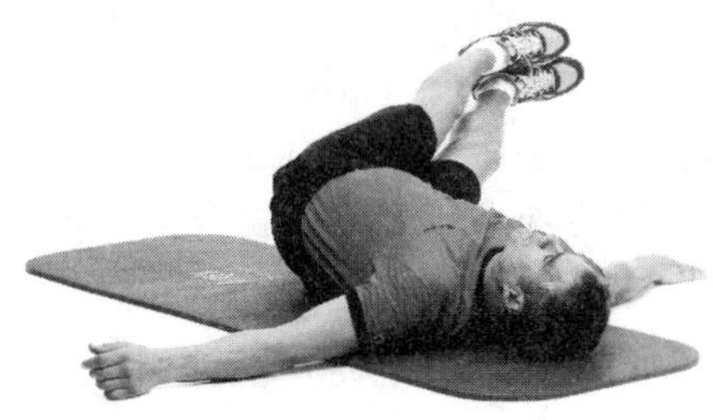

LOWER-BODY ROTATIONAL TEST WITH SUPERIOR ROTATIONAL ABILITY

You can note how far you've gone by using a simple clock reference to gauge your results. Working under the premise that the starting position represents 12 o'clock, allowing your legs to drift over slightly to your right, to 1 o'clock, and slightly left, to 11 o'clock, signals limited rotational ability (see the topmost photo on this page). Further rotation in each direction, to 2 o'clock and 10 o'clock, shows good rotational ability (see the middle photo on this page). Finally, making it to the point where your outer leg is almost touching the floor indicates superior rotational ability (see the bottom photo on this page). This last range of motion would enable you to easily withstand powerful rotational forces like swinging a golf club or transferring a child out of a car seat.

Modified sit and reach. For this test, you'll need a box approximately 1 foot high, a yardstick, and your trusty friend to help record your score. To begin, sit on the floor with your legs stretched out in front of you and the soles of your feet against the box. Next, keeping your shoulders stacked over your hips, stick your arms out in front of you with one hand placed on top of the other. Your helper should then bring the yardstick to meet the tips of your fingers, with the rest of it lying on top of the box. This will be the starting point for your measurement. From here, simply lean forward, sliding your hands along the yardstick and making sure to keep your knees perfectly straight. Do this three times and record the final measurement, in centimeters, as your score. Then compare your results to the norms in the Self-Assessment Score Sheet on page 57.

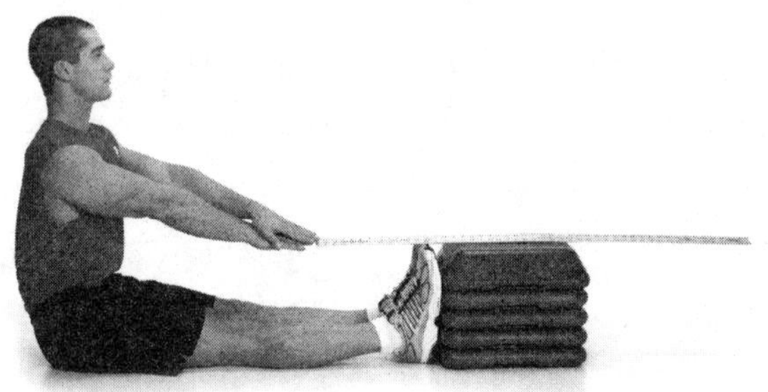

MODIFIED SIT AND REACH

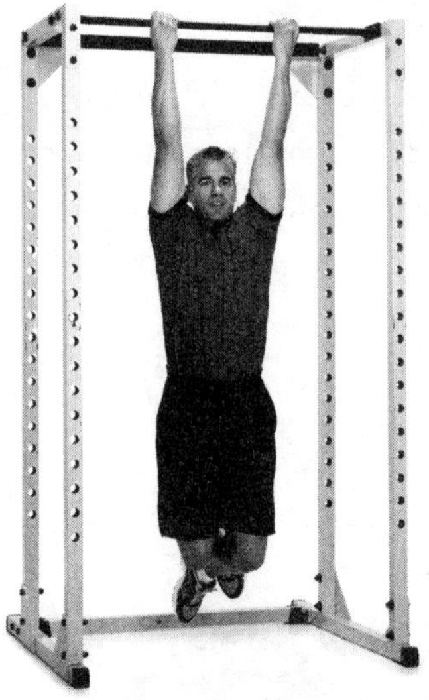

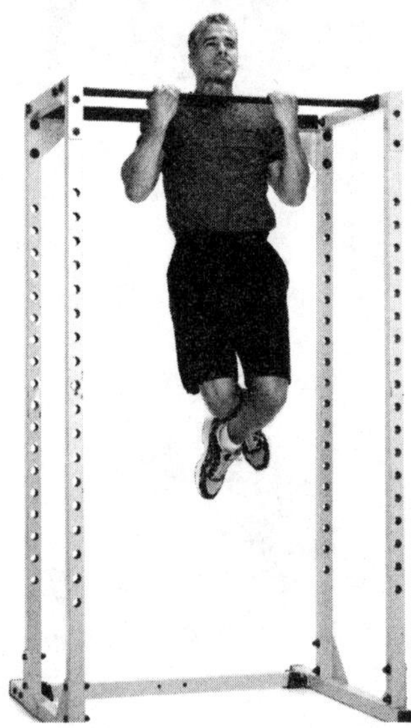

CHINUP

Muscular Strength Assessment

Upper body: chinup. Yeah, I know, chinups aren't exactly what most people consider to be a beginner exercise. I also know that they're one of the best upper-body lifts going and one that every grown man should be able to do at least a couple of times. To begin, hang from a chinning bar with a supinated (palms facing you) grip, with your knees bent and your ankles crossed behind you. Then simply pull yourself up with your chest sticking out until your chin clears the bar. Hold momentarily, lower, and repeat. Record the number of reps you can do. You pass if you can do more than 5.

Lower body: one-leg squat. Yep, here we go again—yet another exercise that you don't often see prescribed for beginners. There's a reason for that: Bilateral lifts (where both limbs work at the same time) don't really offer a reliable gauge of true strength potential—especially if they're done on machines. There are just too many ways for your body to cheat and shift more weight onto the stronger limb, or worse, get joints and connective tissue to pick up more of the stress. With this exercise, though, you either have the strength, flexibility, and balance to do it or you don't. This makes it a perfect choice in my estimation.

Begin by selecting a leg to start with and lifting the other about a foot off the floor out in front of you (see photo A). Next, stick out your arms at about shoulder height and start sitting down and back as you descend towards the floor (see photo B). As you do, you'll find that your back needs to round somewhat in order to allow you reach the desired depth. That's okay: Just remember that the main objective is to bend at the hips and knees, not just allow your torso to completely collapse. Once you get down to the point where your working thigh is at least parallel to the floor, pause for a second before pushing back up to the starting position.

Success on this test is measured by being able to maintain the form I've just described without any of the following happening: your working knee pinching in (see photo C) or bowing out (see photo D), the heel of your working leg coming up off the floor, your back rounding excessively

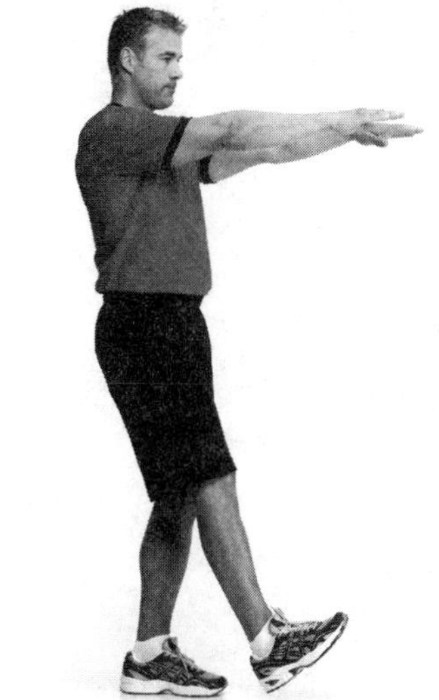

A

ONE-LEG SQUAT STARTING POSITION

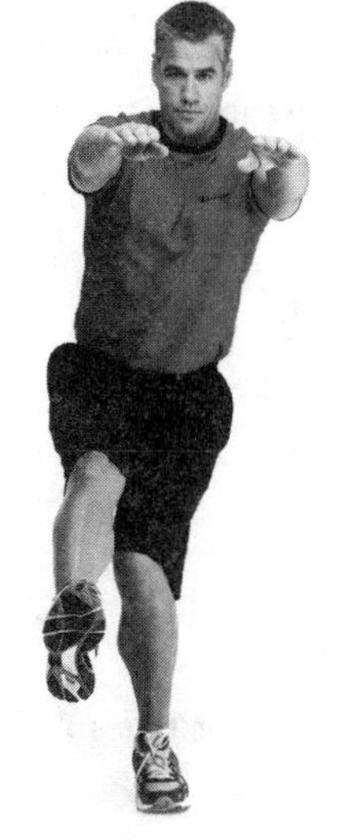

C

ONE-LEG SQUAT WITH KNEE PINCHING IN

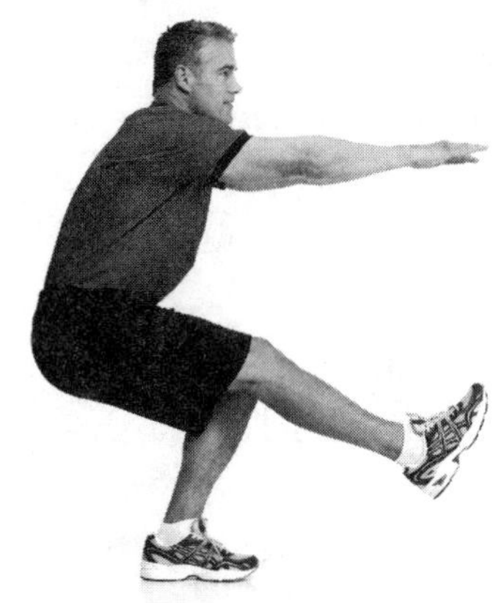

B

IDEAL ONE-LEG SQUAT

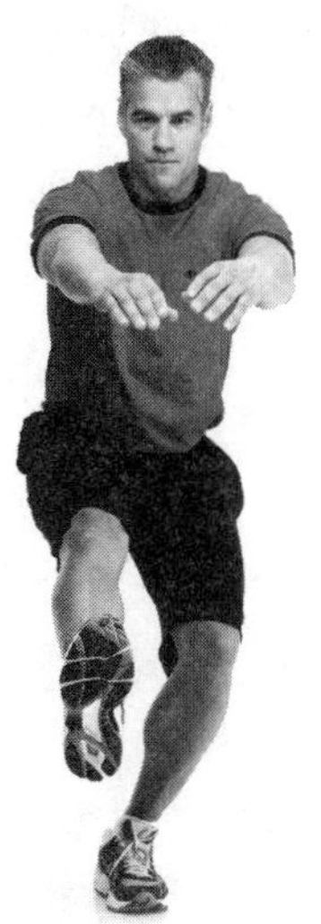

D

ONE-LEG SQUAT WITH KNEE BOWING OUT

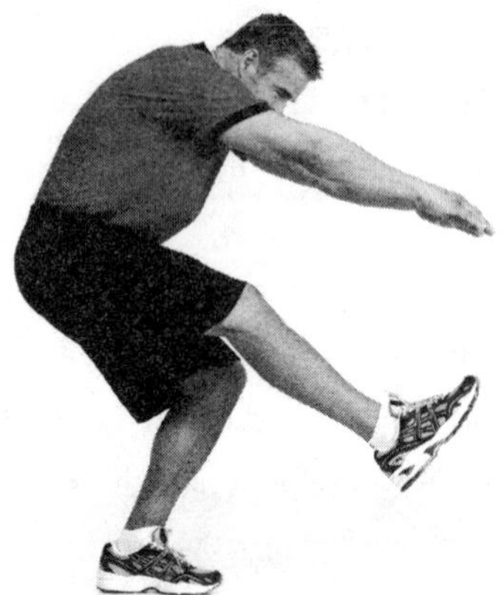

ONE-LEG SQUAT WITH ROUNDED BACK

(see the photo above), or only making it down a few inches for fear of any of the above occurring. If any of it does, you have failed the test and have some work to do.

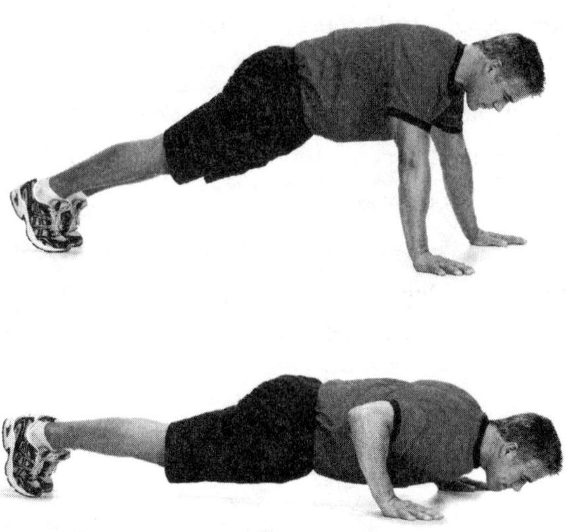

NEUTRAL-SPINE PUSHUP

Muscular Endurance

Neutral-spine pushup. This is in all likelihood a far cry from any pushup that you've ever seen or tried in the past. For starters, because it requires you to hold a neutral spine—a position that I'll explain in a second—it really blasts your core. Second, since you'll be doing it at a specific speed, you won't be able to use momentum or muscle elasticity to get back up.

To begin, get yourself in a basic pushup position with your hands placed slightly wider than shoulder-width apart. Before your descent, pull your belly button in toward your spine and simultaneously contract your glutes. This should result in a disappearance of the arch in your lower back and an immediate awareness that your core musculature is working.

All you have to do now is maintain this position as you descend down for a 2-second count until your body is a couple of inches off the floor. Then pause for a full second before pressing back up and repeating. Do as many reps as you can at this speed and record your results. If you can do more than 10, that's an indication of decent endurance.

Core Tests

The following two tests assess the strength of your core musculature.

Leg lowering. Here's another good exercise recommended by Cressey and Robertson. Lie faceup on a carpet or exercise mat. With your arms folded across your chest and your head remaining in contact with the floor, lift your legs until they're extended straight up over your hips. Tilt your pelvis by pulling your abs in toward your spine and contracting your glutes (the same way you did in the neutral-spine pushup). This should once again eliminate the normal arch in your lower back; strive to maintain this position throughout the duration of this test.

Keeping your legs straight, lower them over a 10-second count as you try to get them as close to the floor as possible without allowing your back to arch. Have a friend observe you to record how far you get down and then compare that to the norms provided in the Self-Assessment Score Sheet on page 59. The point at which your back begins to arch indicates the presence and degree of lordosis.

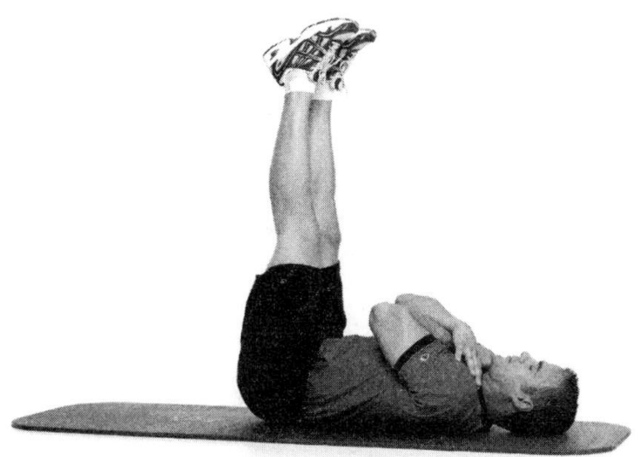

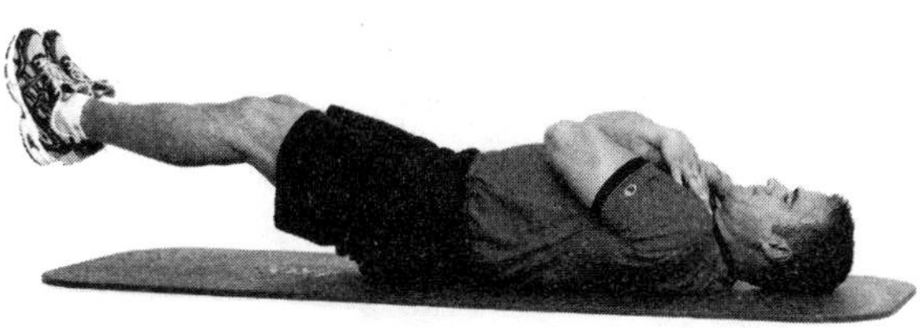

LEG LOWERING

Slow situp. Do this just the way it sounds: Lie faceup on the floor with your knees slightly bent and slowly sit up. Don't laugh—it's not as easy as it sounds. Without the use of momentum, you might find that sitting all the way up at a controlled pace is much harder than you thought it would be. You may notice that you come up only a couple of inches and then just completely stop (a sign of weak abdominals); or that the higher you come up, the more your back arches (an indication of overactive back extensors and/or hip flexors); or that your heels rise up off the floor (evidence of overactive hip flexors). Whatever the case, you'll need to do some specific strengthening and stretching to correct the problem.

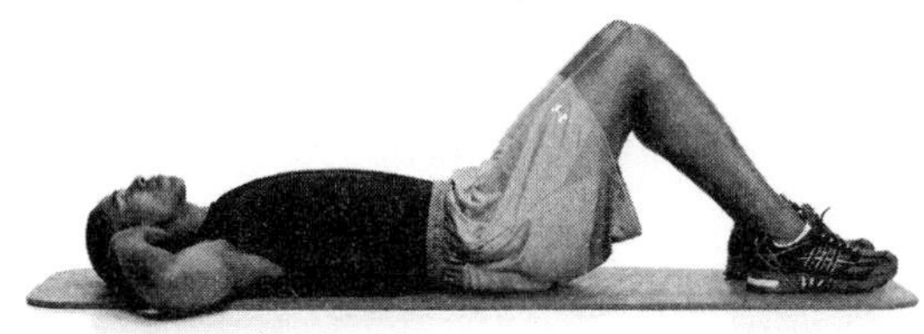

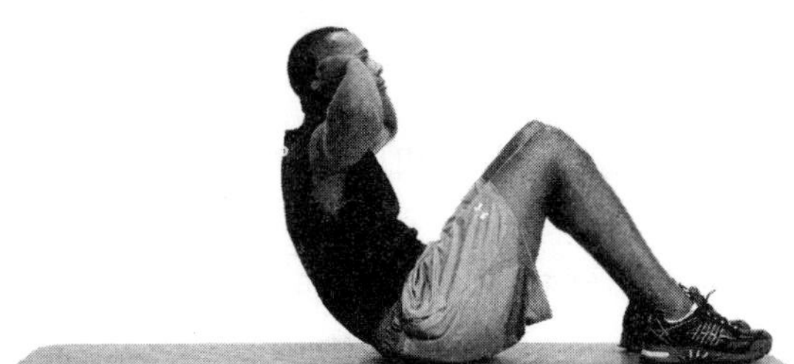

SLOW SITUP

Cardiovascular Tests

Queens College step test. For this test, you'll need a stopwatch and a step that's approximately 16 inches high. Begin stepping at a steady, rhythmic pace (up, up, down, down at a rate of about 24 steps per minute) for 3 minutes straight, being sure to alternate legs every few steps to avoid fatigue. At the end of the three minutes, stop stepping and wait 15 seconds before taking your heart rate (see "Just Beat It" below for instructions on doing this). Then plug your heart rate into the following formula to get your estimated VO_2 max, a measure of the milliliters of oxygen per kilogram of body weight that your body is capable of processing per minute.

111.33 – (0.42 × heart rate in beats per minute) = _____ ml/kg/min VO_2 max

JUST BEAT IT

To determine your heart rate, place your first two fingers either at the thumb side of your opposite wrist (just below the heel of your hand) or alongside your carotid artery (just below the base of your jawbone, on the side of your neck). Count the number of beats you feel in 15 seconds and multiply that number by 4 to give your heart rate in beats per minute (bpm).

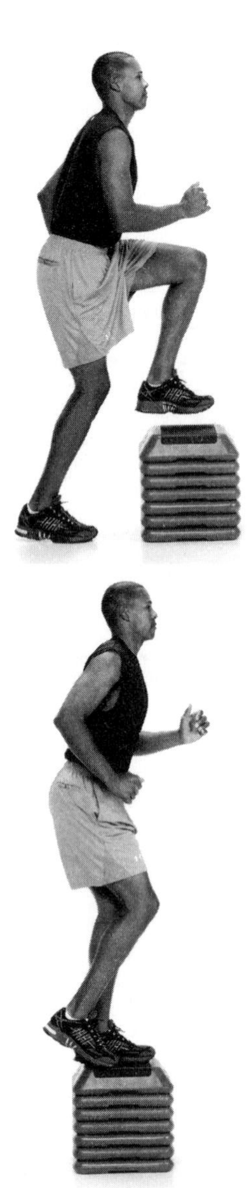

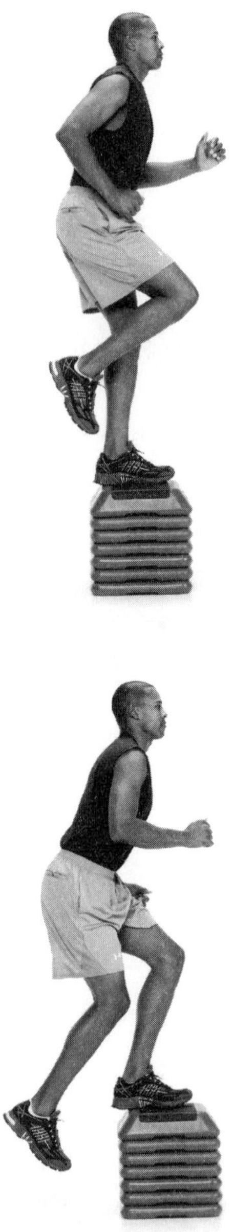

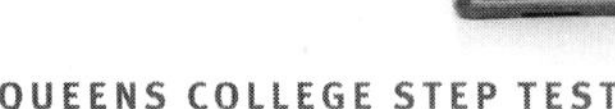

QUEENS COLLEGE STEP TEST

Your VO_2 max is an indication of your aerobic capacity; compare yours to the established norms provided in the Self-Assessment Score Sheet on page 60.

1.5-mile run. I've included this second cardiovascular test because differences in height and limb length can make the Queens College step test difficult for some people to perform. In the event that you're one of them, the 1.5-mile run is a better alternative. After a thorough warmup, run 1.5 miles as fast as possible and record your time. Then convert your run time from minutes and seconds to a decimal figure—for example, 13 minutes and 30 seconds would be 13.5 minutes—and insert this number in the following formula:

$(483 \div \_\_\_\_ \text{min}) = \_\_\_\_ \text{ml/kg/min VO}_2 \text{ max}$

Compare this value to the VO_2 max norms provided in the Self-Assessment Score Sheet on page 60.

BATTLE TESTED

NOW YOU KNOW, YOU'RE GOOD TO GO

At this point, besides feeling incredibly tired, you've also got to be feeling incredibly good about yourself. Not too many people in your shoes would have the discipline and patience to put themselves through what you just did. As I mentioned earlier, most beginners just rush right into a new training program without first thinking things through. You have a decided advantage over them because you now know where your weaknesses lie, so you can implement a specific plan of action to eliminate them. That alone can be the difference between scrapping this whole project a few weeks in and sticking with it for the long haul. I don't know about you, but that's not an opportunity that I'd be willing to waste.

Bear in mind that this isn't something that's going to come easy; you're gonna have to work for it. Because this approach is so different, there'll be plenty of people encouraging you to scrap it and go with something more conventional. You yourself may even question the validity of doing some of the specific exercises and stretches contained in the next chapter. I'm urging you to stay the course anyway. People like to treat exercise like some simple, mindless endeavor, where nothing more than hard work and a little sweat will produce amazing results. Not to overcomplicate things, but there's a little more to it than that. Although hard work and determination may be the foundation on which results are built, you have to give some thought to the best way to apply them. Otherwise, you'll just be spinning your wheels.

SELF-ASSESSMENT SCORE SHEET

Place a check mark in the boxes that apply to the results of each test.

POSTURAL ASSESSMENT

STANDING PROFILE

	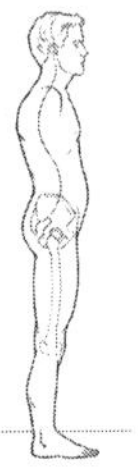 Moderate	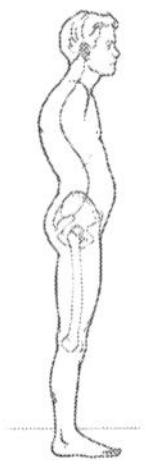 Severe
Lordosis	☐	☐
Kyphosis	☐	☐
Forward head	☐	☐

STANDING FACING FORWARD

Foot Overpronation/External Rotation 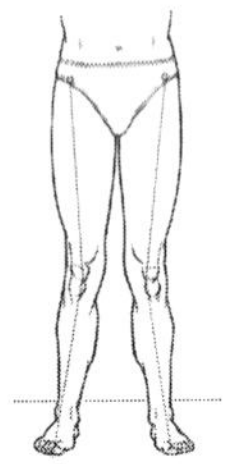	Knee Pinching
Right ☐	Right ☐
Left ☐	Left ☐

STANDING FACING BACKWARD

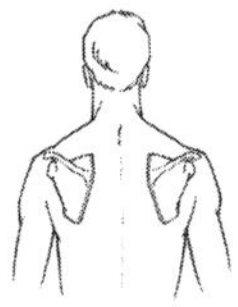 Shoulder Blade Winging	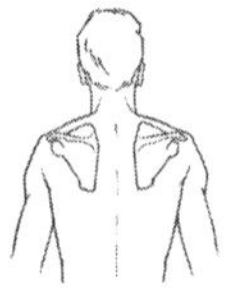 Shoulder Blade Elevation
Right ☐	Right ☐
Left ☐	Left ☐

FLEXIBILITY TESTS

OVERHEAD SQUAT

Foot Overpronation	Foot External Rotation	Knee Pinching	Excessive Arch	Low Back Rounds	Arms Drift Forward
Right ☐	Right ☐	Right ☐	☐	☐	☐
Left ☐	Left ☐	Left ☐	☐	☐	☐

LOWER-BODY ROTATIONAL TEST

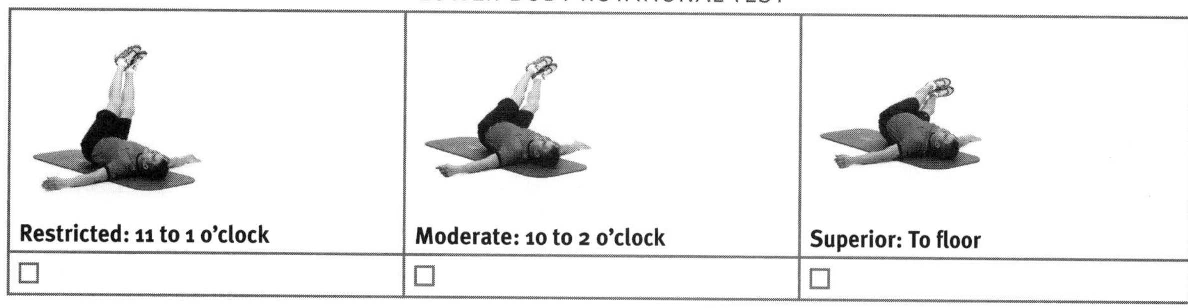

Restricted: 11 to 1 o'clock	Moderate: 10 to 2 o'clock	Superior: To floor
☐	☐	☐

MODIFIED SIT AND REACH

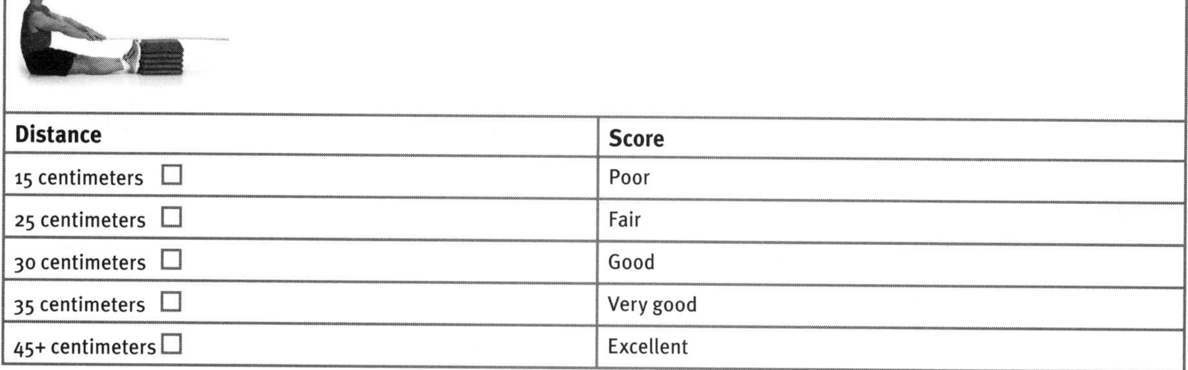

Distance	Score
15 centimeters ☐	Poor
25 centimeters ☐	Fair
30 centimeters ☐	Good
35 centimeters ☐	Very good
45+ centimeters ☐	Excellent

(continued)

MUSCULAR STRENGTH ASSESSMENT

UPPER BODY: CHINUPS

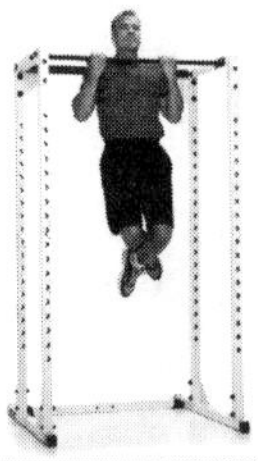

Number of Repetitions	Score
Greater than 5 ☐	Pass ☐
5 or less ☐	Fail ☐

LOWER BODY: ONE-LEG SQUAT

Fail ☐	Pass ☐
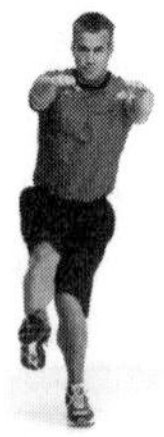 Knee pinching in ☐	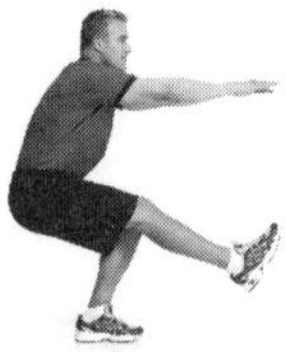
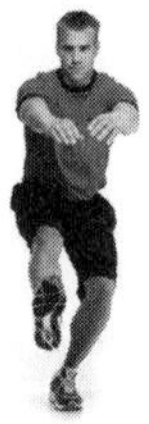 Knee bowing out ☐	
Heel lifting ☐	

LOWER BODY: ONE-LEG SQUAT (cont.)

Fail ☐	
Back rounding ☐	
Squatting only inches ☐	

MUSCULAR ENDURANCE

NEUTRAL-SPINE PUSHUP

Number of Repetitions	**Score**
More than 10	Decent ☐
10 or less	Fail ☐

CORE TESTS

LEG LOWERING

Leg Lowering	**Score**
90 to 75 degrees ☐	Poor (severe lordosis) ☐
75 to 45 degrees ☐	Moderate (moderate lordosis) ☐
45 degrees to floor ☐	Excellent ☐

(continued)

SELF-ASSESSMENT SCORE SHEET *(cont.)*

CORE TESTS (cont.)

SLOW SITUP

Can't Lift Torso Off Floor	Lower Back Arches	Heels Lift Off Floor
☐	☐	☐

CARDIOVASCULAR TEST

QUEENS COLLEGE STEP TEST

Heart Rate: ____________ bpm
VO_2 max: _____ ml/kg/min

1.5-MILE RUN

Time: ________________ min
VO_2 max: _____ ml/kg/min

VO_2 MAX (SCORES IN ML/KG/MIN)

Age	Very Poor	Poor	Fair	Good	Excellent	Superior
18–29	←37.1	37.1–40.9	41.0–44.1	44.2–48.1	48.2–53.9	→53.9
30–39	←35.4	35.4–38.8	38.9–42.3	42.4–46.7	46.8–52.4	→52.4
40–49	←33.0	33.0–36.7	36.8–39.8	39.9–44.0	44.1–50.3	→50.3
50–59	←30.2	30.2–33.7	33.8–36.6	36.7–40.9	41.0–47.0	→47.0
60 and over	←26.5	26.5–30.1	30.2–33.5	33.6–38.0	38.1–45.1	→45.1

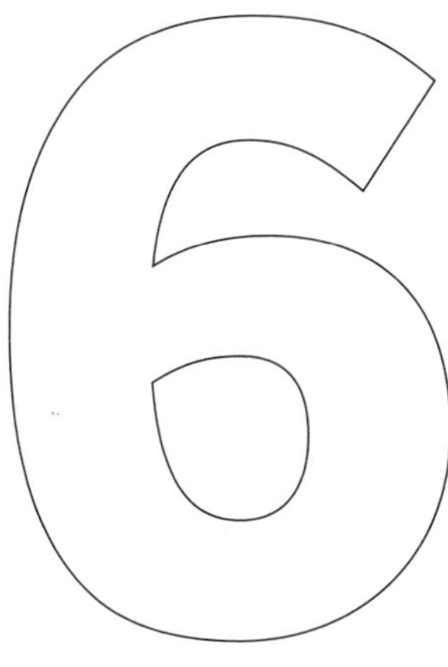

BEGINNER, HEAL THYSELF

PHASE 2: HERE'S YOUR CUSTOM-MADE PLAN FOR HEALING ALL THAT AILS YOU

Now that you're done holding your body up to inspection, it's time to interpret your results and get started on the road to the new you. In your hands you now have a checklist of exactly what you need to work on. For some of you, flexibility will be more of a concern, while others may need to focus more on strengthening. Some of you may even find that core work needs to take precedence over everything else. Regardless of what your needs are, the real comfort comes in knowing that you're addressing *your* specific areas of weakness. This chapter doesn't just contain some cookie-cutter blueprint of a training program. It offers a completely individualized plan that's made just for you. Provided, of course, that you're willing to work for it.

People normally shell out big bucks to have private trainers do this sort of thing for them. So don't think the program is just going to magically fall into your lap. I've gone through the trouble of categorizing specific exercises and stretches according to which weaknesses and imbalances they counteract. All you have to do is pick out the ones that will help correct everything you've checked off on your Self-Assessment Score Sheet, and then I'll show you how to arrange them into a workout based on the schedule you outlined for yourself in Chapter 3. The result will be your own tailor-made plan. Not an entire training program, mind you—more of a first phase designed to get your body back in good working order. I call it the corrective phase and include it in every program I write. I can also say without hesitation that it's what makes my programs so effective. You're actually laying the foundation for making fitness a permanent part of your life. In the process, you're going to learn an awful lot about how your body responds to training.

CORRECTIVE PRESCRIPTION

THE MOVES THAT ARE GOOD FOR WHAT AILS YOU

"Faults and Fixes," beginning on the opposite page, is a list of all of the tests and conditions we covered during the self-assessment, along with the specific exercises and stretches you'll need to correct those conditions. Many of the names of these drills, as well as the pictures and descriptions of them, may seem quite odd at first, especially if you're an ex-jock or seasonal. They're not your typical gym fare. You're bound to get a few strange looks and possibly even a stare or two. Don't let that faze you; it's a good sign. Because if you're doing things differently than most of the other people at your gym, you know you're on the right track.

I know that seems like a gratuitous slap at the gym crowd, but it's one that I take based on years of personal experience and observation. Believe me when I tell you that there's quite a bit of nonsense going on in most gyms. People routinely lift with bad form, use too much weight, and most disturbingly, dispense questionable training advice with the utmost confidence. All of this serves to breed a sort of herd mentality when it comes to fitness, where a few of the more "buff" members set the standard which many of the others try to emulate. This often leads to people doing exercises that are either too advanced or completely inappropriate for them based on their goals and needs. And yet, people usually do them anyway just to fit in with everyone else.

Remember, though, your goal isn't to replicate the same tired old exercises you've seen everybody doing for years. It's to create a strong, flexible, and balanced physique that performs as good as it looks. And doing that is going to require a little bit of creative license when it comes to your exercise selection. I promise the results will be well worth the effort.

Next up beginning on page 67: instructions on how to perform the prescribed exercises and stretches. Note that the number of repetitions will be explained in the individual workouts.

FAULTS AND FIXES

TEST(S)	CONDITION	CORRECTIVE EXERCISES	STATIC STRETCHES
STANDING PROFILE (PAGE 45) 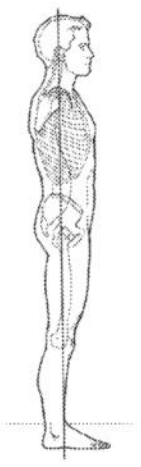	Lordosis 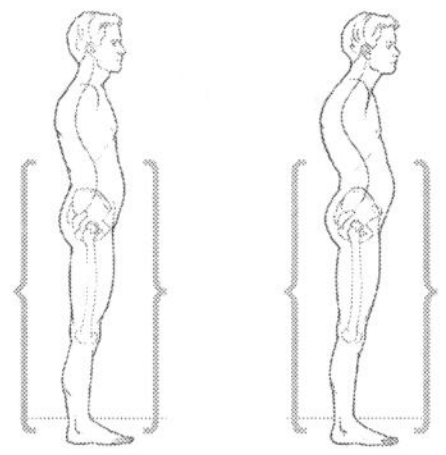	Pelvic tilt (page 67) and plank (page 68)	Hip flexor stretch (page 90) and erector stretch (page 91)
	Kyphosis 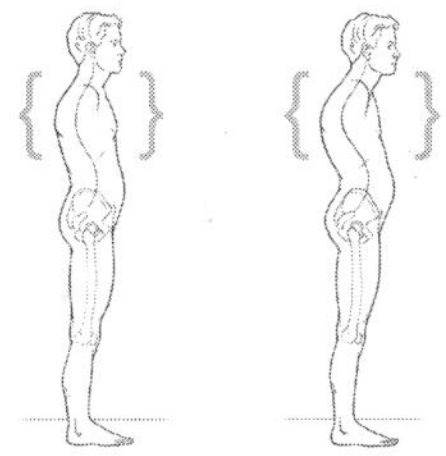	Cable row (page 69), prone dumbbell row with elbows out (page 70), reverse fly (page 71), and side-lying external rotation (page 72)	Pec wall stretch (page 92), lat stretch (page 93), and internal rotator broomstick stretch (page 94)
	Forward head 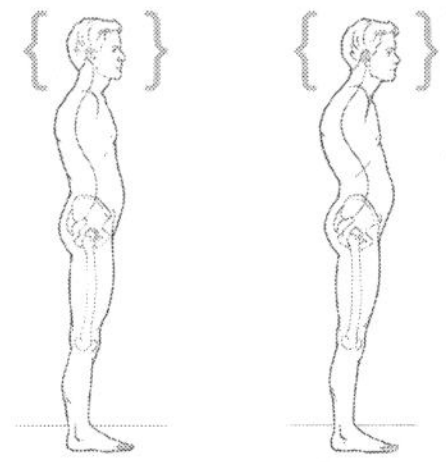		Wall chin tuck (page 95) and corner stretch (page 96)
STANDING FACING FORWARD (PAGE 46) AND OVERHEAD SQUAT (PAGE 47) 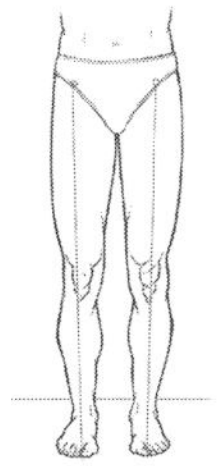 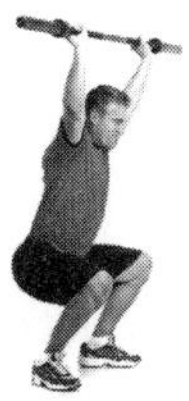	Foot overpronation 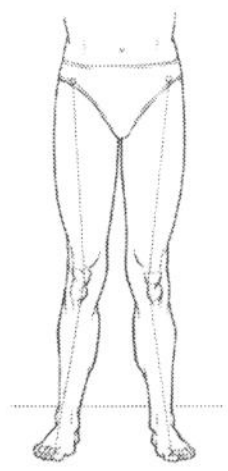		Pike calf stretch (page 97), hamstring doorway stretch (page 98), and glutes and piriformis stretch (page 99)

(continued)

TEST(S)	CONDITION	CORRECTIVE EXERCISES	STATIC STRETCHES
STANDING FACING FORWARD (PAGE 46) AND OVERHEAD SQUAT (PAGE 47) (cont.)	External rotation 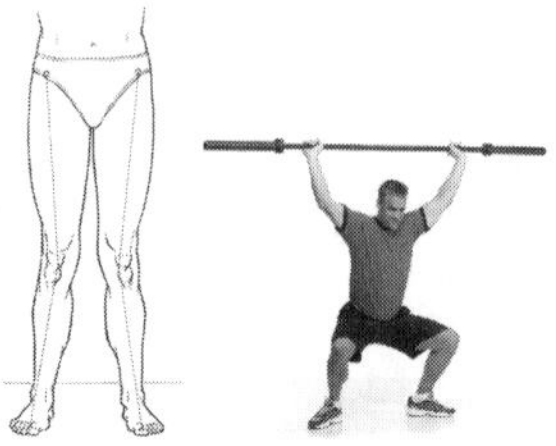	Supine bridge hip extension (page 73), Swiss ball hip extension (page 74), and cable hip abduction (page 75)	
	Knee pinching	Supine bridge hip extension (page 73) and cable hip abduction (page 75)	Butterfly adductor stretch (page 100)
STANDING FACING BACKWARD (PAGE 46) 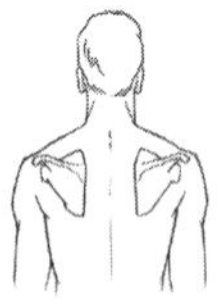	Shoulder blade winging 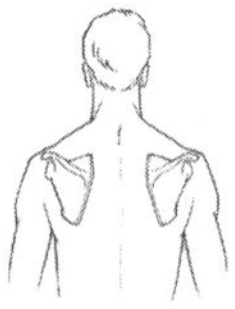	Cable row (page 69), prone dumbbell row with elbows out (page 70), reverse fly (page 71), and side-lying external rotation (page 72)	Pec wall stretch (page 92), lat stretch (page 93), and internal rotator broomstick stretch (page 94)
	Shoulder blade elevation 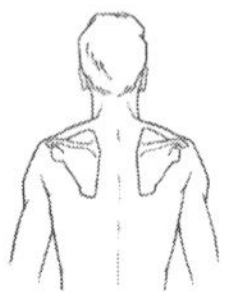	Prone front raise (page 77) and reverse shrug on lat pulldown machine (page 78)	Trapezius stretch (page 101) and prisoner stretch on wall (page 102)
OVERHEAD SQUAT (PAGE 47) 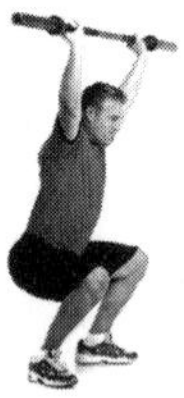	Lower back rounding 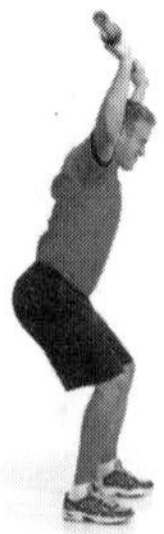	Swiss ball back extension (page 79) and Superman (page 80)	Hamstring doorway stretch (page 98)

TEST(S)	CONDITION	CORRECTIVE EXERCISES	STATIC STRETCHES
OVERHEAD SQUAT (PAGE 47) (cont.)	Arms drift forward	Prone dumbbell row with elbows out (page 70), prone front raise (page 77), and side-lying external rotation (page 72)	Pec wall stretch (page 92) and lat stretch (page 93)
LOWER-BODY ROTATIONAL TEST (PAGE 49)	Restricted or moderate	Russian twist (page 81) and medicine ball wall rotation (page 82)	Seated rotational stretch (page 103)
MODIFIED SIT AND REACH (PAGE 49)	Poor to good	Unilateral Romanian deadlift (page 83)	Hamstring doorway stretch (page 98)
CHINUP (PAGE 50)	0 to 4 reps	Negative chinup (page 84)	Pec wall stretch (page 92) and lat stretch (page 93)

(continued)

FAULTS AND FIXES *(cont.)*

TEST(S)	CONDITION	CORRECTIVE EXERCISES	STATIC STRETCHES
ONE-LEG SQUAT (PAGE 50)	Failed	Unilateral dumbbell touch (page 85), side-lying hip abduction (page 76), and cable hip abduction (page 75)	Pike calf stretch (page 97) and hamstring doorway stretch (page 98)
NEUTRAL-SPINE PUSHUP (PAGE 52)	10 or less	Plank (page 68), negative situp (page 86), and negative neutral-spine pushup (page 87)	Hip flexor stretch (page 90) and erector stretch (page 91)
LEG LOWERING (PAGE 52)	90 to 45 degrees		Hip flexor stretch (page 90) and erector stretch (page 91)
SLOW SITUP (PAGE 53)	Heels lift off floor, lower back arches, or can't lift torso off floor	Pelvic tilt (page 63), negative situp (page 86), crunch with pelvic tilt (page 88), and bird dog (page 89)	
QUEENS COLLEGE STEP TEST (PAGE 53)		See page 118 for instructions on doing cardio during the corrective phase.	
1.5-MILE RUN (PAGE 54)		See page 118 for instructions on doing cardio during the corrective phase.	

PELVIC TILT

Lie faceup on the floor with your knees bent and your feet flat.

Beginning with a normal spine arch, exhale as you pull your belly button toward your spine while simultaneously contracting your glutes so that your lower back presses against the floor. Hold for 3 to 5 seconds and release.

A

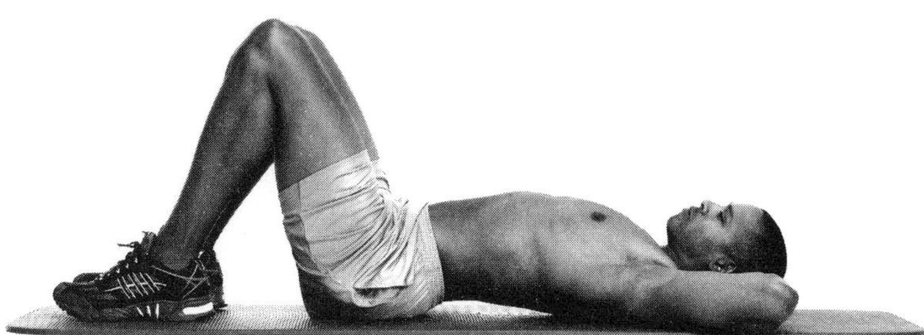

B

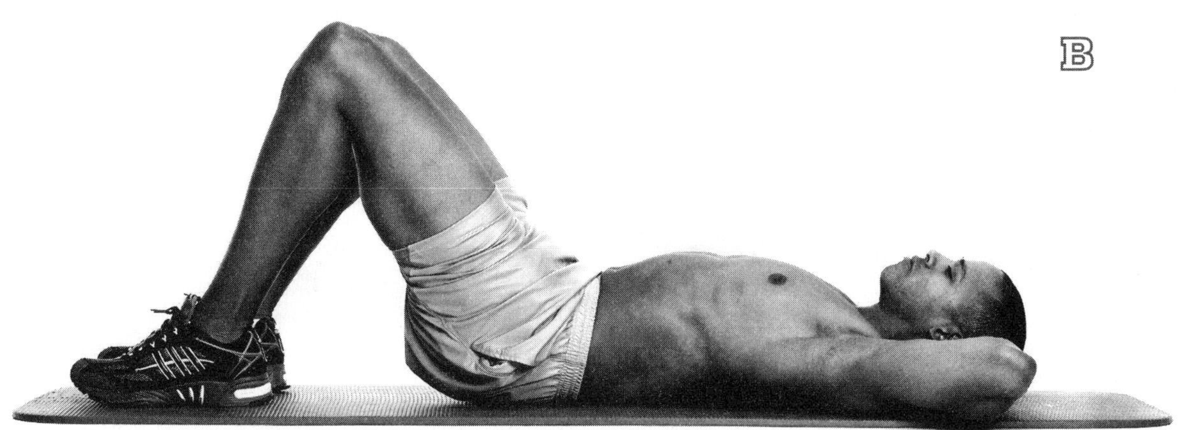

PLANK

Assume a pushup position, but instead of having your arms straight, rest your weight on your forearms. Suck in your belly button and contract your glutes to flatten the arch in your lower back. Hold for 20 to 30 seconds and release.

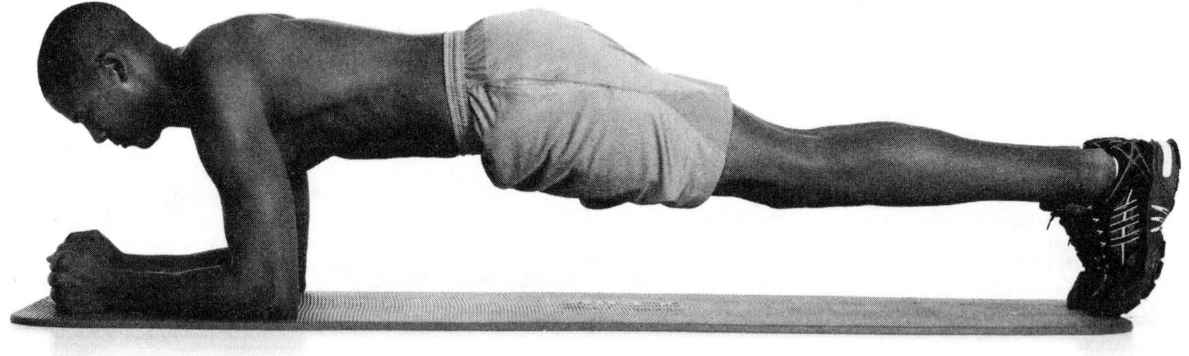

CABLE ROW

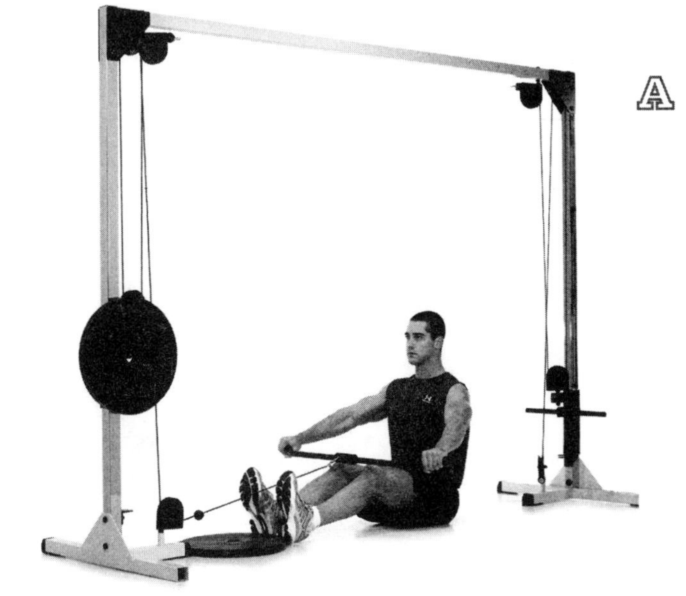

Attach a long, straight bar to the low pulley of a cable station and position yourself in the machine. Grab the bar with an overhand grip that's just beyond shoulder width. Sit up straight with your shoulders stacked over your hips.

Pull your shoulders back and then follow through with your arms until the bar almost touches your torso. Pause for a second and return the bar to the starting position.

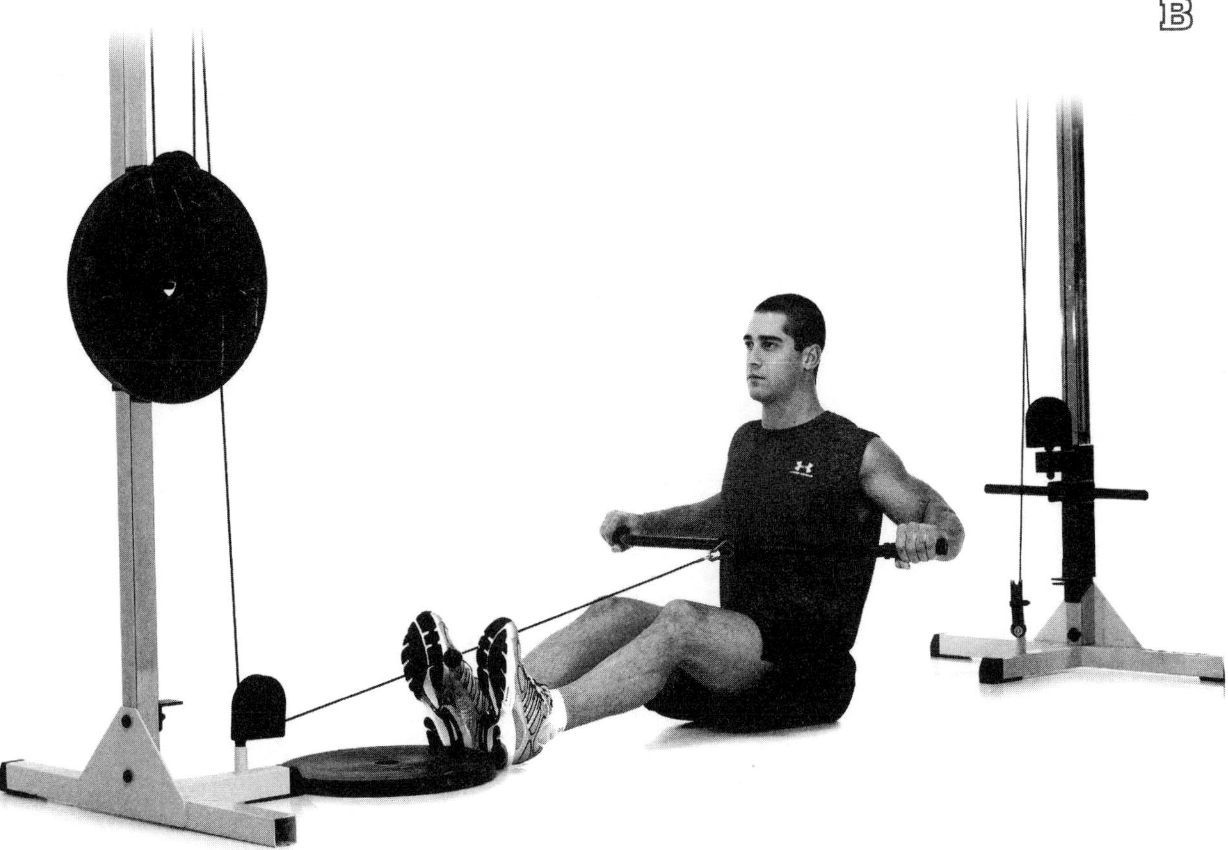

PRONE DUMBBELL ROW WITH ELBOWS OUT

Set an incline bench to a 30-degree angle. Grab a pair of dumbbells and lie with your chest against the pad. Let your arms hang straight down from your shoulders and turn your palms so that your thumbs are facing each other.

Lift your upper arms as high as you can by bending your elbows and squeezing your shoulder blades together. At the top of the move, your upper arms should be perpendicular to your body and your lower arms should be pointing toward the floor. Pause, then slowly lower the weights to the starting position.

A

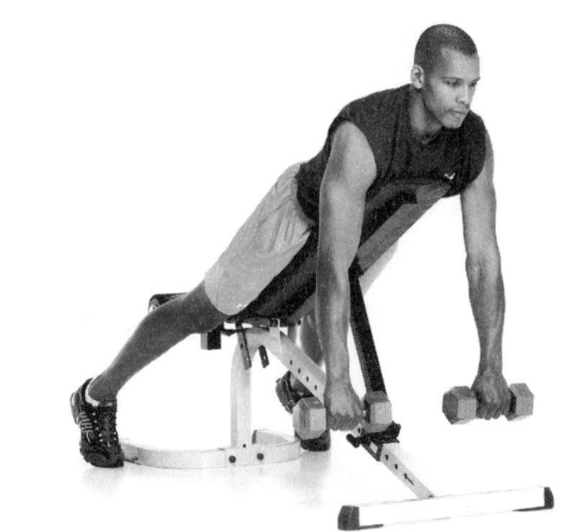

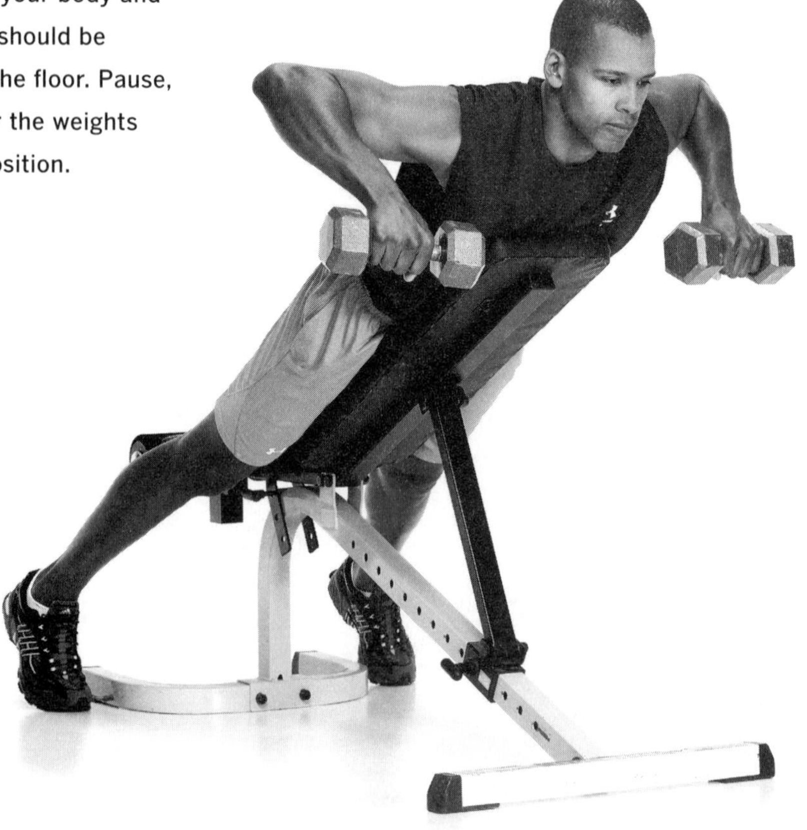

REVERSE FLY

Lie facedown on a 45-degree incline bench holding a pair of dumbbells at arm's length with your palms facing each other.

Keeping a slight bend in your elbows, pinch your shoulder blades together and work your arms up in a wide, arcing motion. At the top of the movement, your elbows should remain slightly bent and you should see the weights out of the corners of your eyes.

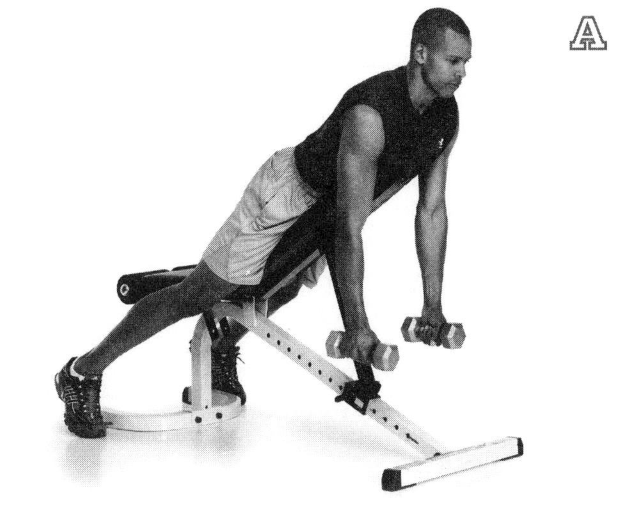

A

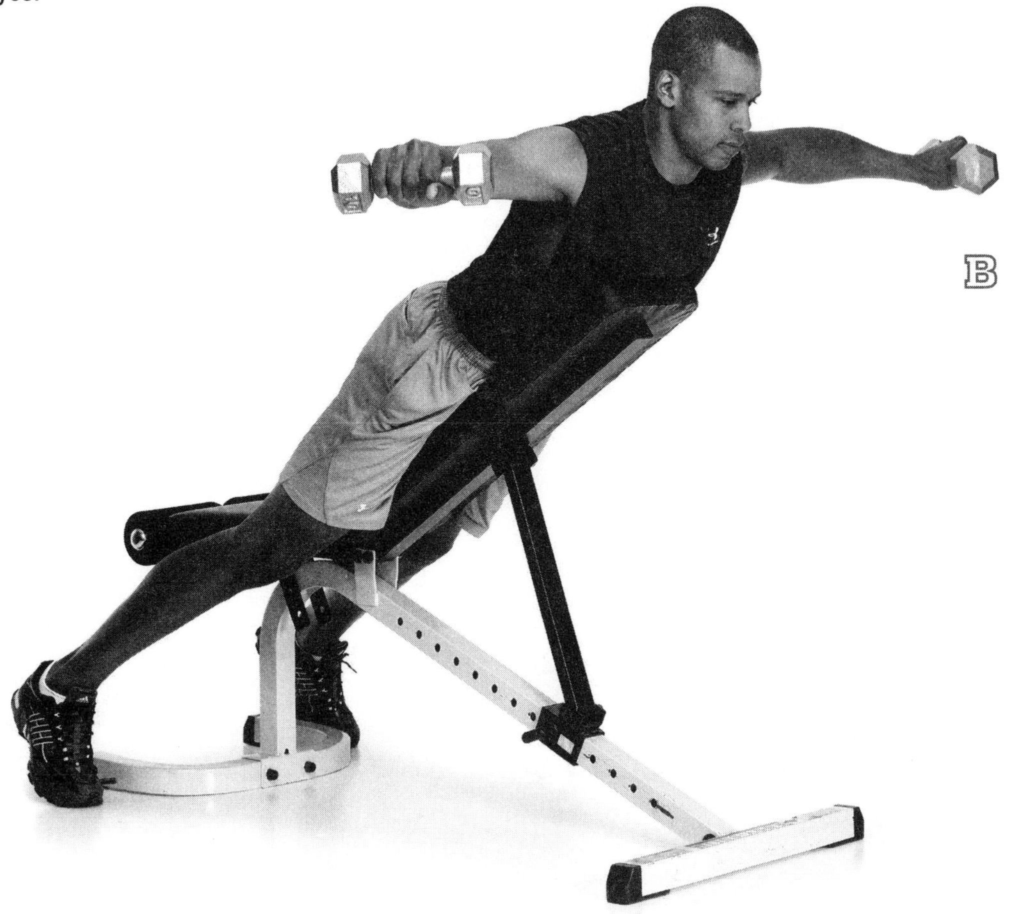

B

SIDE-LYING EXTERNAL ROTATION

Lie on your side on the floor or a bench with your supporting elbow bent 90 degrees and one rolled-up towel between your hip and the inside of your upper elbow and another between your knees.

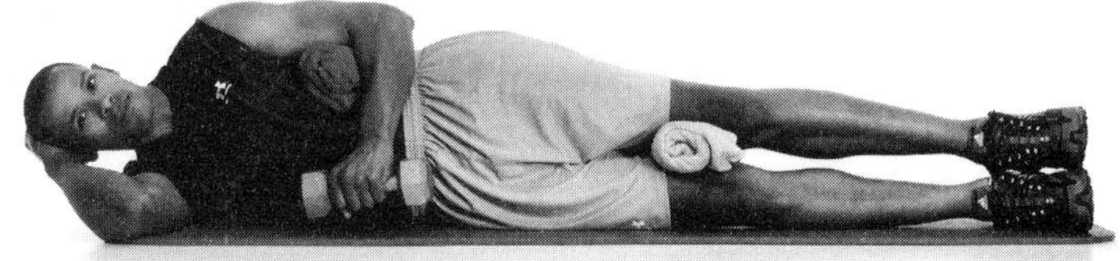

Holding a light dumbbell in your upper hand, rotate your forearm until your arm is as close to perpendicular to the floor as you can get it. Be sure to maintain a neutral wrist and avoid cocking your hand back in an attempt to increase your range of motion. Pause for a second and then rotate your arm back down. Finish your set and then do the same number of reps with your other arm.

B

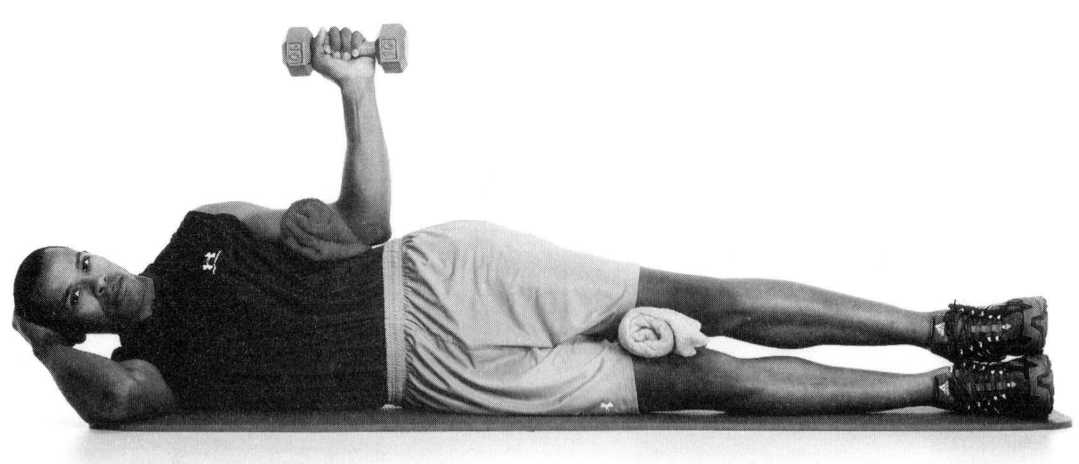

SUPINE BRIDGE HIP EXTENSION

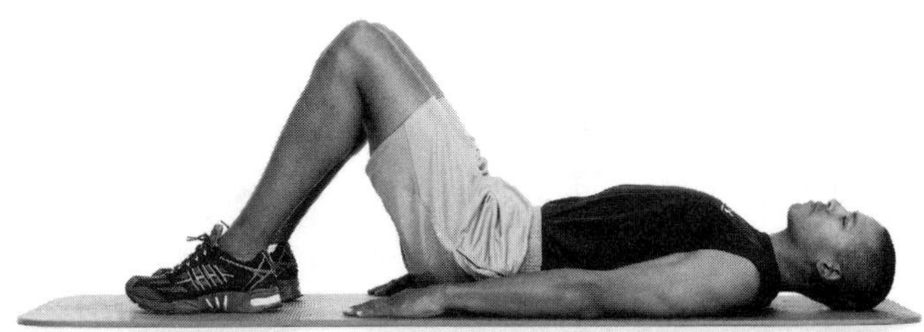

Lie faceup on the floor with your knees bent about 90 degrees and your feet pressed into the floor.

Keeping your arms at your sides, press both heels into the floor and lift your hips until your body forms a straight line from your shoulders to your knees. Hold for a second or two and lower back down.

To increase the difficulty, you can also do this with one leg at a time, extending the nonworking leg directly above your hips. Just make sure that both hips press up toward the ceiling; do not allow the nonworking side to droop down.

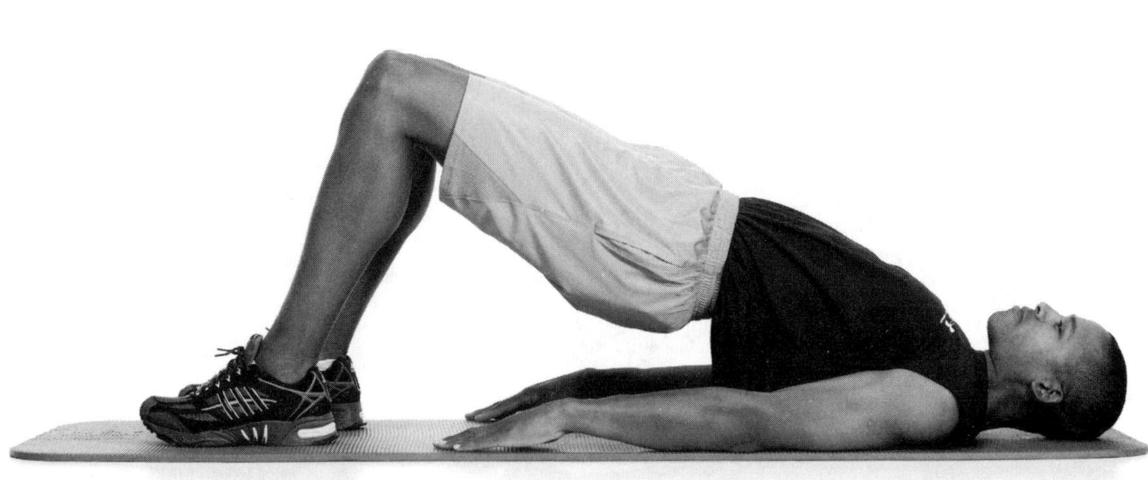

SWISS BALL HIP EXTENSION

Lie faceup on the floor with your legs straight and the backs of your heels and lower calves on top of a Swiss ball.

Keeping your arms flat on the floor to help you balance, brace your core muscles tightly as you press your legs into the ball and lift your hips. In the top position your body should form a diagonal line from your shoulders to your feet. Pause for a second and then lower back down.

A

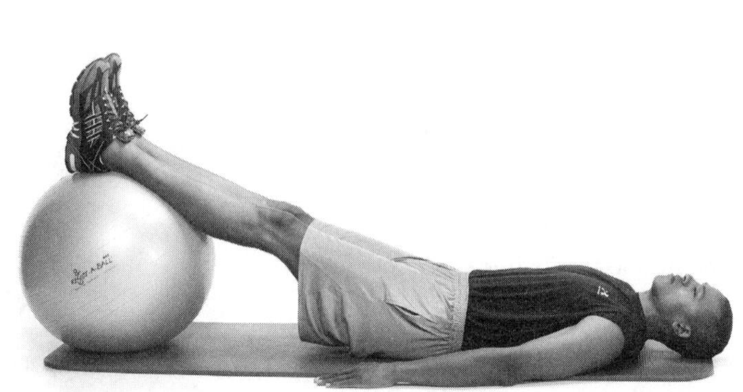

B

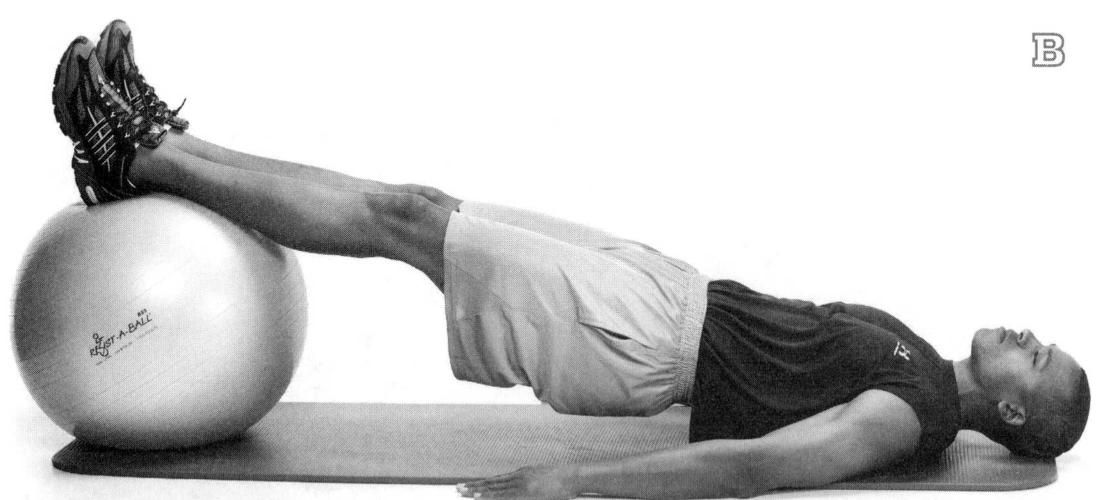

CABLE HIP ABDUCTION

Attach an ankle strap to the low pulley of a cable station and then secure the strap to one ankle. Stand with your opposite side facing the weight stack, holding on to the station upright for balance. Lift your working foot a few inches off the floor and extend it just in front of your supporting foot.

Keeping your knees and back completely straight, move your working leg out to the side, lifting it as far as you can. Hold for a second or two and then lower. Finish your set and then repeat with your other leg.

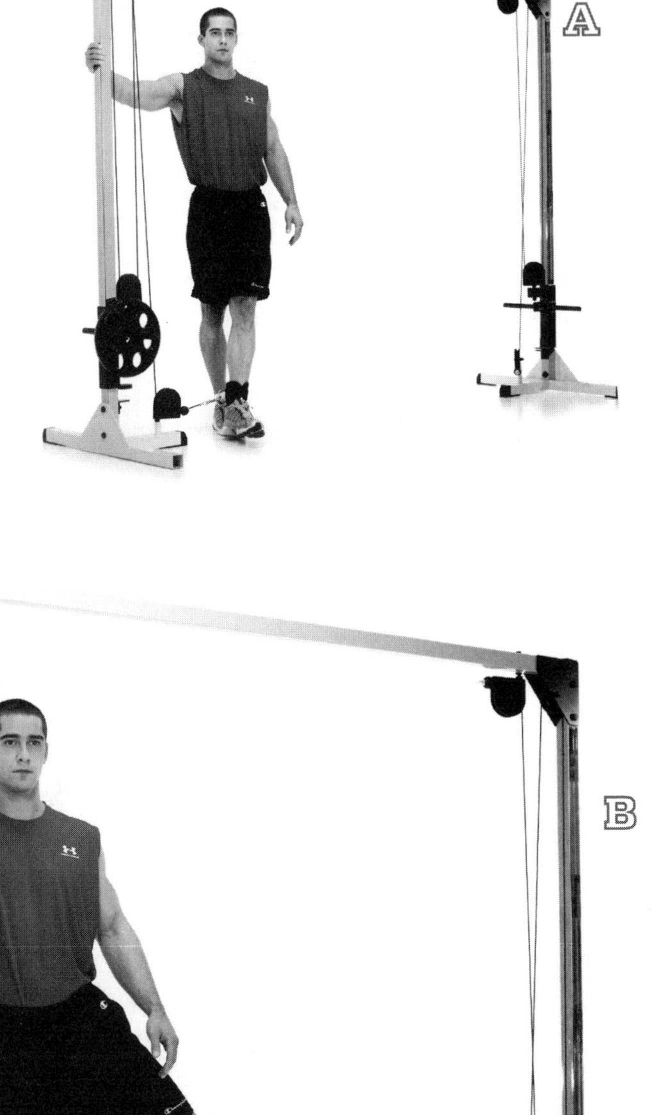

SIDE-LYING HIP ABDUCTION

Lie on your side so that your shoulders, hips, and knees are stacked over each other. Next, bend your bottom knee about 45 degrees and bring it toward your chest.

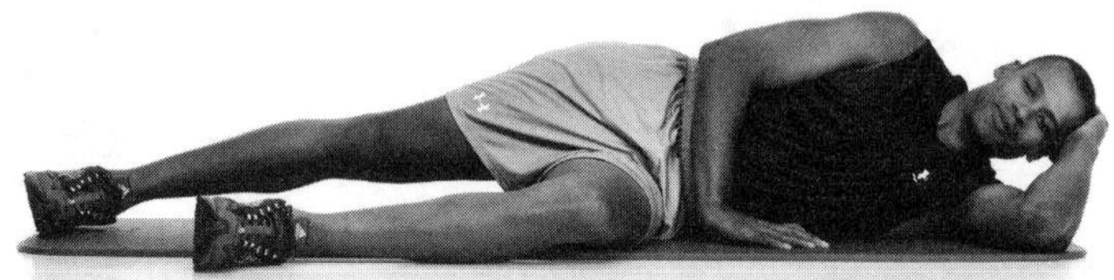

Keeping your top leg straight, lift it toward the ceiling, leading with the outside portion of your foot, not with your toes. When the leg reaches an angle of approximately 45 degrees to the floor, hold for a second, then lower it back down. Finish your set and then do the same number of reps on your other side.

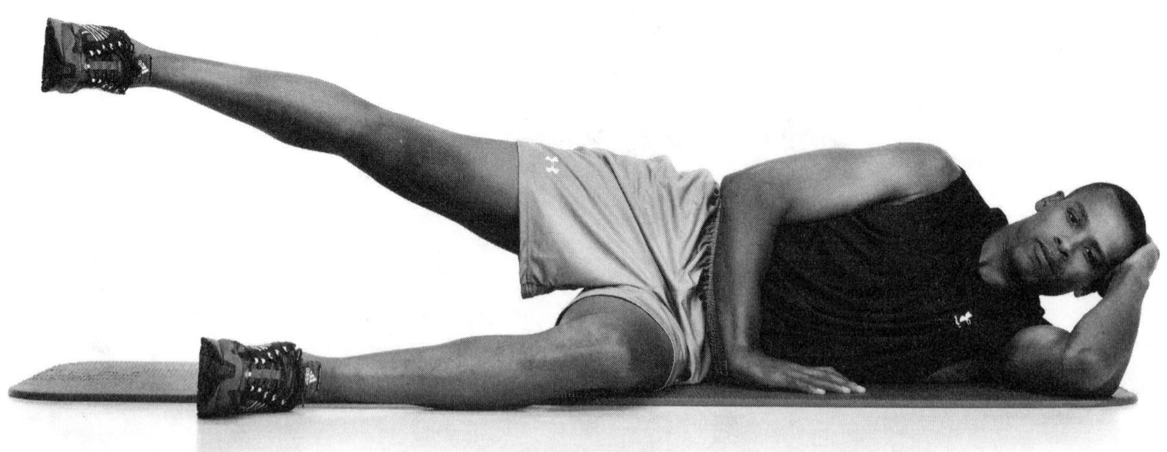

PRONE FRONT RAISE

Holding a pair of dumbbells with your palms facing each other, lie facedown on an exercise bench set to a 45-degree angle.

Keeping your arms completely straight, lift the dumbbells, keeping your arms in a V position. Keep your shoulder blades together until you get to the point where your arms are parallel to the floor. Hold for a second and then lower the weights back to the starting position.

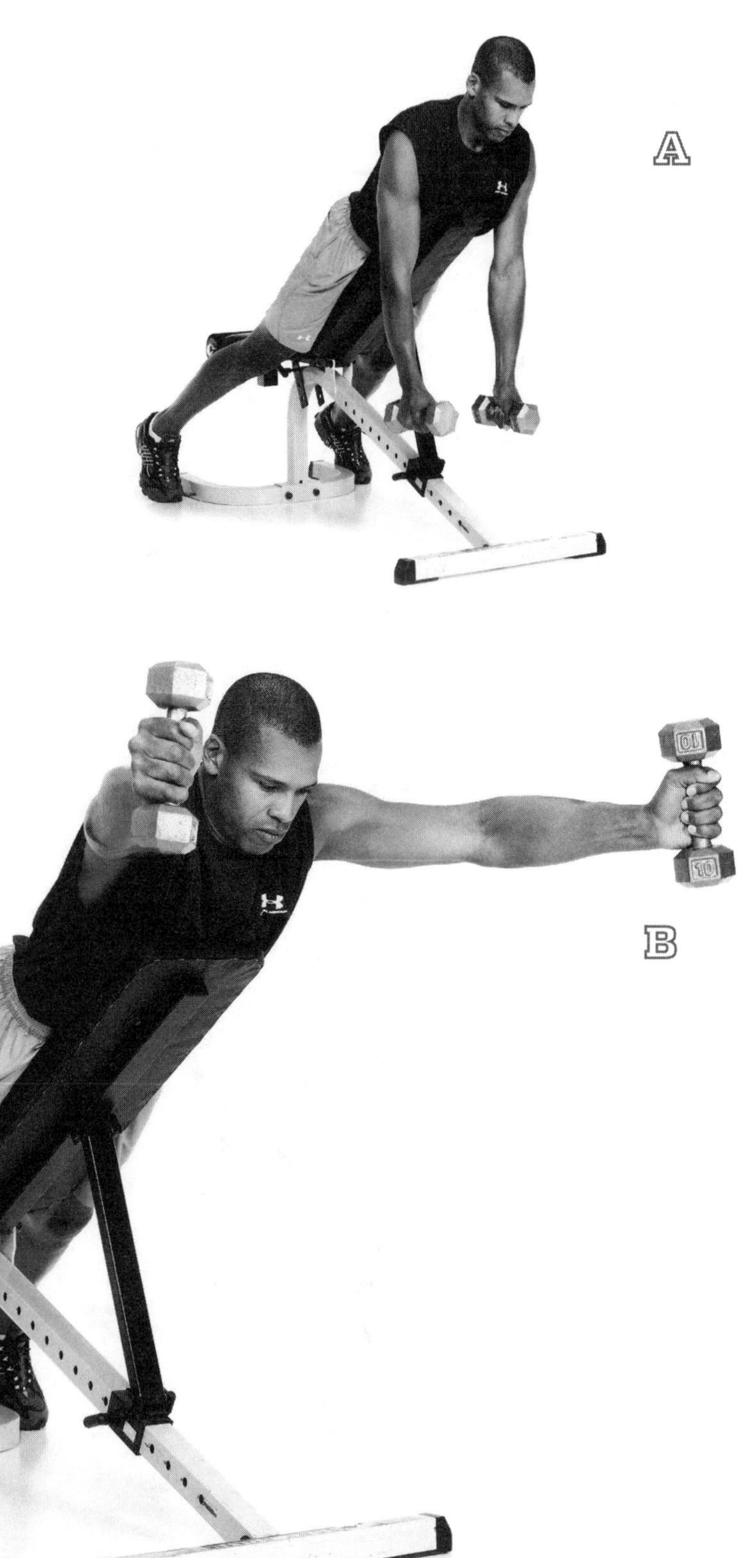

REVERSE SHRUG ON LAT PULLDOWN MACHINE

Load a lat pulldown or a cable station with a relatively light weight (no more than half of your body weight to start) and sit with your feet flat on the floor. Next, lean back at the waist slightly and hold the bar with a shoulder-width, overhand grip.

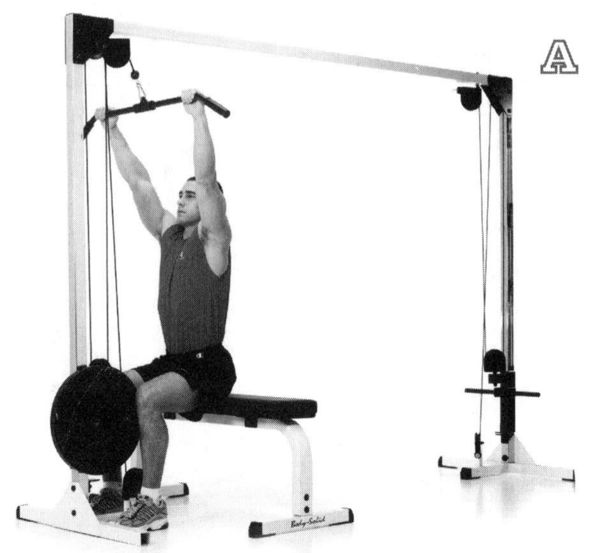
A

Keep your arms straight as you "pinch" your shoulder blades down and in toward your spine. Hold for a second and then bring the weight back to the starting position.

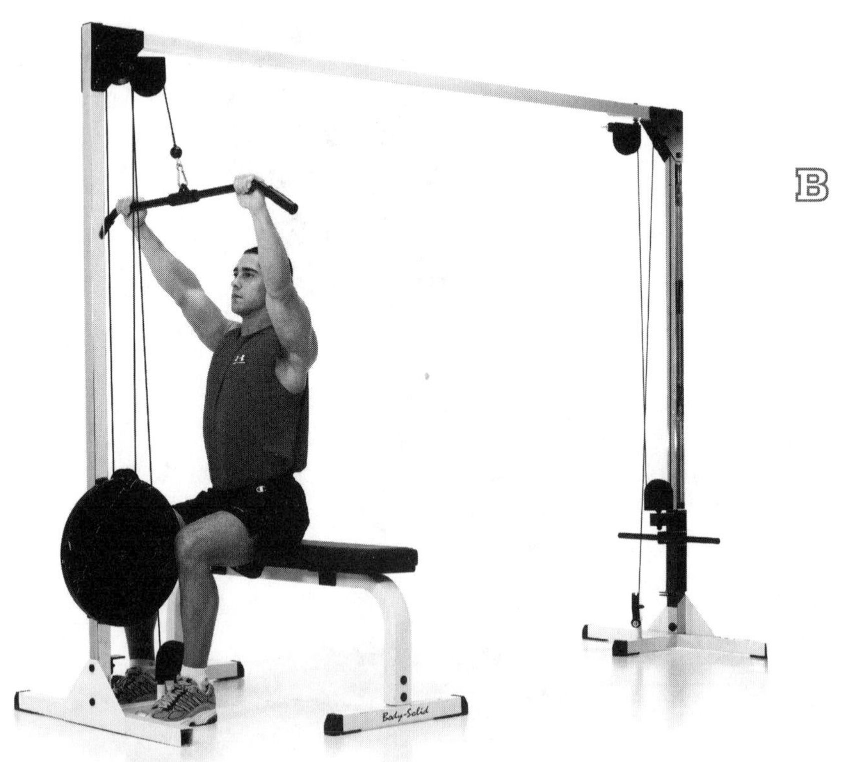
B

SWISS BALL BACK EXTENSION

Lie facedown with your torso rounded over a Swiss ball, your legs straight, and your hands folded behind your back.

Using the muscles that run up and down your spine, extend your spine and lift your chest completely off the ball. Hold for 20 to 30 seconds and release.

A

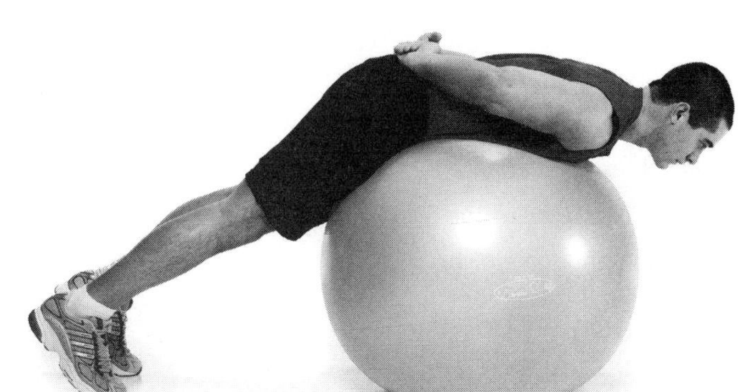

B

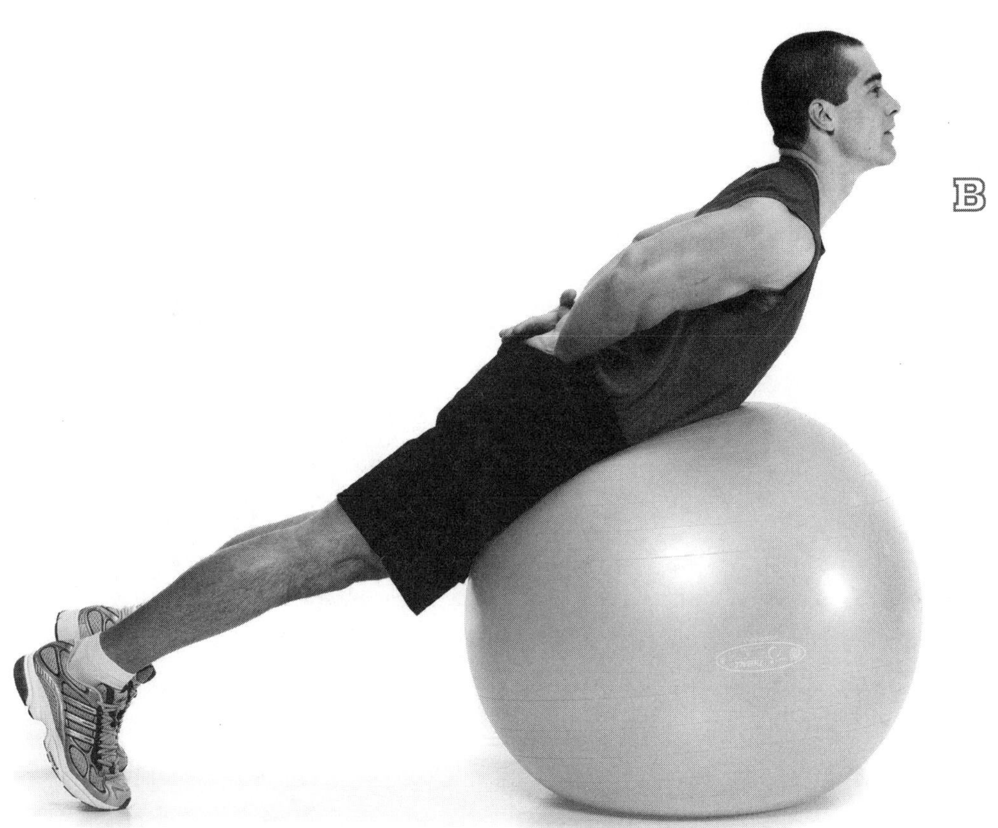

SUPERMAN

Lie facedown on the floor with your legs straight and your arms extended over your head.

Using the muscles that run up and down your spine, simultaneously lift your chest, arms, and both legs off the floor. Hold for a second in the top position and then lower back down.

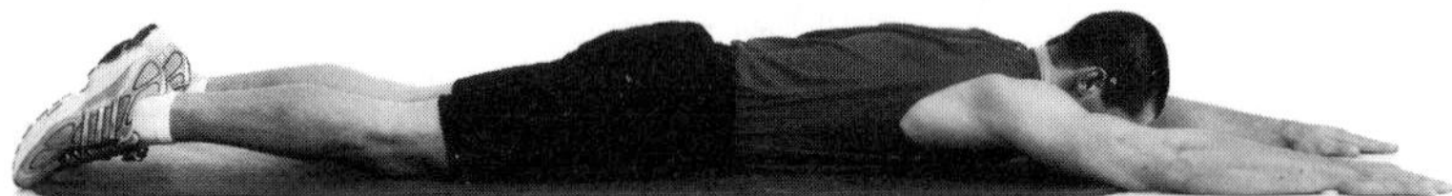

B

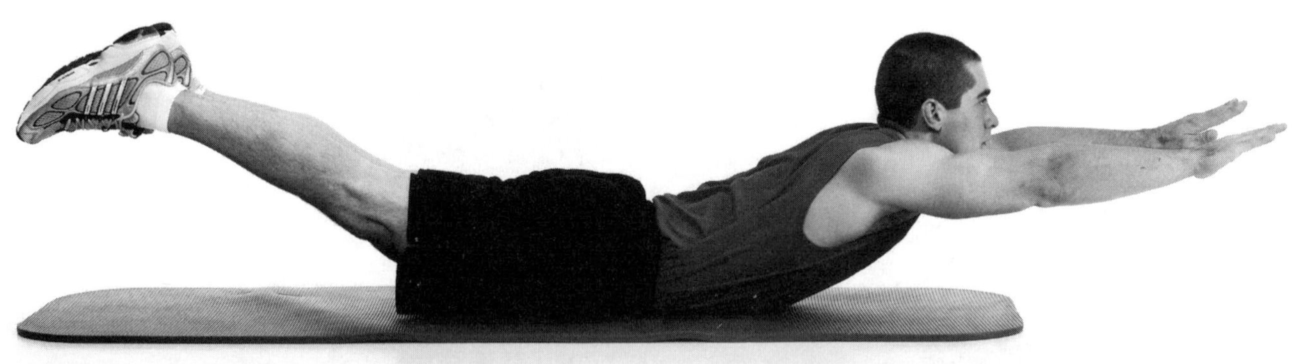

RUSSIAN TWIST

Sit on the floor with your knees bent about 90 degrees and your feet flat on the floor. Next, extend your arms and lean back until your wrists line up over your knees.

Hold this same trunk angle as you twist as far as possible to one side and then the other.

A

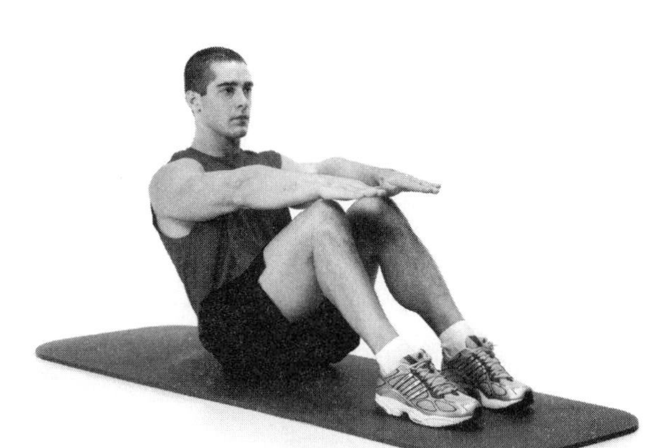

B

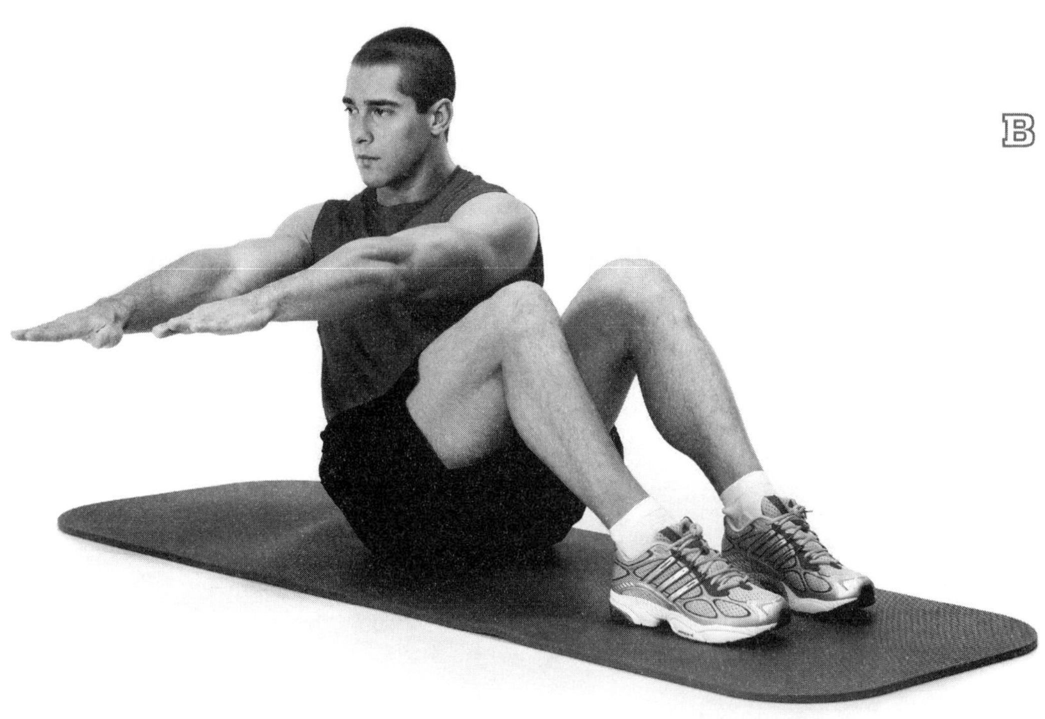

MEDICINE BALL WALL ROTATION

Stand 2 to 2½ feet from a wall, with your back to it, and hold a light medicine ball at arm's length in front of your chest.

Keep your arms as straight as possible as you attempt to touch the wall with the ball. Keep your feet pointed forward and your knees slightly bent as you do this—no pivoting to try to get farther around. Keep turning slowly from side to side, trying to go a little farther with each rotation.

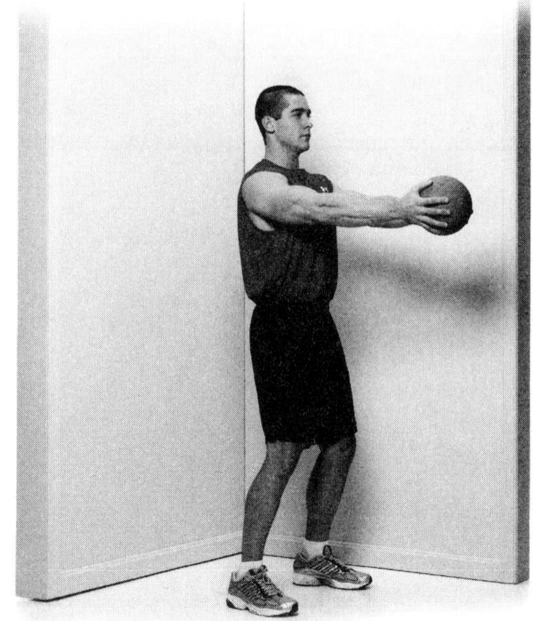

A

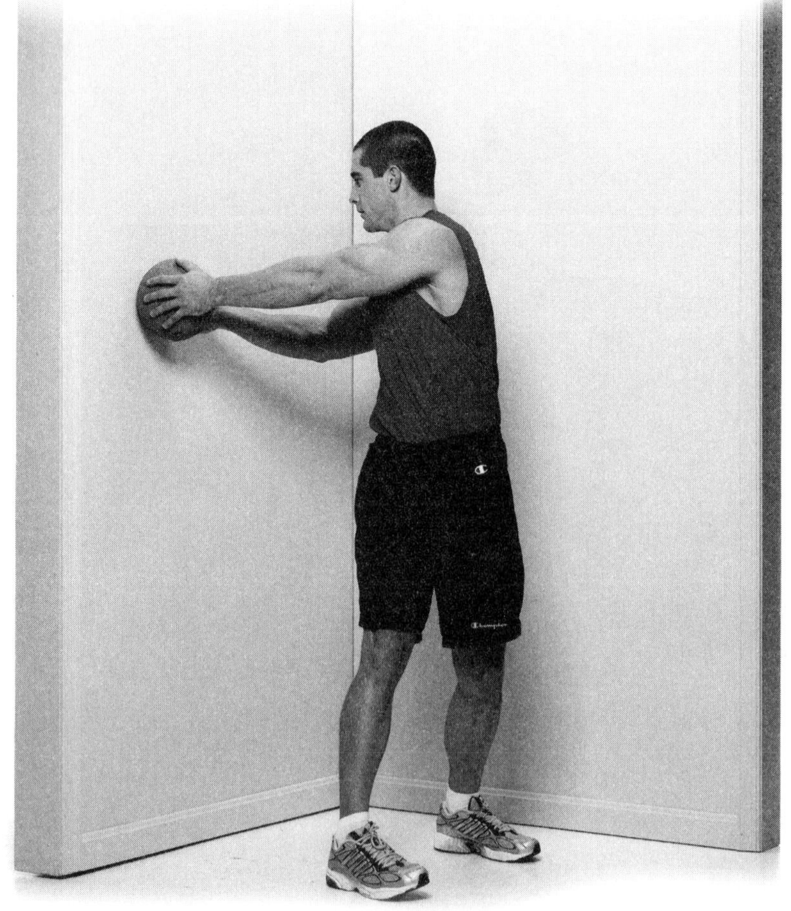

B

UNILATERAL ROMANIAN DEADLIFT

From a standing position, lift one foot an inch or two off the floor while maintaining a slight bend in your supporting knee.

Drive your hips back as you begin to lean forward until your torso is as close to parallel to the floor as possible. As you lower yourself forward, be sure your supporting knee doesn't bend any more and your back doesn't round. Return to the starting position. Finish your set and then do the same number of reps with your other foot lifted.

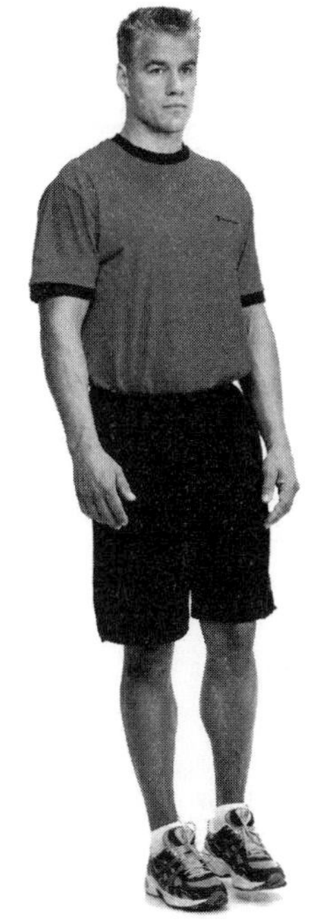

B

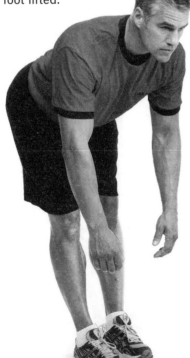

NEGATIVE CHINUP

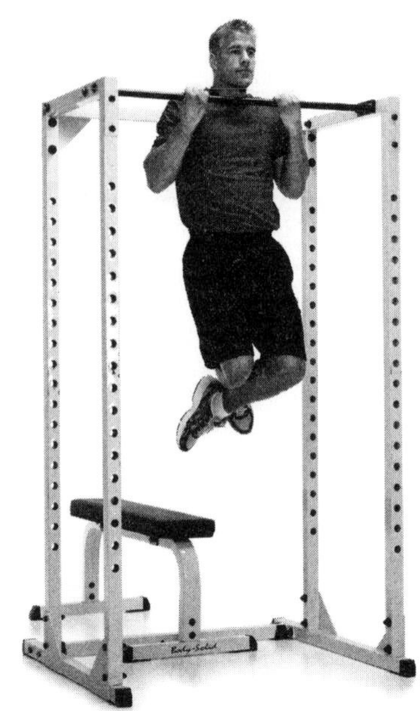

Position a bench or high step underneath a chinning bar, about one foot behind it. Next, standing on the bench, grab the bar with a supinated (palms facing you) grip that's about shoulder width. Boost yourself up so that your chin is over the bar, your legs are bent about 90 degrees behind you, and your ankles are crossed.

Without allowing your legs to swing, begin to lower yourself down for a count of 5 seconds. Once your arms are just about completely straight, place your feet on the bench or step and once again prop yourself up into the starting position.

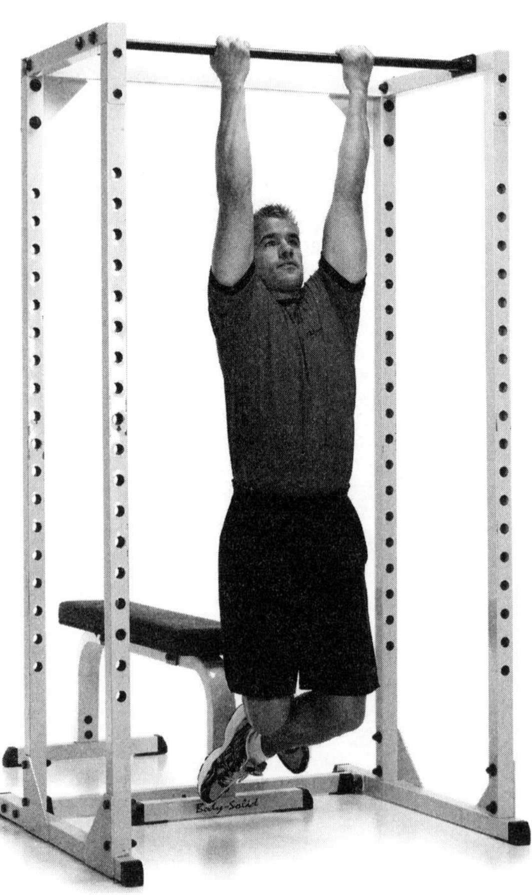

B

UNILATERAL DUMBBELL TOUCH

Stand a dumbbell (or another object, such as a water bottle) on its end on the floor about 1½ feet in front of you. Next, bend your right leg about 90 degrees and hold it behind you.

Sit down and back into your left hip as you bend your knee and reach forward with both hands to touch the dumbbell. Once your working knee has reached a 90-degree angle, lightly touch the dumbbell with both hands and push back up to the starting position. Finish your set and then do the same number of reps with your left leg lifted.

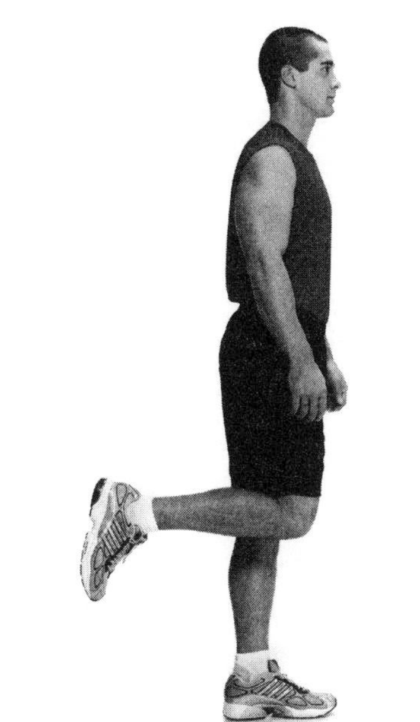

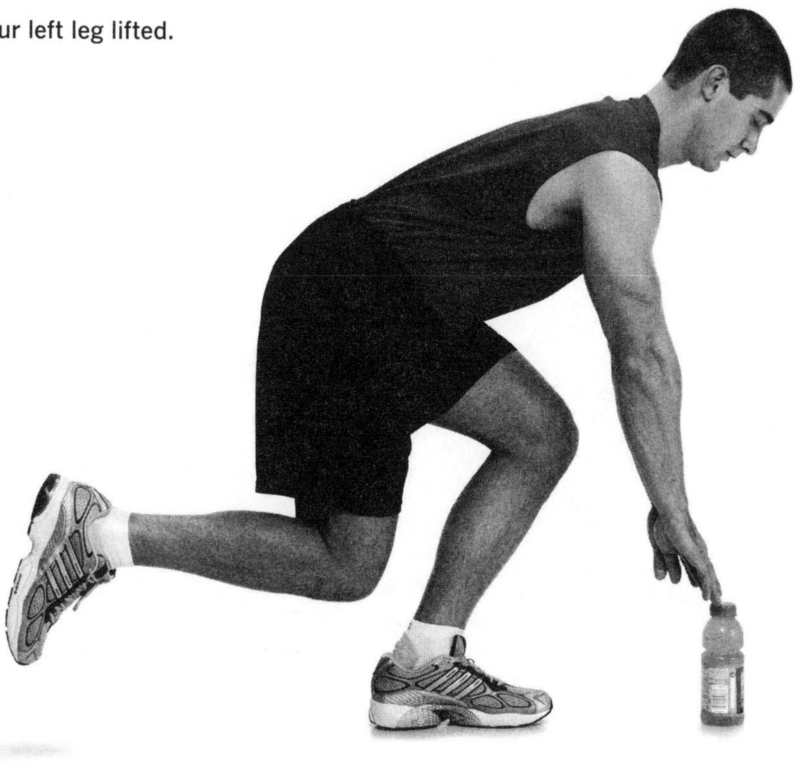

B

NEGATIVE SITUP

Sit on the floor with your knees bent slightly and your feet flat. The degree of bend in your knees will determine the difficulty of this exercise. Start with a slight bend to maintain the desired tempo, and as you get stronger, work your feet in closer, increasing the amount of knee bend.

Slowly begin to lower yourself toward the floor, using your core muscles to resist the pull of gravity. It should take a full 5 seconds before your shoulder blades and head touch the floor. You can then grab one knee to "roll" yourself back up to the starting position.

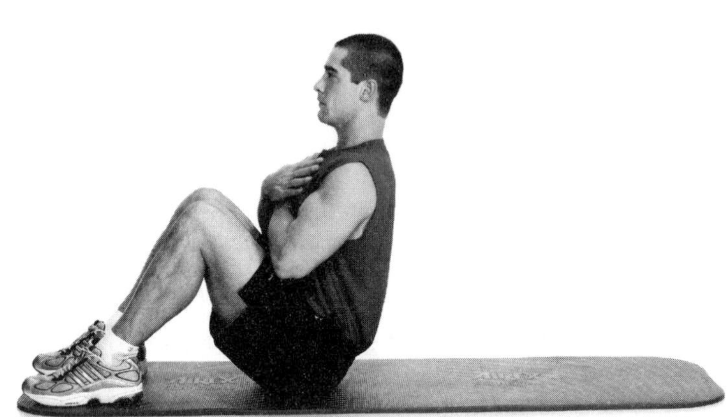

B

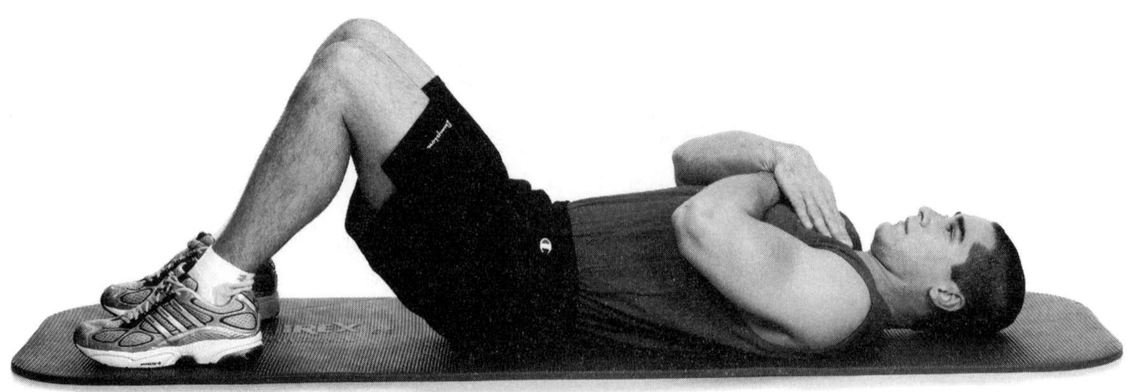

NEGATIVE NEUTRAL-SPINE PUSHUP

Get into a basic pushup position with your body a couple of inches off the floor and your hands placed slightly wider than shoulder-width apart. Pull your belly button in toward your spine and simultaneously contract your glutes. This should result in a disappearance of the arch in your lower back and an immediate awareness that your core musculature is working.

Maintain this position as you push yourself up for a 2-second count. Then pause for a full second before lowering and repeating.

A

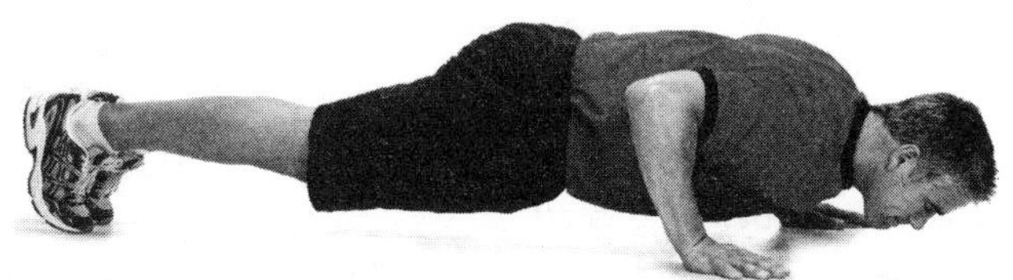

B

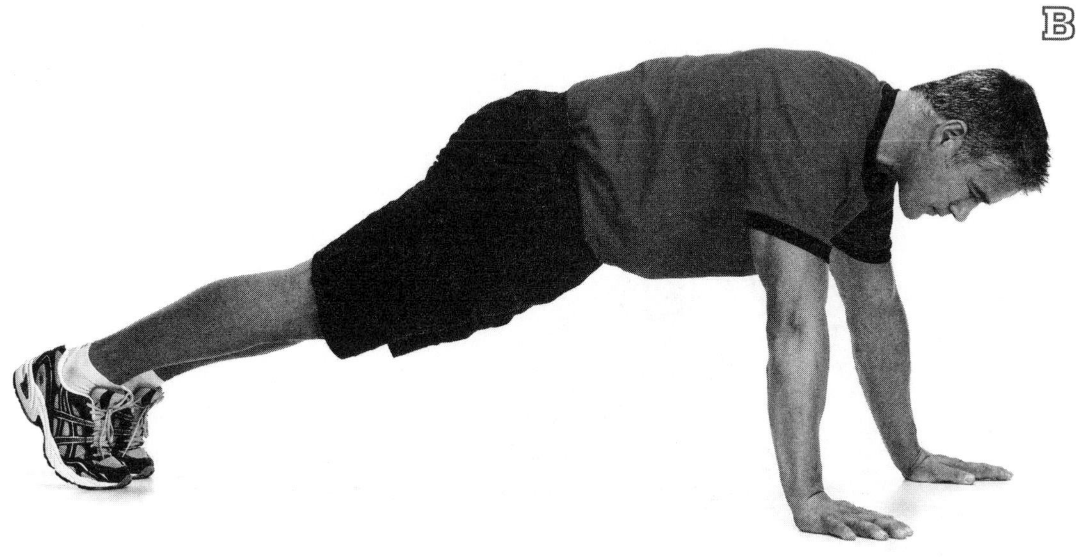

CRUNCH WITH PELVIC TILT

A

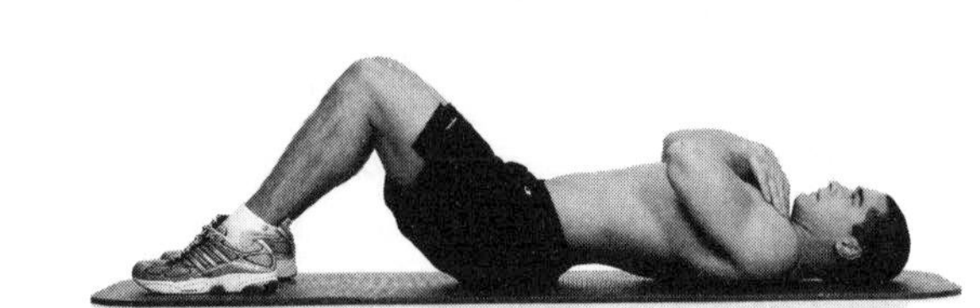

Lie faceup on the floor with your knees bent about 90 degrees and your feet flat.

Eliminate your normal spine arch by tilting your pelvis (bringing your belly button in and contracting your glutes).

B

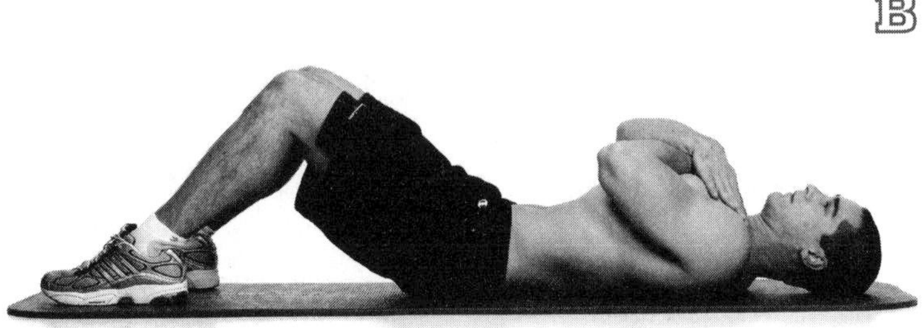

With your arms crossed on your chest, lift your shoulder blades off the floor. Hold for a second, then lower and repeat.

C

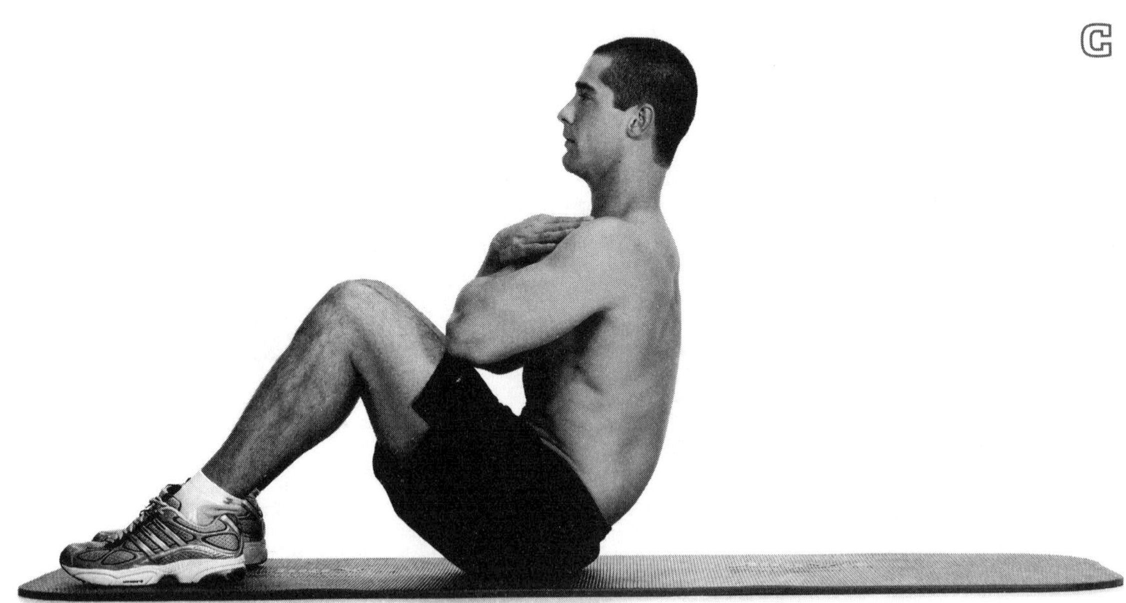

BIRD DOG

Get down on all fours with your knees bent 90 degrees and your arms directly beneath your shoulders.

Bracing your core muscles tightly, lift one arm and the opposite leg out (in front and in back of you, respectively) until they're parallel to the floor. In doing so, try to keep your torso and hips as still as possible; don't allow them to tilt over to one side. Hold for a second and then lower and repeat with the other side.

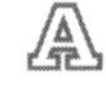

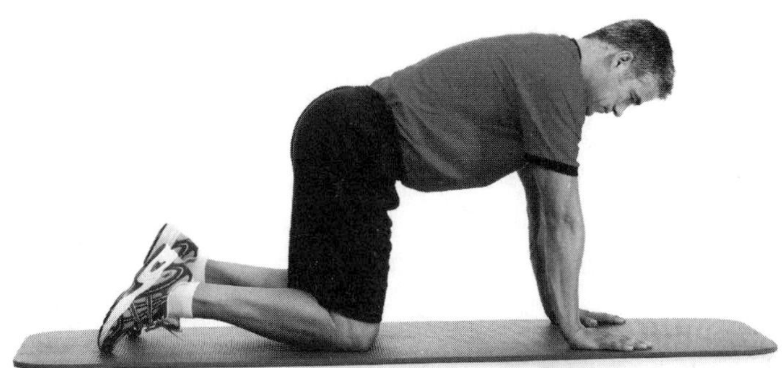

B

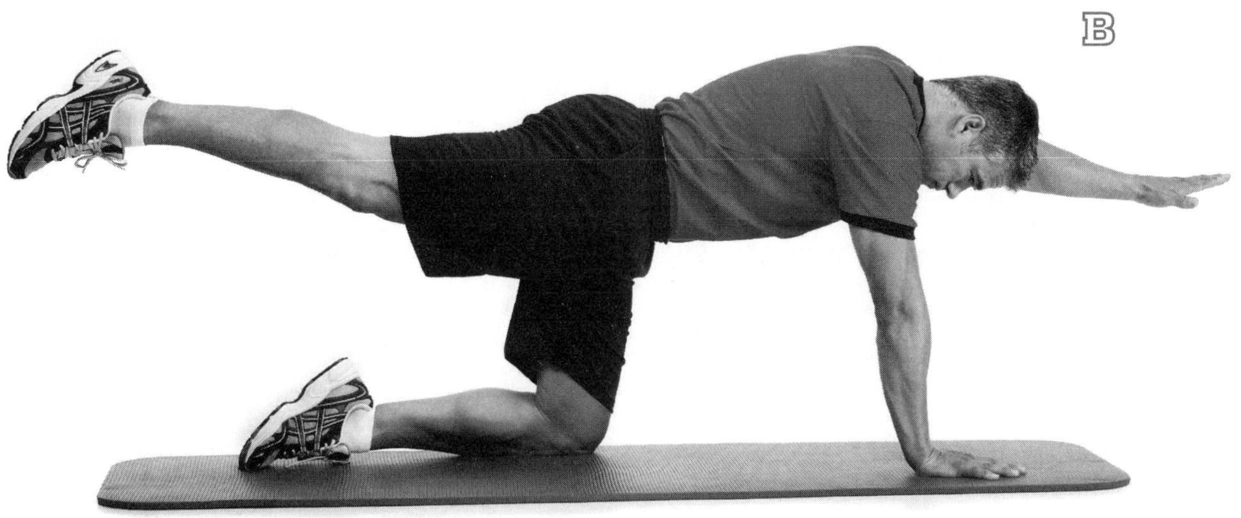

HIP FLEXOR STRETCH

Kneel on the floor and place one foot in front of your body with your knee bent approximately 90 degrees. Keeping your back straight and your belly button pulled in toward your spine, lean your hips forward, being sure to keep your back knee in contact with the floor. You should feel the stretch in your back leg. Hold for 20 to 30 seconds and repeat with the opposite leg.

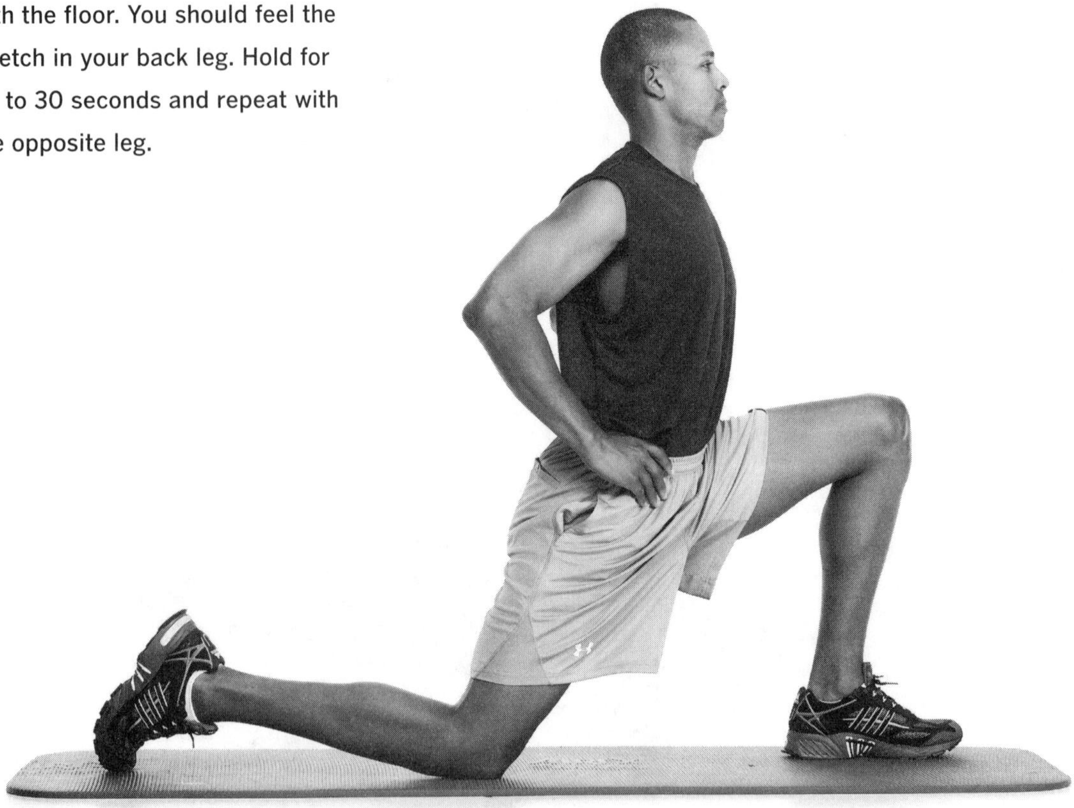

ERECTOR STRETCH

Lie faceup on the floor and hug your knees to your chest as you simultaneously bring your shoulders off the floor and your head toward your knees. Hold for 20 to 30 seconds and release.

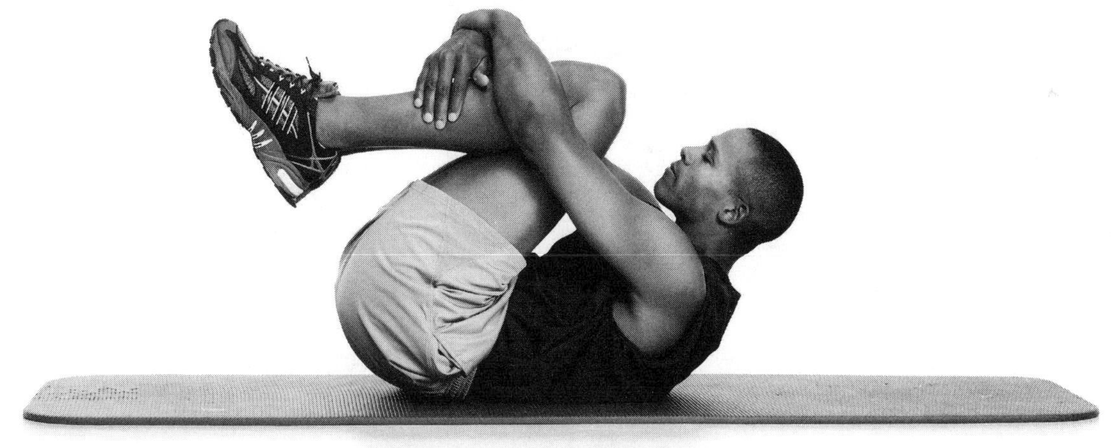

PEC WALL STRETCH

Stand sideways next to a wall and place the arm and shoulder closest to it up on it with your palm opened up. Keeping your shoulder and arm completely in contact with the wall, step the corresponding leg forward and turn away from the wall. Hold for 20 to 30 seconds and release. Repeat with your other arm on the wall.

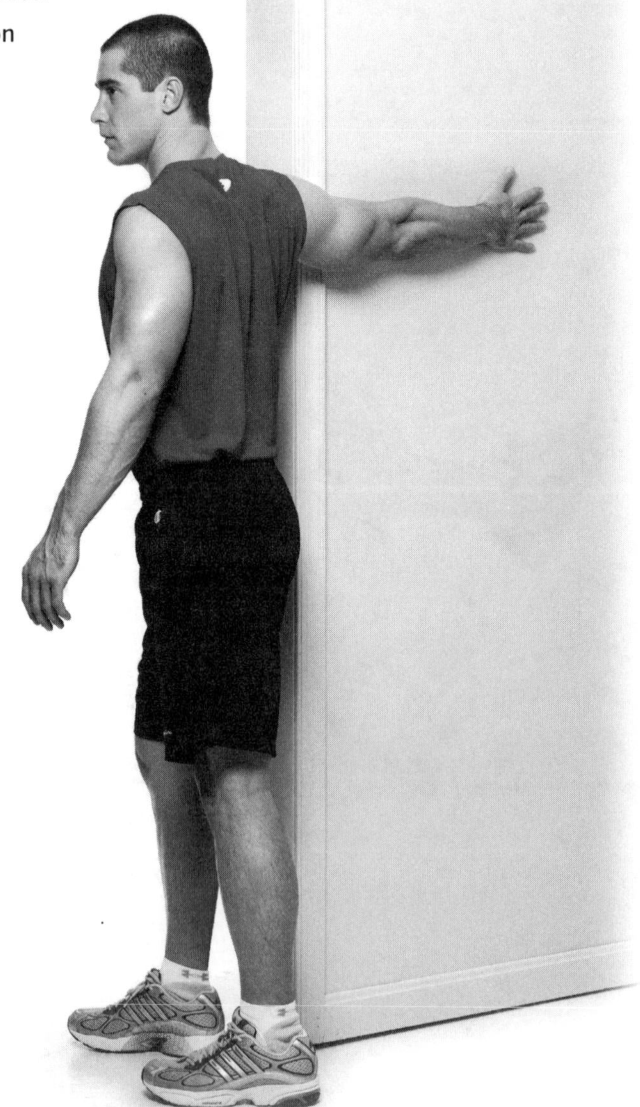

LAT STRETCH

Stand in front of a sturdy object that won't move and grab it with both hands at about hip level. You can use a squat rack if you're at the gym or the banister of your staircase at home. Bend over and sit back into your hips until your arms are completely straight. Hold for 20 to 30 seconds and release.

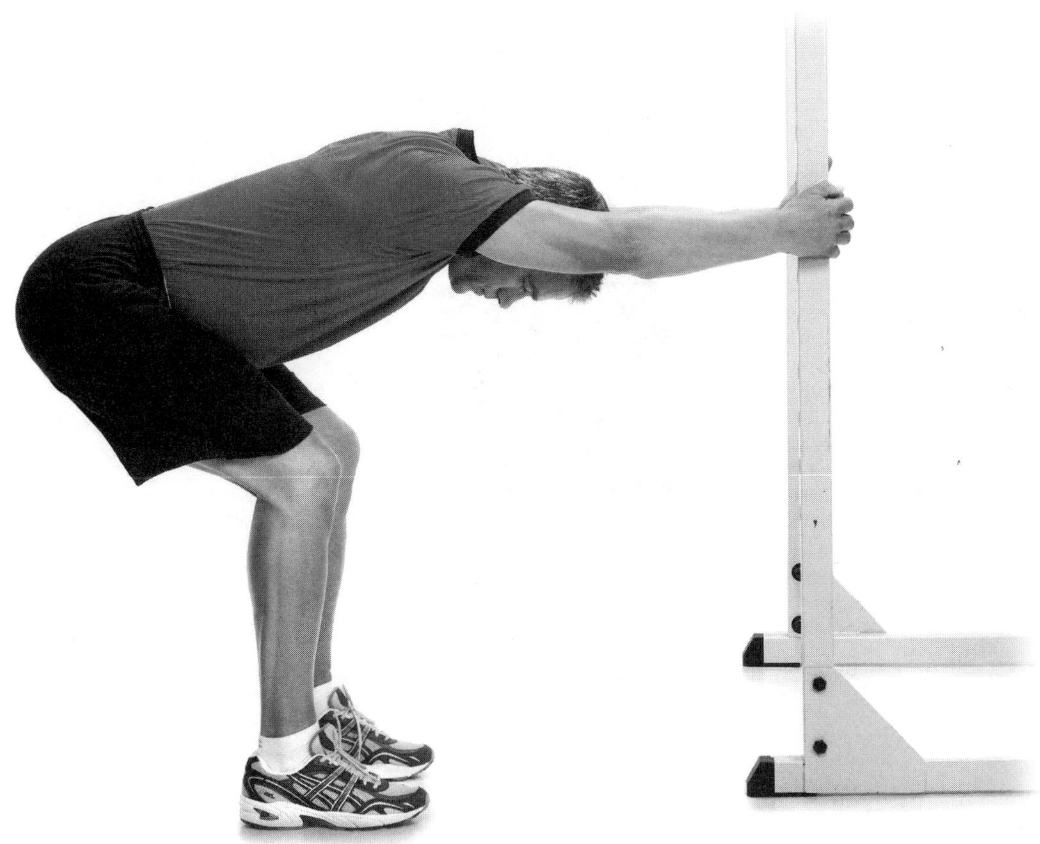

INTERNAL ROTATOR BROOMSTICK STRETCH

Hold a broomstick over your left shoulder as shown. With your right hand, pull the bottom of the broomstick forward until you feel a stretch in your left shoulder. Hold for 20 to 30 seconds and release. Repeat with the broomstick over your right shoulder.

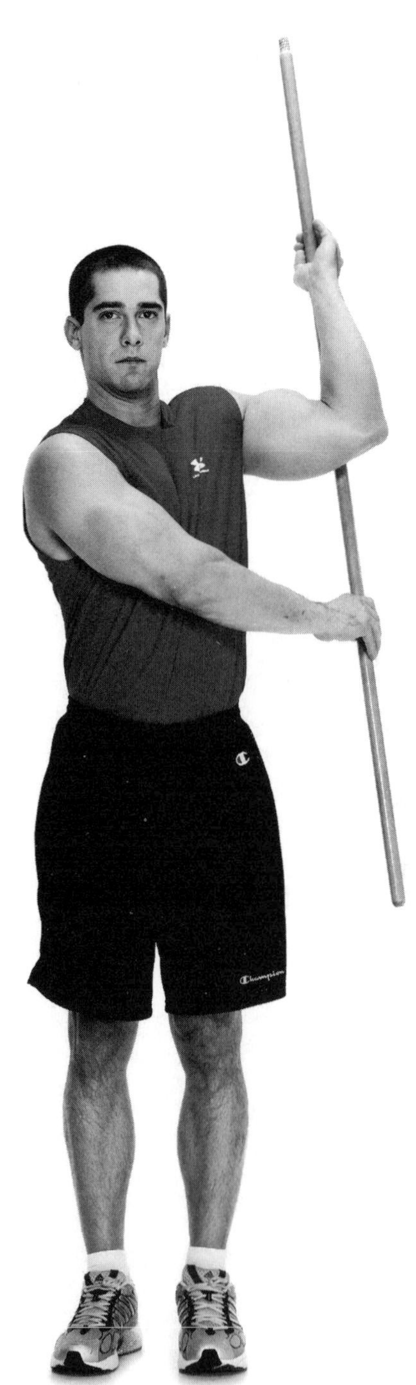

WALL CHIN TUCK

Stand with the back of your head and your entire back in contact with a wall.

Retract, or pull back, your jaw, trying to make a "double chin." This will cause the back of your head to press into the wall slightly. Hold this position for 3 to 5 seconds and release.

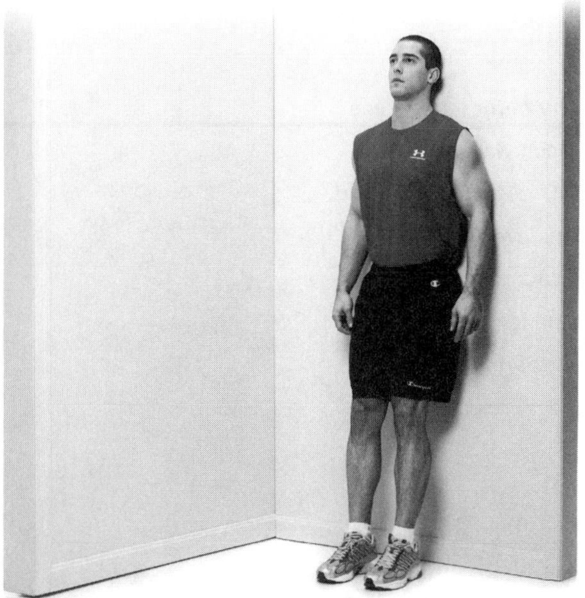

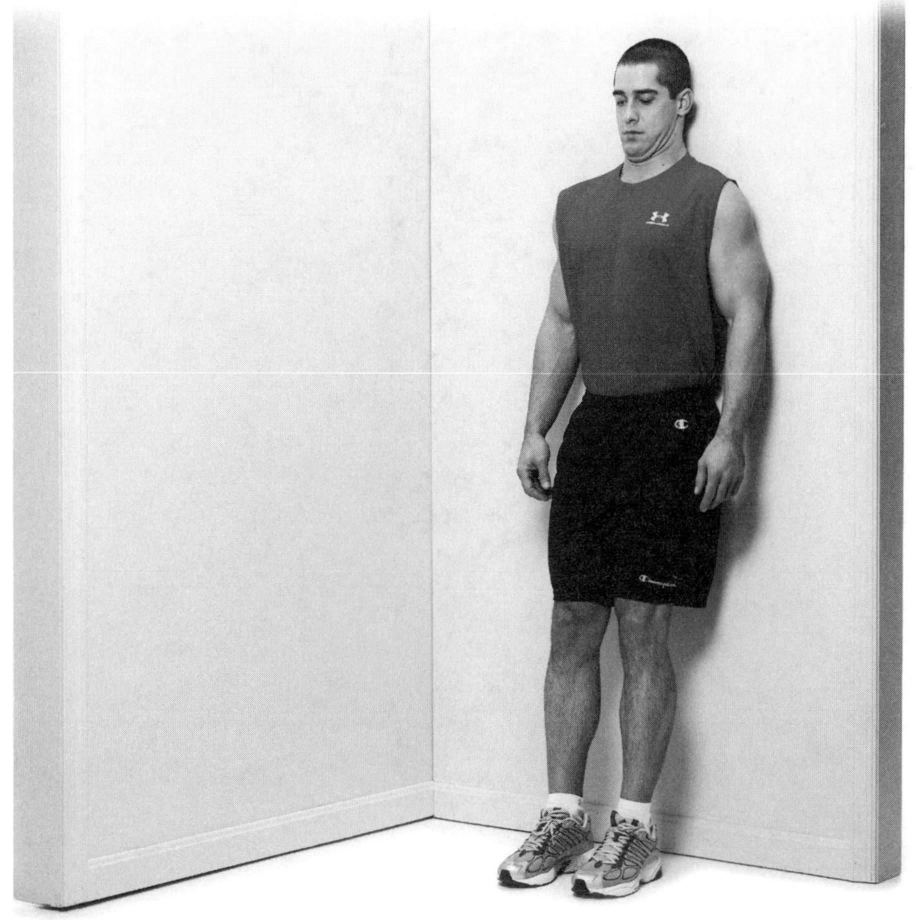

B

CORNER STRETCH

Walk over to any corner and place a forearm on each wall with your arms bent at 90-degree angles and your upper arms even with or slightly below your shoulders. Step forward with one leg and lean your body into the stretch. Hold for 20 to 30 seconds and release.

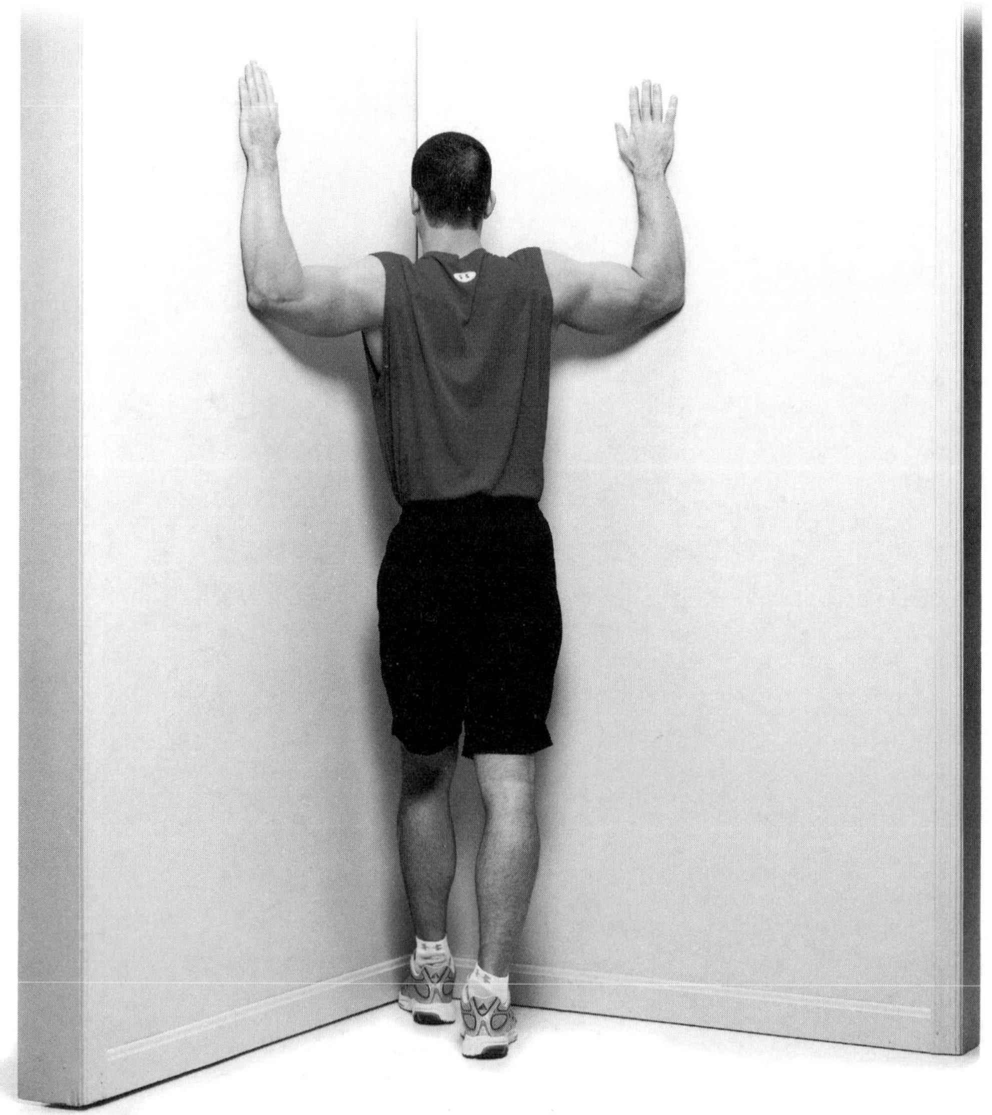

PIKE CALF STRETCH

In a pike position (hands and feet somewhat close together on the floor, hips in the air), place the ball of your right foot on the floor and rest the top of your left foot against the back of your right calf. Next, lower your right heel and try to get it as close to the floor as possible while keeping your right knee straight. Hold for 20 to 30 seconds and release. Repeat with the ball of your left foot on the floor.

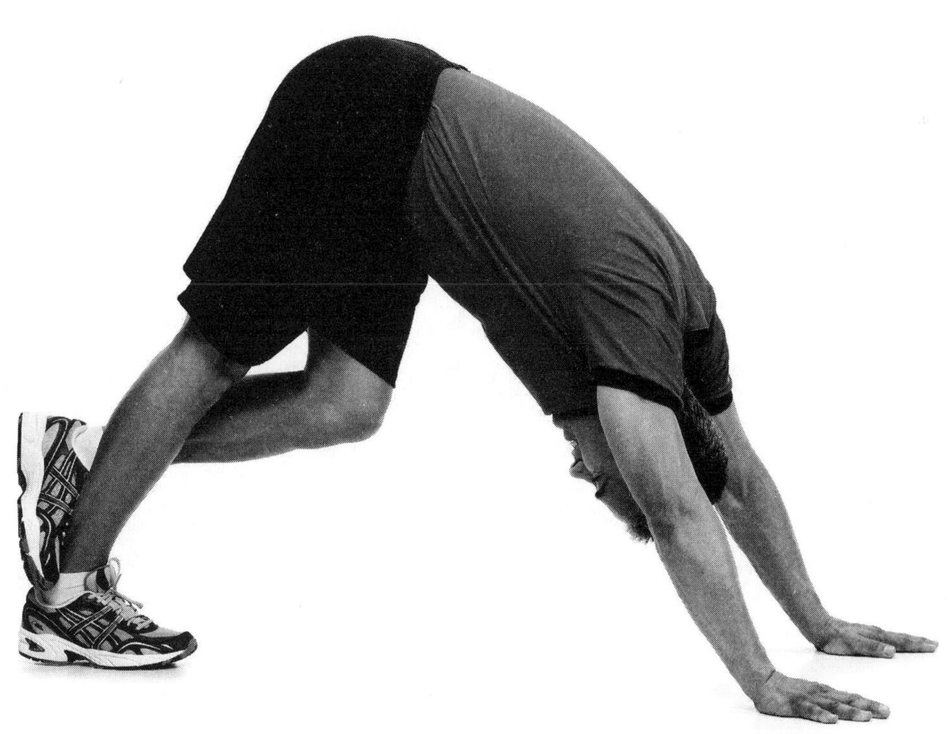

HAMSTRING DOORWAY STRETCH

Lie faceup on the floor inside a door frame and place the leg closest to the wall up on the wall, trying to get your leg as close to perpendicular to the floor as possible. Try to get your hips as close to the wall as possible while keeping your legs straight. Hold for 20 to 30 seconds and release. Repeat with your other leg on the wall.

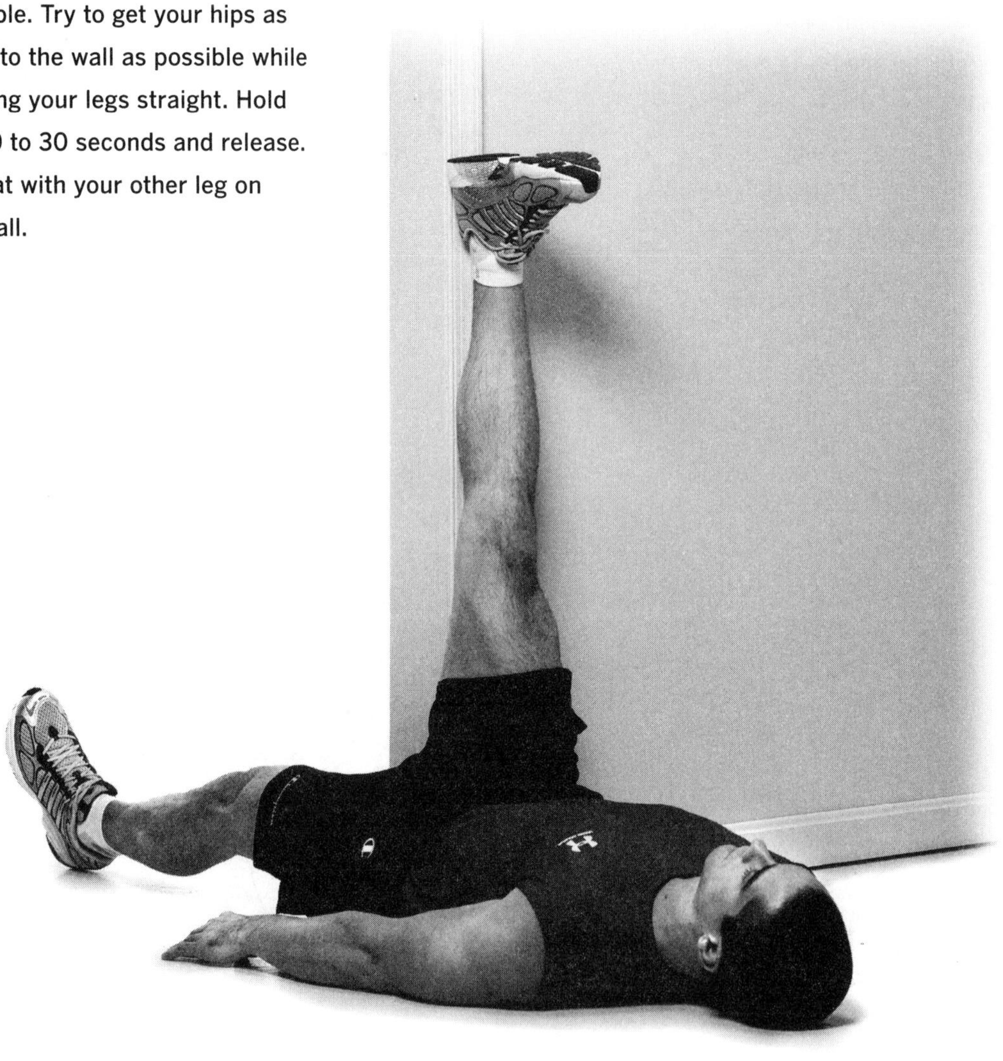

GLUTES AND PIRIFORMIS STRETCH

Sit on the floor with your left leg extended and your right leg bent 90 degrees as shown. Bend your left leg back behind you and lean your torso over your right knee. Repeat with your right leg behind you, leaning to your left.

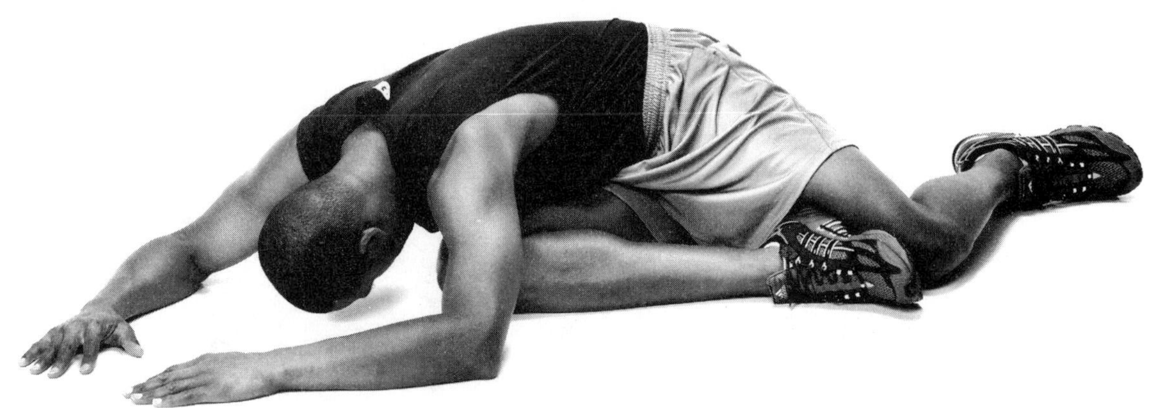

BUTTERFLY ADDUCTOR STRETCH

Sit with your back to a wall and bring the soles of your feet together. With your back as straight as possible, lower your knees as close to the floor as you can.

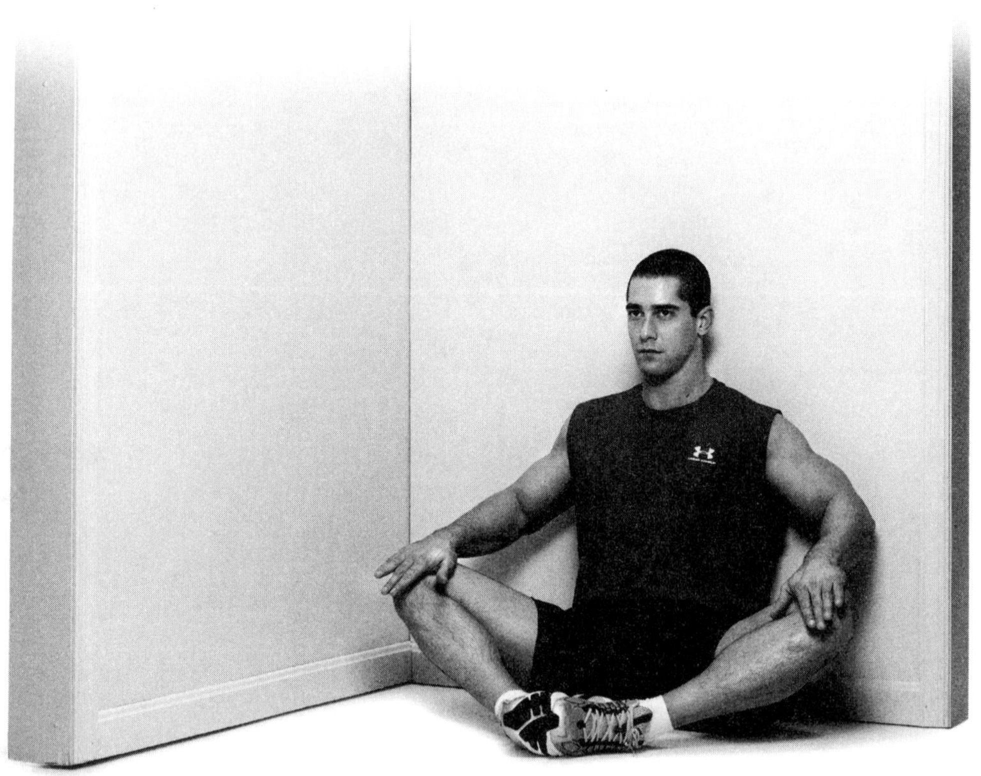

TRAPEZIUS STRETCH

Sit on a chair and hold the bottom of the seat with your left hand. Next, bring your right hand over your head and lightly grab the left side of it, just above your ear. Keeping your back straight, gently pull your head to the right by trying to bring your right ear toward your right shoulder. Hold for 20 to 30 seconds and repeat toward the other side.

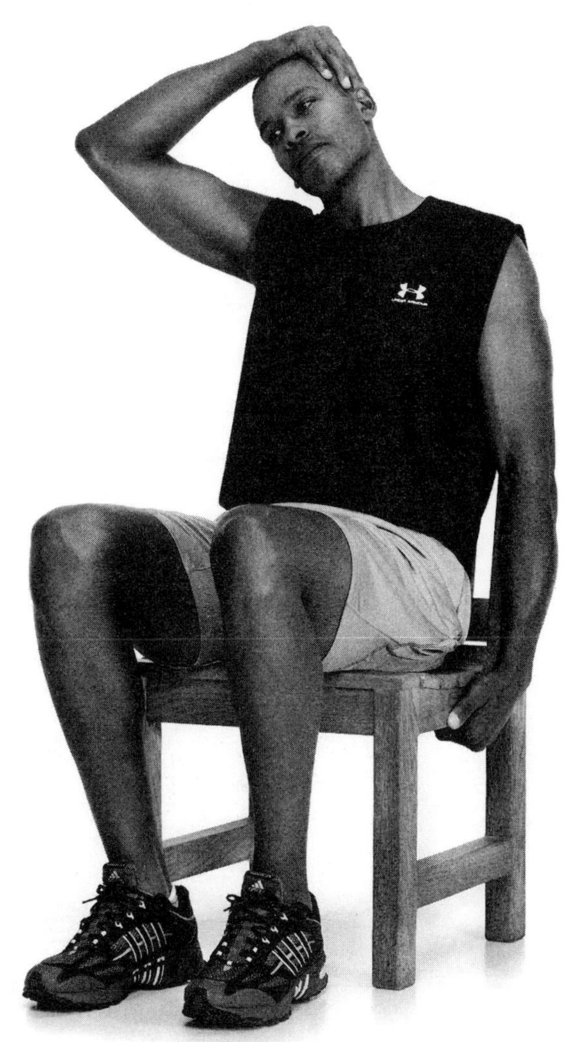

PRISONER STRETCH ON WALL

Stand a couple of feet from a wall and lean your back against it. Begin by tilting your pelvis to eliminate your normal spine arch and bring your arms up in line with your shoulders so the backs of them are in contact with the wall at a 90-degree angle. Next, without allowing any part of your back to come away from the wall, slowly start to straighten your arms as you slide them up against the wall. Be sure that both your arms and wrists maintain contact with the wall at all times. Go as high as you can and then hold for 20 to 30 seconds.

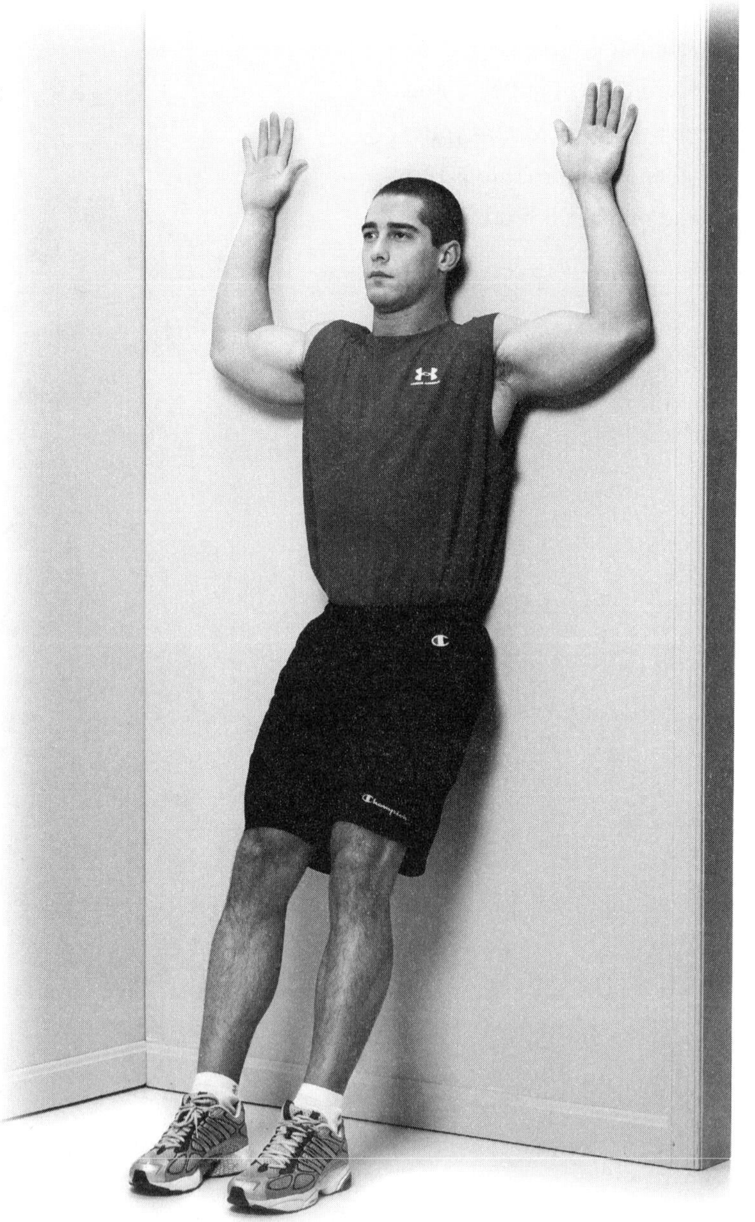

SEATED ROTATIONAL STRETCH

Sit in a chair with your legs bent 90 degrees and turn to one side as you attempt to grab the back of the chair. Hold for 20 to 30 seconds and release. Repeat to the other side.

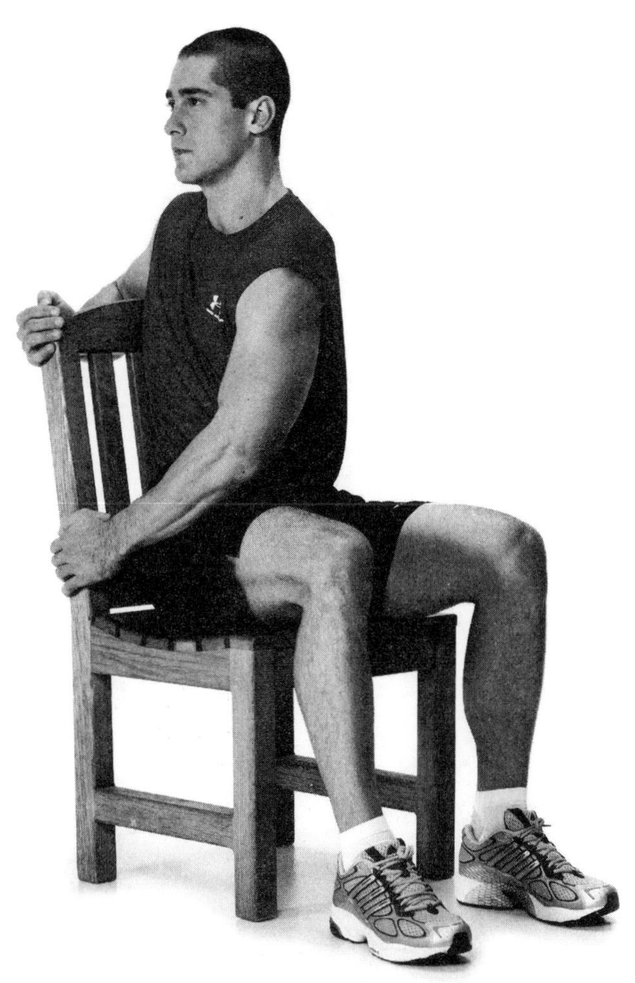

Dynamic Flexibility Drills

That takes care of all of the specific exercises and static stretches. The final piece of the puzzle in terms of getting your body back on track is the inclusion of dynamic flexibility drills. These differ from static stretches in that they involve *gradually* and actively working your muscles through an increasing range of motion.

This second type of stretching is necessary because flexibility is, without question, one of the most important aspects of fitness. When you increase the range of motion of the muscles that act on a particular joint, you gain more freedom of motion. And when you can move more freely, just about any physical activity you engage in, both inside and outside of the gym, becomes much easier.

Allow me to qualify that last statement. Improving your range of motion *doesn't* always lead to improvements in movement efficiency; it depends on how you go about it. Static stretching, the kind where you place the muscle to be stretched in an elongated position and hold it for at least 15 seconds, can indeed help increase the length of a given muscle. But does increased muscle length translate into improved movement efficiency when that muscle is asked to work with other muscles to produce movement? Researchers, coaches, and trainers have begun to question the benefit of static stretching, particularly when it's done prior to physical activity. Some of the more interesting findings are that static stretching prior to exercise does not reduce injury potential but can reduce the ability of your muscles to generate force. In fact, a 2004 study published in the *Journal of Strength and Conditioning Research* showed that static stretching added a statistically significant half second to 20-meter sprint times. This is particularly interesting considering that dynamic stretching (where you gradually move your muscles through a large range of motion to limber them up, as opposed to just holding the stretched position) resulted in more than a half-second improvement.

Another failing of static stretching is that it's useless to increase a muscle's length and the range of motion of the joint(s) that muscle acts upon unless you also develop strength through that improved range of motion. For instance, both the quadriceps (front thighs) and hip flexors (located at the tops of your thighs, right below your waist) are muscle groups that are chronically tight in many people. Those who work at desk jobs can attest to the fact that sitting all day shortens the hip flexors like nobody's business. If tight enough, these muscles can disallow your getting into a deep lunge position. This can be overcome with some targeted stretching of this area. Let's assume you decide to go exclusively with static stretching to help alleviate this problem. Let's also assume that after a few weeks you notice a marked improvement in flexibility in these muscles. Chances are, if you need to get into this lunging position during the course of daily living, it won't be to show off how flexible you are. It'll probably be to bend down to pick up something. While your improved range of motion may allow you to get down into this position, your failure to build strength through this newfound range leaves you extremely susceptible to an injury.

Just because a muscle (or group of muscles) has the capacity to move through a specific range of motion doesn't mean it can apply strength through that entire range. If all you ever do is gently bring your muscles into a specific position and then hold it for several seconds, all they learn to do is relax when they're in said position. Asking them to suddenly generate strength from this position, often rather quickly in response to some immediate situation, dramatically increases your chances of injury. The point being that static flexibility alone simply isn't enough. You also need to include some form of dynamic flexibility training, preferably with additional weight, to best meet the demands of daily living. So I'm providing 10 dynamic stretching drills you should do prior to strength training or intensive cardio exercise. You'll see them included in many of the workouts going forward.

Don't misinterpret these dynamic drills to mean that you should be aggressively swinging limbs all over the place. Regardless of which drill you're doing, start slowly and allow your muscles to "open up" at their own pace.

In addition to increasing your core temperature and the bloodflow to your working muscles, these drills also offer the added bonus of firing up your body for activity. This is the exact opposite of what occurs when you perform static stretching, where you're trying to relax your muscles. So don't be surprised if incorporating these dynamic drills into your routine ultimately allows you to lift a little more weight or push a little harder than usual. Note that the number of repetitions will be explained in the individual workouts.

QUAD STRETCH WALK

From a standing position, grab your right instep and pull your heel toward your butt.

Hold for a second, then take a step and do the same with the other leg. Continue this way until you've covered the desired distance.

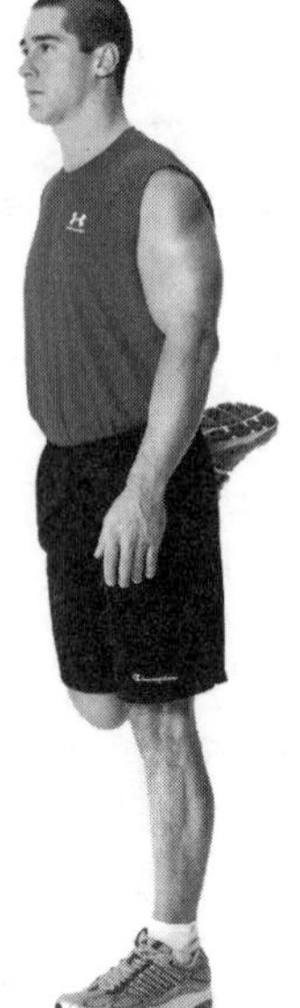

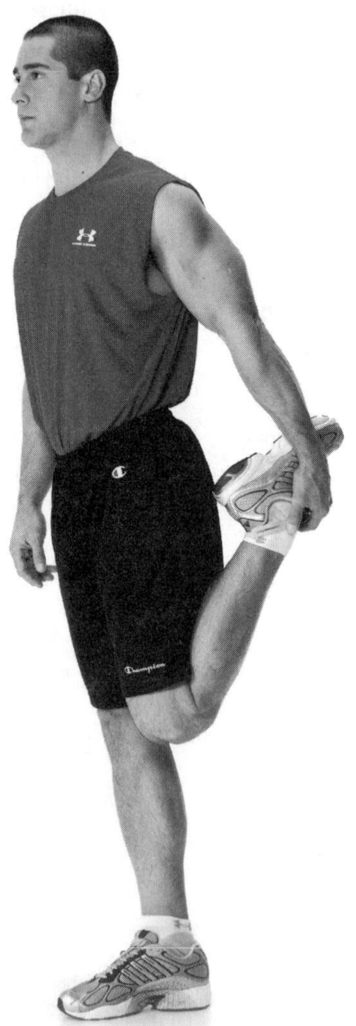

B

FRANKENSTEIN

Stand with your arms extended out in front of you.

Kick one leg straight up toward your hands without dropping your chest or rounding your back. Repeat with the other leg and continue for the desired number of reps.

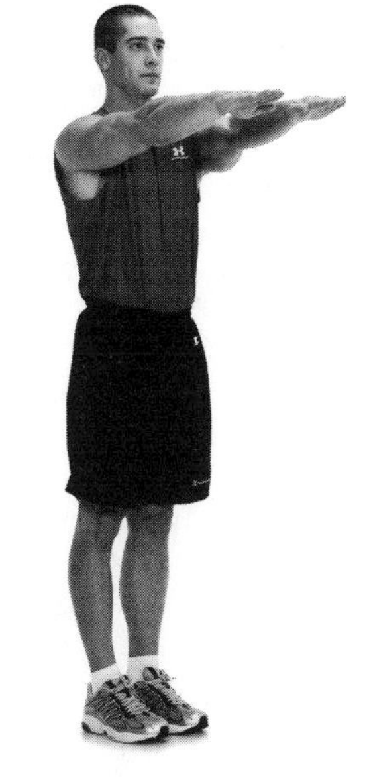

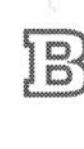

GATE SWING

From a standing position, lift one knee out to the side until it's just above your belt line.

Once it's there, swing that leg around in front of you and lower it forward. Repeat the same sequence with the other leg.

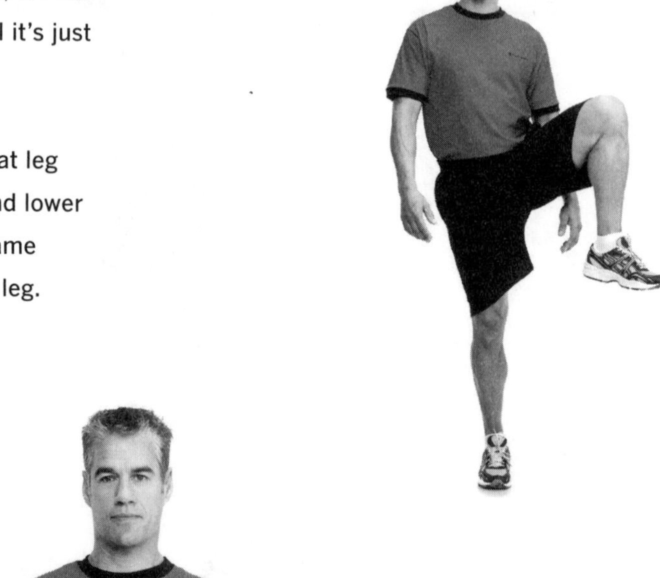

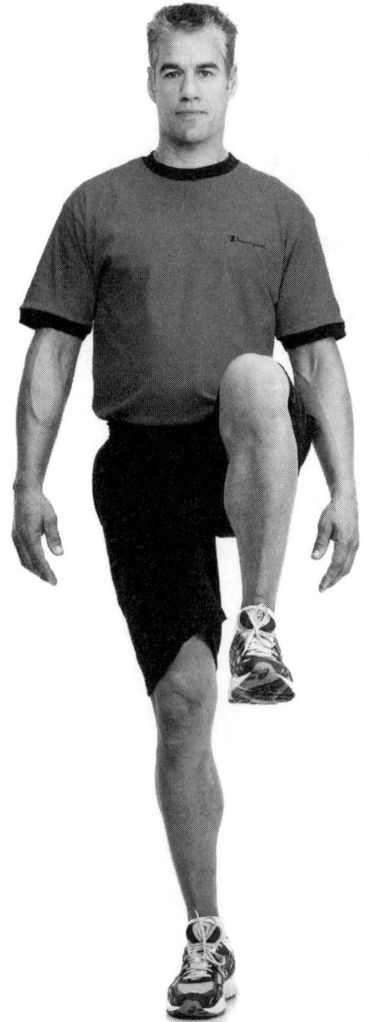

B

REVERSE GATE SWING

From a standing position, lift one leg directly out in front of you, just above your belt line, by bending your knee 90 degrees.

Hold this knee angle as you swing your hip open and step back behind you. Repeat with the other leg.

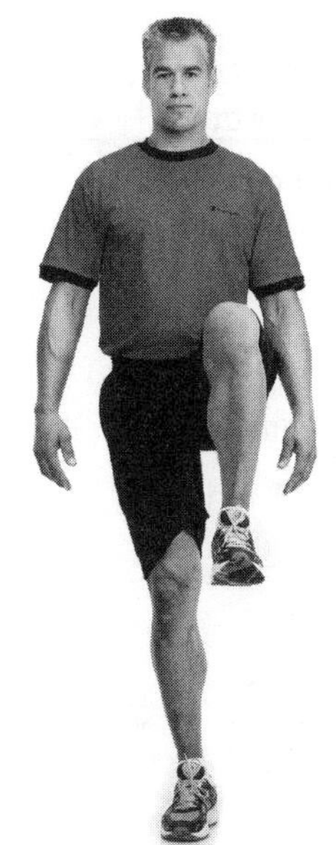

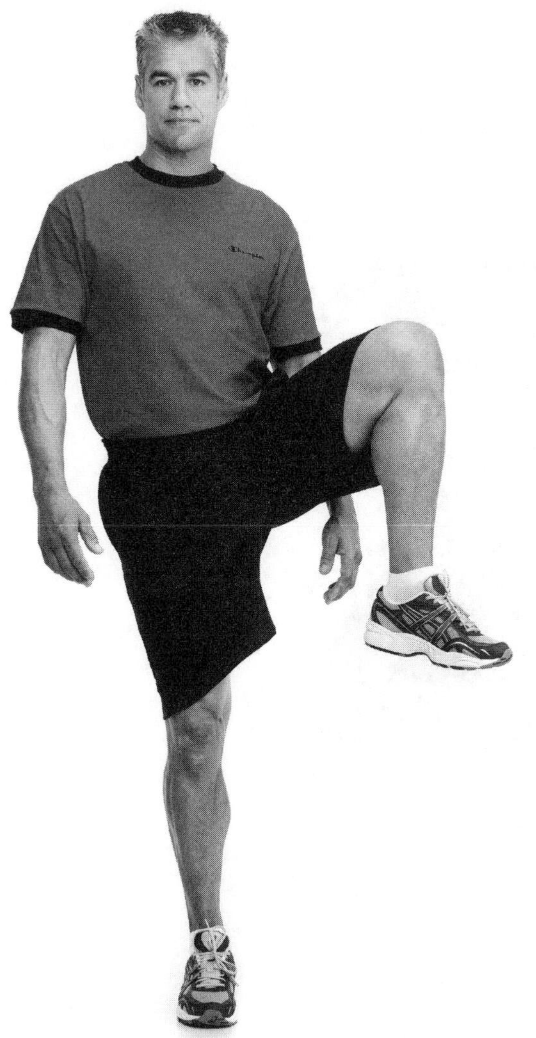

B

MEDICINE BALL WRAPAROUND

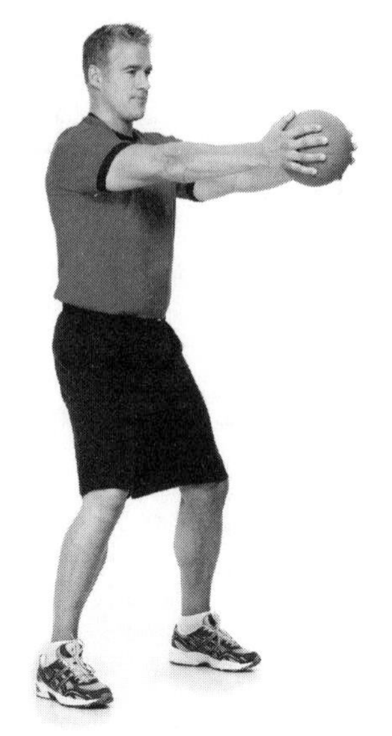

Stand with your feet shoulder-width apart and your knees slightly bent, holding a light medicine ball at arm's length in front of you.

Begin by cradling the ball in one hand and bringing it back past your torso, holding your other hand out in front of your chest. Once there, immediately swing it around and switch hands, bringing the ball around to the other side.

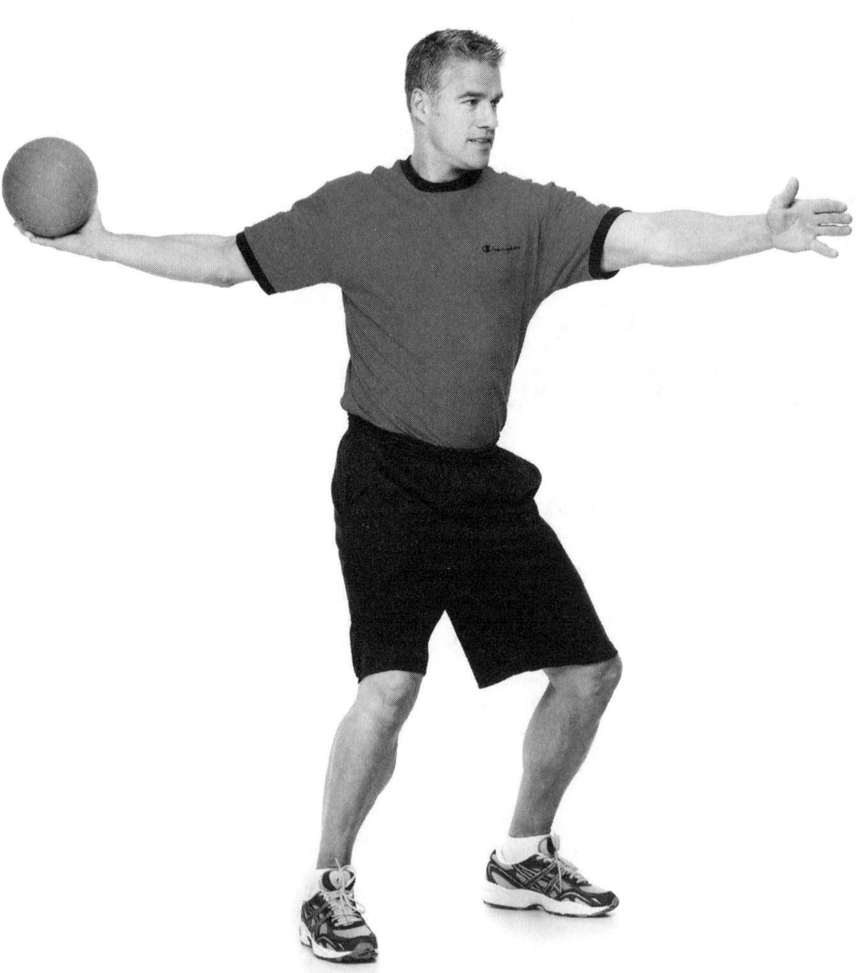

B

MEDICINE BALL WOODCHOPPER

Stand with your feet shoulder-width apart and your knees slightly bent, holding a medicine ball with your arms outstretched over your left shoulder.

Using your core to initiate the movement, "chop" the ball down using a long, sweeping stroke so that you finish with the ball outside your right calf. Be sure to bend your knees and round your back slightly as you chop downward. Bring the ball back to the starting position and repeat. When you've finished a set, repeat on the other side.

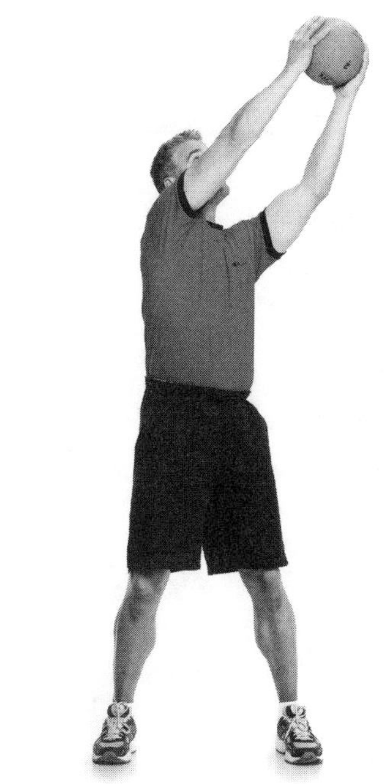

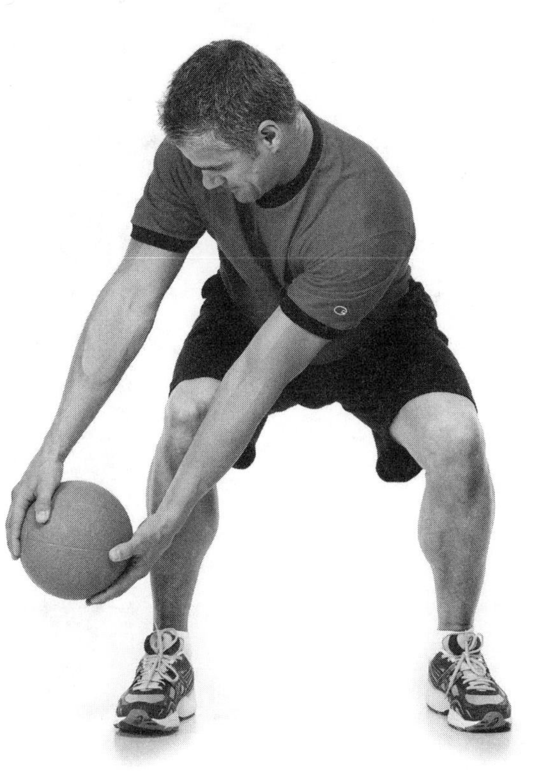

B

HIP WALK

From a standing position, raise one leg across the front of your body and grab that shin. Once you have it, simultaneously pull up so the shin ends up parallel to the floor, and come up on the ball of your opposite foot. Lower, step forward, and repeat with the other leg.

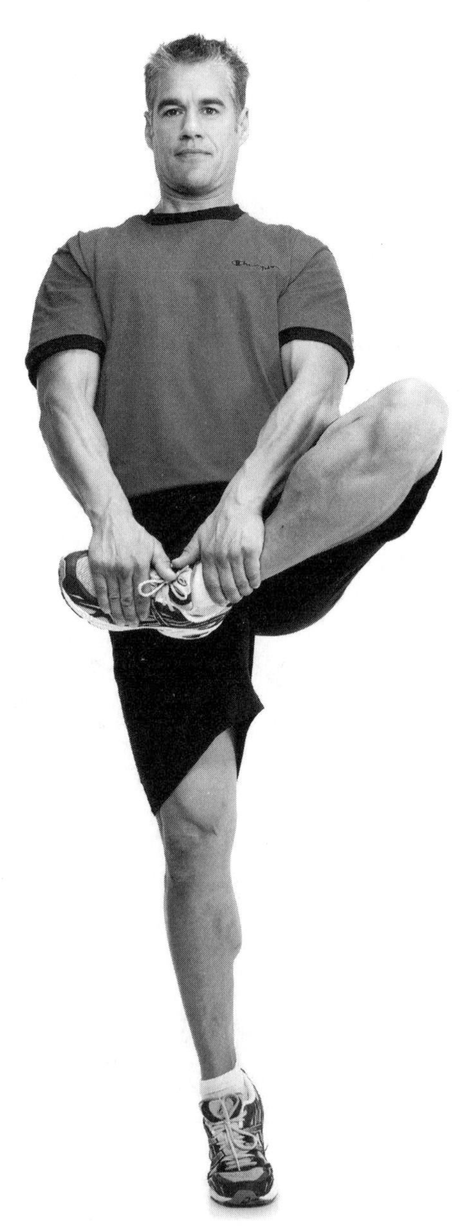

REVERSE LUNGE WITH ROTATION

Stand with your feet shoulder-width apart and your arms at your sides.

Begin by striding backward with one leg into a lunge position by allowing only the ball of your back foot to come in contact with the floor. As you do so, bend your back knee until it almost touches the floor and allow your front knee to bend to a 90-degree angle. Once in this lunge position, rotate your torso and arms toward the same side as your forward leg (if you stepped back with your left, rotate your arms and torso to the right) and lean back slightly at the waist. Slowly reverse the process and repeat to the other side.

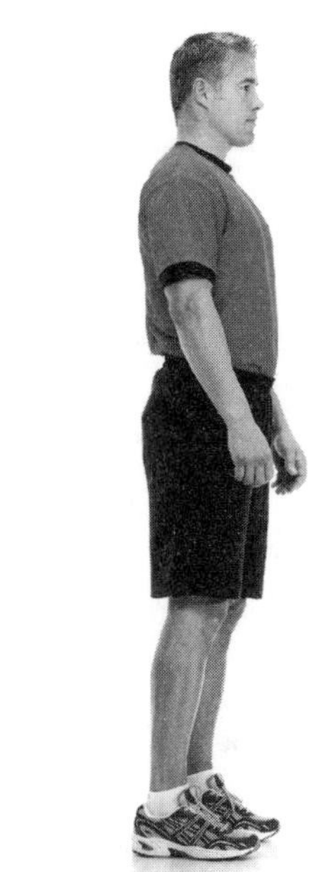

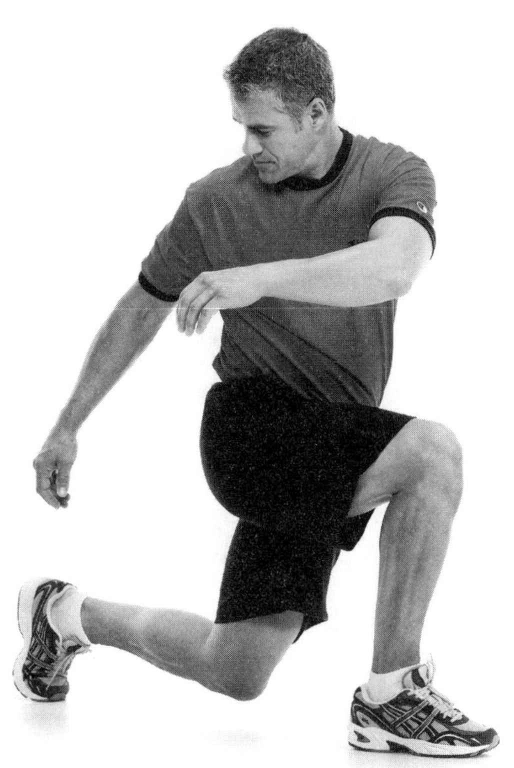

B

SPIDERMAN

Get into a standard pushup position with your hands slightly wider than shoulder-width apart.

Raise one foot and bring it around until it plants softly right next to the corresponding hand. Simultaneously pick up that hand and drop that elbow toward the floor, with your forearm perpendicular to your shin. As you do so, drop your opposite hip and knee toward the floor. Return to a pushup position and repeat on the other side.

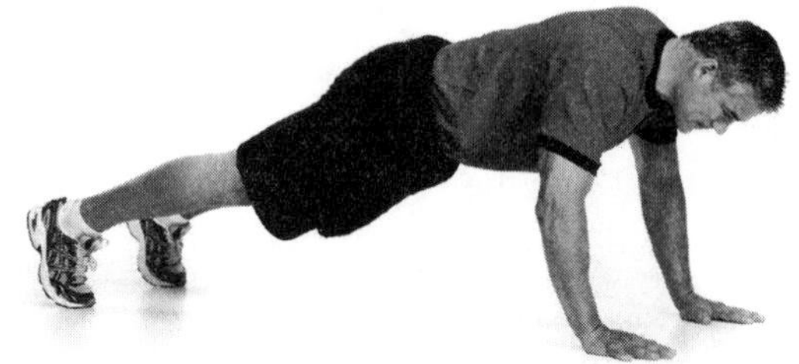

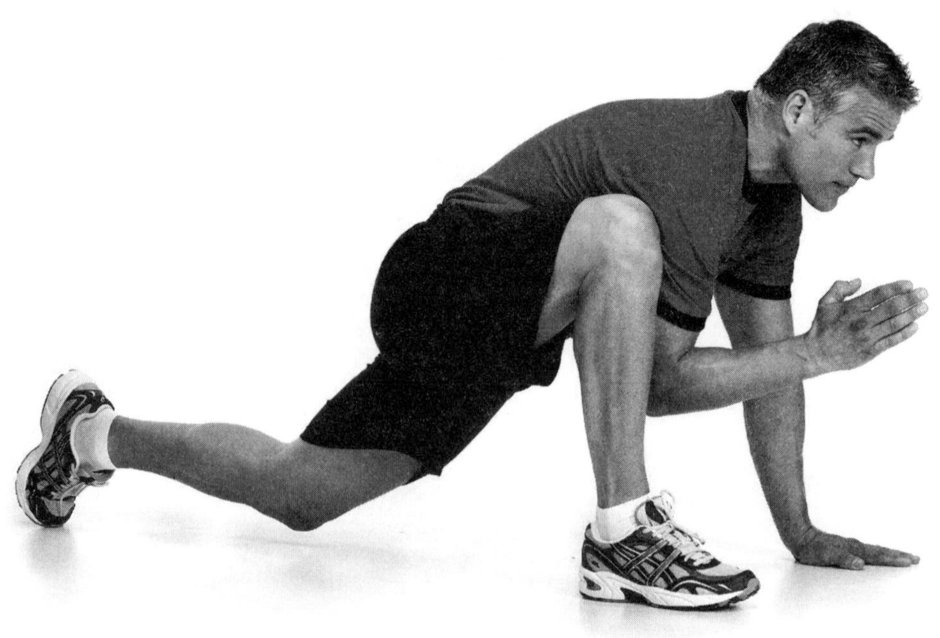

SIDE LUNGE AND TOUCH

Stand with your feet shoulder-width apart and your knees slightly bent. Begin by stepping out to one side, making sure that your foot and knee continue to point straight ahead as you lower yourself into the side lunge position.

Lean forward at the waist slightly to reach your arms toward the floor—just be sure not to round your back excessively. In the bottom position, your working thigh should be parallel to the floor and your other leg should be completely straight. Push back to the starting position and repeat on the other side.

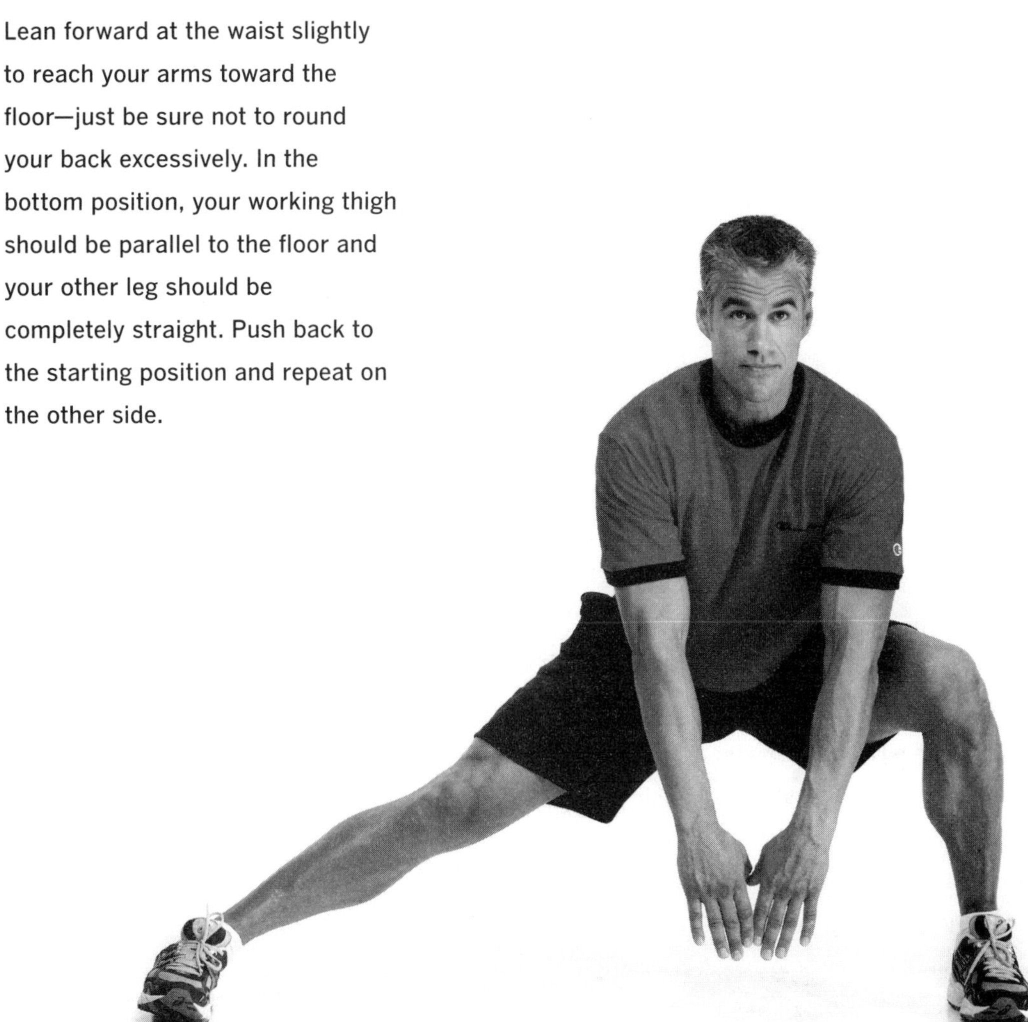

MR. FIX-IT

THE DO-IT-YOURSELF APPROACH YIELDS MORE LASTING RESULTS

All right, let's get to it! Remember a while back when I said your corrective program wasn't just going to be dumped in your lap? Well, I wasn't kidding. Instead of putting together *your* specific program, which would be impossible to do, I'm going to show you how to do it yourself. Putting together your own custom-designed workout is not as tough as you might think. It really just comes down to identifying your biggest areas of concern, picking out the appropriate exercises and stretches, organizing them into workouts, and fitting those workouts into a realistic schedule that you know you can commit to. The following worksheet should help simplify the process for you. Just fill in the blanks and by the end you'll have a complete 4-week corrective phase that will rival anything a high-priced personal trainer could have put together for you.

Areas of Concern

In the numbered spaces that follow, prioritize your specific weaknesses, as identified in your self-assessment, from most important (your greatest weakness) to least (your strongest point). This will be the order in which you address them during your workouts. So if the leg lowering test revealed that you have poor core strength and you also have kyphosis (rounded upper back), but only to a moderate degree, your core would be a higher priority than the kyphosis. If you're equally weak in most areas, prioritize according to which type of training you like the least. If you hate stretching, for instance, doing it first virtually guarantees it will always get done, and you won't blow it off at the end of your workout. By that same logic, placing your favorite activity at or near the bottom of the list ensures that you'll include every aspect of fitness in your workout.

1. ____________________

2. ____________________

3. ____________________

4. ____________________

5. ____________________

When choosing specific exercises, be sure to select more stretches and exercises for the more severe conditions and fewer for those that exist to a more moderate degree. Here's a helpful guideline: If a weakness or flexibility imbalance is moderate, select one exercise and one stretch for the affected area. If it's severe, do two exercises and two stretches. The exception is if there are a limited number of corrective drills for your particular problem (as is the case with the forward head posture). In that case, just do more sets of the appropriate exercise(s) and more repetitions of the available stretch(es). Keep in mind that certain drills can help address more than one problem. For instance, if you have moderate kyphosis and can perform zero chinups, the pec wall stretch (or the lat stretch) could help correct both, allowing you to correct two problems with one stretch and thereby streamlining your workout. List the exercises and static stretches to correct your weaknesses and imbalances here.

Exercises

1. ____________________

2. ____________________

3. ___________________________________

4. ___________________________________

5. ___________________________________

6. ___________________________________

7. ___________________________________

8. ___________________________________

9. ___________________________________

10. ___________________________________

Static Stretches

1. ___________________________________

2. ___________________________________

3. ___________________________________

4. ___________________________________

5. ___________________________________

6. ___________________________________

7. ___________________________________

8. ___________________________________

9. ___________________________________

10. ___________________________________

Training Frequency per Week

Strength training (also addresses posture and muscular endurance concerns): 2 or 3 days per week, with at least 1 day off between workouts

Core training: 2 or 3 days per week, along with strength training

Cardio training: 3 to 5 days per week

Flexibility training (also addresses posture and muscular endurance concerns): Daily

Organizing Your Workout

Start off by allotting a specific amount for each training variable according to your individual needs. If you have the scheduling flexibility to break up your training into different segments so you don't have to include all training variables in every workout, you can assign even more time to those areas that might require additional time. So it's possible that adding up the minutes for all areas could give you a total higher than your available training time for a single day. Also keep in mind that the order presented here may not be consistent with your priorities, so feel free to alter it.

Say you allot 15 minutes for strength training, as in the example below. Let's also say that you'll be doing six strength-training exercises. At an average length of 30 to 45 seconds per set and with a rest interval of 30 to 60 seconds between sets, you can basically do 1 or 2 sets of each exercise. So staying within your available training time is a matter of carefully timing your rest intervals. It's just strength and core work where you have to plan things out a bit in advance. I've found that doing so really prevents overtraining. It's a little easier with flexibility and cardio work: Just stretch for 5 to 7 minutes or stay on the aerobic modality of your choice for 12 to 15 minutes.

Here's an example of how your workouts might shake out.

Available training time: 35 to 45 minutes per day

Flexibility training: 5 to 7 minutes per day

Strength training: 12 to 15 minutes per day

Core training: 6 to 8 minutes per day

Cardio training: 12 to 15 minutes per day

Since your cardio work will be somewhat unstructured and won't be taking up too much time, there's no need to establish any specific guidelines at this point. You don't necessarily need to worry about maintaining a particular heart rate as a means of gauging your intensity. During this early stage, the "talk test" should suffice: As you're doing the cardiovascular segment of your workout, you should be slightly winded but able to carry on a conversation with someone standing next to you. Converse too easily and you're probably not working hard enough; on

A SORE SUBJECT

What causes muscle soreness?

A word of warning before you get started with your workouts: You're going to get sore. Not because they're especially tough, although you certainly will know you're working. The reason you're going to be sore is because your body simply isn't used to what you're doing, and soreness is the result of unfamiliar, somewhat intensive activity.

A little soreness is okay and can often be an indication of a good workout. Too much, however, is a sign that you overdid things a tad and exceeded your body's ability to recover from the exercise stimulus. In fact, push yourself hard enough and you might find that achiness lingering on for several days after the workout. Contrary to popular belief, this is not necessarily a good thing, since your level of soreness isn't an indication of how effective your workout was.

Realizing that most people aren't thrilled by the prospect of wincing every time they attempt to sit or dress themselves, I thought it might be helpful to identify some of the potential causes of muscle soreness, along with some strategies for minimizing it.

Delayed-onset muscle soreness (DOMS). This dull, aching pain, usually accompanied by stiffness or tenderness, develops during the first 24 to 48 hours after exercise. Although it can last as long as a week, it usually peaks within 24 to 72 hours. The severity and duration of the pain depend on a variety of factors, including how hard you trained, your level of training experience, your training volume (number of sets, reps, and exercises), and most important, your familiarity with the exercise stimulus. The more foreign an exercise is to you, the greater your chances of being sore a day or so after you do it. Obviously this means a newbie can expect to be quite sore early on, but even the fittest individuals experience some soreness when engaging in new exercises or activities.

Microtrauma (small tears) to individual muscle fibers. Intense training actually causes structural damage to your muscle fibers at the cellular level. It is your body's ability to recover from and repair this damage (through increased protein synthesis) that ultimately determines how much muscle you can build. It's kind of like having to tear yourself down before you can build back up. However, if the damage to your muscle fibers is too severe, your recovery capacity will be diminished and your gains virtually nonexistent. This is why it's so important to start out slowly and avoid doing too much in the beginning. This can mean using lighter weights or doing fewer sets and exercises or perhaps doing cardio activities for a shorter time frame than you originally wanted to. Such strategies give your body a chance to ease into the exercise stimulus. As long as the training stimulus is manageable,

the other hand, if you're gasping for air between words, you might want to take things down a bit.

As far as flexibility goes, make sure you save enough time to perform the dynamic drills in the beginning of your workout, as part of the warmup, and the particular static stretches you need (as determined by your assessment) at the end of your workout. As a general rule, static stretches should be held for anywhere between 15 and 30 seconds and should be performed two or three times (with each limb, where applicable).

your body will be able to adapt and adequately recover. Don't worry; there'll be plenty of chances to up the intensity down the road.

Connective tissue damage. Besides your muscle fibers, connective tissue (tendons and ligaments) is also placed under tremendous stress during intensive activities like strength training and running. In fact, because it lacks the elasticity of skeletal muscle, connective tissue may be even more susceptible to injury. This is especially true when you perform exercises that allow you to work your muscles through, and sometimes beyond, their full range of motion. A common chest exercise called a dumbbell fly is a perfect example of this. In an attempt to get "as big a stretch as possible," many lifters allow the dumbbells to drift out too far and exceed the optimal range of motion for keeping tension on the chest. Once this happens, the tendons and ligaments that help support the shoulder are placed under more strain than they're able to quickly recover from, and the resulting soreness lingers for several days. As long as you stick to the exercise instructions provided in this book, you should be fine in this regard.

Muscle spasms. Sometimes muscles can actually go into spasm following intense exercise. One of the best ways to combat this is to try to return the muscles to their resting length through static stretching at the end of your workout. This not only helps increase the availability of blood and oxygen to the muscles but also sends them a signal to relax and stop firing.

Accumulation of metabolic waste. Another proposed reason for post-workout soreness is that intense exercise brings an accumulation of metabolic waste products that causes swelling in and around the muscles. This swelling, in turn, stimulates sensory nerve endings, causing pain. Sounds good in theory, but most experts give it little credence. Still, in my own experience, I've found that the following remedy may help: At the end of your workout, try doing some light cardio work such as 5 to 10 easy minutes on an exercise bike or rower. Besides flushing away any metabolic waste that may have accumulated, the increased bloodflow can help augment the recovery process by transporting oxygen and nutrients to those tired muscles.

So how do you avoid soreness? The truth is, you can't. The discomfort may get more tolerable, but when you change your training on a regular basis, as is proposed in this book, you're going to experience some soreness from time to time. That's okay; a little soreness lets you know you've challenged your body enough to induce change. The trick is keeping that soreness to manageable levels so you can continue to make gains.

The strength-training portion of your workout, on the other hand, will be a little bit tougher to put together. During this corrective phase you need to be sure that you're doing the specific exercises that will help address your particular areas of weakness. The following guidelines should provide you with all of the assistance you need.

Exercise order: Begin by listing all of the exercises you've selected. Then, giving priority to those areas that need it the most, arrange the exercises accordingly. It's not as simple as always starting with large muscle groups first, or doing your cardio work immediately following your workout to maximize fat loss, as is often recommended. This workout is specifically designed for your body and, as such, needs to deviate from the norm if need be. So don't be afraid to do core work first, devote a large chunk of your workout time to flexibility training, or do what seems like an inordinate number of certain types of exercises at the expense of others. The whole idea here is to fix what's wrong.

Here are a few tips that may help in putting your strength workouts together.

- When severe imbalances are present, perform stretching drills before, during, and after your workout—not to mention on off days as well. This would entail doing dynamic flexibility drills both as part of your warmup and even between sets of strength work, during your rest intervals. You would also do static stretches immediately following your workout.

- Always give priority to those exercises that are specifically aimed at correcting a strength imbalance; for instance, perform upper-back exercises like cable rows and reverse flies if you suffer from a round-shouldered (kyphotic) posture.

- Normally, do core work toward the end of a workout, since fatiguing the core musculature can lead to subpar performance on other lifts. The exception is if you have severe weakness of your core muscles, as evidenced by a poor result on the leg lowering test and on the slow situp test. In that case, make core strength a priority instead. Besides, none of the other lifts will be heavy enough anyway to worry that core fatigue will in some way compromise performance.

- Stick to total-body workouts with no more than 8 to 10 exercises. Avoid the kind of volume-laden "split" routines you see in the muscle magazines.

- Repetition is key during the corrective phase, so doing two to three total-body workouts composed essentially of the same exercises doesn't present a problem.

As far as how the individual workouts themselves should be constructed, here's a template you can follow. Keep in mind that there are no hard and fast rules. I'm merely establishing what I feel are appropriate ranges for you to fall into. If, for instance, you select eight exercises for your first workout and afterward feel that they weren't enough, go back to the list and add another one or two that are pertinent to your situation. This works both ways: If you select the higher number for a given training variable and then feel it was too much, simply back off and do less next time. After all, this is your body: Only you know how much it can tolerate. You're going to have to take an active role in this process in order for the program to be successful.

Here are a few more helpful hints on designing your workout.

Number of exercises per workout: 8 to 10

Number of sets per exercise: 1 or 2

Number of reps per exercise: If you're a newbie or weak in almost all areas of your self-assessment, do 6 to 10 straight sets (do all the sets of a given exercise before moving on to the next). If you're an ex-jock or seasonal and performed better in the self-assessment, do 8 to 12 for circuits (do one set of all of the 8 to 10 exercises in succession with minimal rest in between before resting 90 to 120 seconds and, if doing a second set, repeating the same order of exercises).

Rest intervals: 60 seconds between straight sets or 30 seconds between circuits

Estimated workout time: Assuming an average set length of 30 to 40 seconds and a 60-second rest interval between sets:

If you're doing 1 set per exercise: 13½ minutes

If you're doing 2 sets per exercise: 26½ minutes

Right about now you're probably wondering how much weight you should use. Once again, there are no inviolable rules, as everyone is different. Suffice it to say that it will take a little bit of trial and error on your part before you get the weight down just right. At most, it shouldn't take you more than one or two workouts to get your initial poundages right. The first thing you want to do is ensure that the weight you select allows you to maintain proper form. There's no sense in risking injury by performing the exercises the wrong way. Secondly, make sure that the weight challenges you to meet the repetition goal of the set. If the recommended rep range is 10 to 12 and you can do 12 reps with ease, choose something a little heavier; if you start fatiguing around rep 5 or 6, back off on the weight a little.

Now that I've provided you with general guidelines, let me give you two specific examples based on different scenarios. Assuming certain results from the self-assessment, I will custom-design a program to meet two hypothetical guys' specific needs.

Scenario #1

Status: Newbie, under age 35

Workout frequency: 2 days per week/45 to 50 minutes total per session

Areas of concern:

- Severe forward head posture
- Severe kyphosis
- Moderate lower-back rounding and arms drifting forward during overhead squats
- Zero chinups
- Zero one-leg squats
- 2 neutral-spine pushups
- Leg lowering to only 45 degrees (poor)
- Failed slow situp test
- Cardiovascular capacity measured as poor by Queens College step test
- Mild knee pinch
- Mild shoulder blade winging

With this many weaknesses and only 2 days to work out, this guy is obviously going to have his work cut out for him. The first thing I would do is address the biggest areas of concern: his obvious flexibility issues and glaring lack of body strength. Forget the fact that this guy's main goals are to gain some muscle mass and trim down his waistline a bit. There are much bigger fish to fry here! Yet despite the fact that his goals won't be the primary focus, he may in fact notice some progress toward them due to the comprehensive nature of the program.

Basing my approach on his needs rather than his wants, the first area I'd concentrate on is flexibility, because doing so will help improve his severe posture issues and free up range of motion that will get his muscles firing better, thus increasing his strength potential. Even before that, however, I'd have to warm him up. So I'd start him off with some nice, easy, continuous forms of cardiovascular exercise like cycling, jogging, or some light calisthenics. Nothing too structured, mind you. I wouldn't have him shoot for a particular heart rate or anything like that, just a little something he could easily manage for 10 to 12 minutes. This would in essence allow me to kill two birds with one stone, as it would also take care of his cardio work for the time being.

Why the seemingly easy pass considering that his cardiovascular capacity tested so poorly? I've always been of the mind-set that in order to get an accurate assessment of someone's cardio capabilities, their body has to be in good working order. Seeing as how this guy is so weak and the Queens College step test is pretty tough, it's possible that muscular fatigue got to him before his lack of cardiovascular stamina did. Throw in his poor flexibility, which likely restricted his ability to move efficiently, and cardio isn't his biggest concern right now. I'd much rather get him to correct all of his little imbalances and increase his strength a bit before going after his cardiovascular system in the subsequent phases.

Once he was properly warmed up, I could really concentrate on improving his flexibility. This would include a heavy dose of dynamic flexibility drills prior to lifting, followed by some static stretching at the end of the workout. I prefer this approach because the dynamic flexibility exercises help him limber up for the weight training, while saving the static stretches for the end relaxes and elongates the muscles he's just pounded during his workout. This might mean devoting as much as 15 minutes to flexibility work, which is a far cry from the amount of time most beginners usually set aside for stretching. I'd also highly recommend that he do some static stretching for at least 10 minutes on the days he doesn't exercise.

Based on the results of his assessment, here is the sequence of dynamic flexibility drills I would choose.

Quad stretch walk (10 to 12 paces)
Gate swing (10 to 12 paces)
Spiderman (5 to 6 each leg)
Medicine ball wraparound (10 to 12 each arm)
Medicine ball woodchopper (6 to 8 each side)
Do all exercises in succession and repeat one to two more times.

Once he was good and limber, I'd hit him with the strength work. Given the severe postural issues, in addition to some more specific stretching he could do during his recovery intervals between sets (pec wall stretch and internal rotator broomstick stretch), he also needs to choose two exercises from among those that will help strengthen that upper back. There'll also be plenty of core work and some unilateral lower-body strengthening exercises. His lower-back rounding also indicates weak, tight hamstrings. That being the case, here's what I'd prescribe.

Exercise(s)	Condition(s)
Unilateral Romanian deadlift	Lower-body strength
Unilateral dumbbell touch	One-leg squat failure
Prone dumbbell row with elbow out and reverse fly	Kyphosis, shoulder blade winging, and overhead squat arms drifting forward
Negative situp	Slow-situp failure
Plank	Lordosis
Bird dog	Slow-situp failure
Negative chinup	Zero chinups
Standing cable abduction	Knee pinching

Note that this chart does not include exercises applicable to this newbie's forward head and poor leg-lowering test, therefore he should do additional stretches for these conditions (see pages 63 and 66).

These exercises would be performed in the same order they're listed, two times per week. Given his novice status and the fact that these exercises are pretty tough, I'd also recommend separating the workouts, with at least 2 days' rest between them. So, he could work out on, say, Mondays and Thursdays, or Tuesdays and Saturdays. As per the general guidelines, he should keep his sets to no more than two per exercise and his repetitions in the 6 to 10 range, with 60 seconds of rest between sets.

Following the workout and on off days, he would perform the following battery of static stretches. Each stretch should be held for 20 to 30 seconds and done two to three times (per side, if applicable).

Stretch(es)	Condition(s)
Wall chin tuck and corner stretch (3 sets of each; 8 to 10 reps of the tucks and two 20-to-30-second holds on each leg for the stretch)	Forward head
Lat stretch (3 x 20–30 seconds) and internal rotator broomstick stretch (3 x 20–30 seconds)	Kyphosis, overhead squat arms drifting forward, shoulder blade winging, and zero chinups
Hip flexor stretch (3 x 20–30 seconds)	Lordosis and poor leg lowering
Butterfly adductor stretch (2 x 20–30 seconds)	Knee pinch
Pike calf stretch (2 x 20–30 seconds)	One-leg squat failure

Under these guidelines, a complete total-body strength workout should take no more than 25 minutes. When added to the warmup/flexibility and cardio exercise, this should bring this person right around the allotted 45- to 50-minute time frame.

Scenario #2

Status: Seasonal exerciser, under age 35

Workout frequency: 5 days (3 strength and 2 cardio workouts) per week (45 and 20 minutes per workout, respectively)

Areas of concern:

- Severe lordosis when standing, as well as during overhead squat and both core tests, most likely due to tight, overactive hip flexors. (This is evidenced by back arching when attempting to perform these tests.)
- Knee pinching on one-leg and overhead squats, and arms drifting forward on the latter.
- Poor strength levels across the board
- Good cardiovascular capacity as measured by 1.5-mile run

Without question, the first thing I'd target here is the severe lordosis, to help reduce strain on the lower-back region. I'd also combine this with an aggressive core-strengthening program. Aside from that, some glute strengthening and adductor stretching is definitely in order to help correct the knee pinch, and there's obviously a need for improving total-body strength as well. Here's how I envision the program laying out.

This guy should do three total-body strength workouts per week with two cardio workouts on off days, as well as daily flexibility drills. To kick things off, after a good general warmup (5 minutes of light cardio exercise followed by two to three rounds of dynamic flexibility drills), I'd go with the core-strengthening drills. As previously mentioned, I generally advise that core work be done toward the end of a workout, since fatiguing the core musculature can detract from your performance on other lifts. However, given that a stronger core is a real need for this guy, I've opted to make it a priority instead. Besides, none of the other lifts will be heavy enough anyway to worry that core fatigue will in some way compromise performance.

After the stretching and core work, I'd go with unilateral lower-body strength work to help correct the knee pinch, as well as upper-body exercises that promote balanced development, particularly of the muscles that act on the front and rear shoulders.

As far as how the 3-day training week would break down, since there wouldn't be a large number of exercises and because repetition is key to bringing about improvements in the corrective phase, I would go with the same total-body workout performed three times per week. To keep things interesting, I would prescribe two of the days to be performed as straight sets in the 6- to 10-rep range, resting 60 to 90 seconds between sets, with the other day performed circuit style, increasing the reps to 8 to 12 per set. For all workouts, I'd limit the strength work to two sets per exercise, or two complete circuits. Starting with dynamic flexibility, here's how I'd arrange the exercise order for each workout.

Reverse lunge with rotation (10 to 12 reps)
Reverse gate swing (10 to 12 paces)
Side lunge and touch (10 to 12 reps)
Medicine ball wraparound (10 to 12)
Medicine ball woodchopper (10 to 12)
Do two to three rounds total. He should do all exercises in succession and repeat one to two more times for both dynamic stretches and strength workouts.

Here's what I prescribe for workouts 1 and 3: straight sets.

Exercise(s)	**Condition(s)**
Crunch with a pelvic tilt	Slow-situp failure
Plank*	Lordosis
Pelvic tilt	Lordosis
Unilateral dumbbell touch	One-leg squat failure
Standing cable hip abduction	Standing facing forward and overhead squat external rotation and knee pinching
Supine bridge hip extension	Knee pinching
Prone dumbbell row with elbow out	Overall structural balance
Negative neutral-spine pushup	Fewer than 10 neutral-spine pushups
Side-lying external rotation	Overhead squat arms drifting forward

*Planks are to be held for 20 to 30 seconds at a time and not done for reps.

Here's what I prescribe for workouts 2 and 4: circuit style.

Exercise(s)	**Condition(s)**
Plank*	Lordosis
Unilateral dumbbell touch	One-leg squat failure
Negative situp**	Slow-situp failure
Prone dumbbell row with elbows out	Overall structural balance
Crunch with pelvic tilt	Slow-situp failure
Machine hip abduction	Standing facing forward and overhead squat external rotation and knee pinching
Supine bridge hip extension	Knee pinching
Negative neutral-spine pushup	Fewer than 10 neutral-spine pushups
Side-lying external rotation	Overhead squat arms drifting forward

*Planks are to be held for 20 to 30 seconds at a time and not done for reps.
**Remember that negative situps are performed with a 5-second lowering phase.

The following static stretches should also be done both after workouts and on nonworkout days.

Stretch	**Condition(s)**
Hip flexor stretch (3 x 20–30 seconds)	Lordosis and poor leg lowering
Erector stretch (3 x 20–30 seconds)	Lordosis and poor leg lowering
Butterfly adductor stretch (3 x 20–30 seconds)	Knee pinch
Pike calf stretch (3 x 20–30 seconds)	One-leg squat failure

Seeing as how this person has the ability to break up cardio and strength workouts, he can afford to work a little harder than the first guy. I still don't want to get too finite with the guidelines here, though. Remember, the objective during this phase of the program is to fix all of things that are hampering your ability to perform. Believe me, in the subsequent phases plenty of attention will be paid to improving cardiovascular function and burning fat. So I wouldn't look to overload anyone with too much right off the bat. The strength and flexibility work is going to pose enough of a challenge for now. That means, just like in our first example, all I'd have him do is low-intensity cardio, albeit for a slightly longer duration (15 to 20 minutes). This might include running (on either the road or a treadmill), bike riding, swimming, or hiking. I'd also strongly recommend he throw in some additional static flexibility work on off days and then look to build strength through that improved range of motion when he lifts.

JUST EAT IT

NUTRITIONAL BASICS TO GET YOU STARTED

From a nutritional standpoint, your best bet is to keep things as simple as possible. I've just hit you with a tremendous amount of information—far more than beginners are usually subjected to. To get really intricate with nutritional guidelines at this point would be a mistake. Therefore, all I want you to do is institute the principles of energy balance, hydration, and meal frequency that were established in Chapter 3. Drinking more water and eating smaller meals on a more frequent basis will give you the energy you need to carry out these workouts successfully. So for now, just make sure you're taking in the appropriate number of calories to meet your energy needs and get your digestive system used to processing nutrients more efficiently.

Simple changes like these, when combined with all the extra physical activity, will probably result in a weight loss of several pounds just by the nature of your body trying to adapt to all of the changes you're putting it through. In the event that you're one of the rare few for whom a weight loss of any type would be completely undesirable, you can offset it by adding a few more calories, specifically from the types of foods provided in the food choice list in Chapter 8.

CORRECTED DEVELOPMENT

LAYING THE FOUNDATION FOR YOUR FITNESS FUTURE

I realize that I'm asking an awful lot of you here. Rest assured that this information is the very best available to someone in your shoes. Taking the time to understand and implement it will be invaluable to your ability to progress beyond the beginner stage and finally build the body you've always wanted.

In the phases that follow, I'll provide you with a variety of workout plans to choose from based on what type of beginner you are. This is the only phase of your training where you need to process so much new information to be properly prepared. There's a good reason for that, though: There's simply no way to correct your individual weaknesses and imbalances with a bunch of preplanned workouts, regardless of how well they're designed. Sure, it would be a lot easier to pull a Nike and "just do it." And I'm sure there are plenty of people who would advise you to do exactly that. Unfortunately, catchy ad slogans don't make the best advice when starting an exercise program. Remember, the main reason so many people fail to make exercise a regular commitment is frustration with their lack of results. Well, their inability to achieve results is related to the fact that they're going about things the wrong way.

The bottom line is, working out doesn't have to be rocket science, but it isn't just some mindless activity either. Expending a little mental effort along with your physical effort will produce results you'll be more than happy with over the long haul. So for now, just do what I ask of you. I promise you'll thank me for it later.

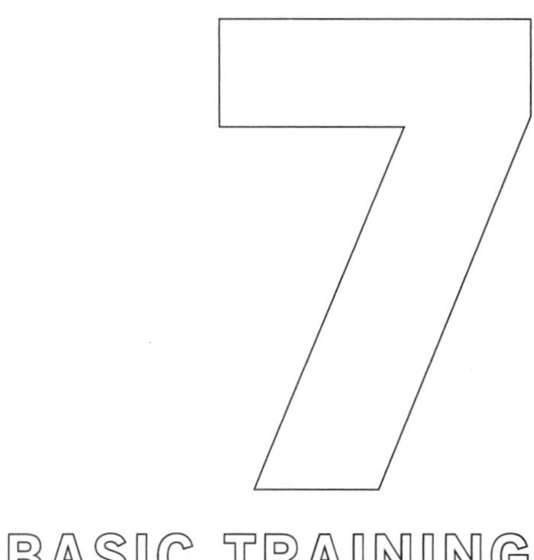

BASIC TRAINING

PHASE 3: YOU'VE GOT TO GET THE FUNDAMENTALS DOWN FIRST

I'm willing to bet that up to this point, this whole process hasn't been anything near what you expected it to be. You probably figured you'd be asked to take a few measurements and maybe weigh yourself before getting right down to the business of burning fat and building muscle. Instead, you were browbeaten into putting yourself through a grueling battery of tests that damaged your self-esteem. You were then asked to train in a manner that seemed completely bizarre, to say the least. Not to mention, pretty darn difficult.

Well, it's time to be rewarded for all of your patience. The workouts contained in this phase are nothing like the ones you experienced for the past few weeks. In fact, they're probably much more along the lines of what you thought you were signing up for in the first place. This will be your first taste of what could be considered a "traditional" training program.

Why the radical shift? Because now that you've fixed all the little things that needed fixing, it's time to get your body conditioned for what it's going to have to endure later on down the road. The workouts you're going to encounter in the latter phases of this program will require you to do some serious work. Nothing beyond your capabilities, mind you, but you'll definitely be challenged. This isn't something you can just rush right into. It's one thing to eliminate weak links in the way your body performs, but that alone isn't enough to ensure your physical readiness once you encounter more difficult forms of training.

Where the corrective phase was all about isolating

your weaknesses with specific exercises designed to eliminate them, this phase is all about integration. Instead of isolation and unilateral exercises (those that work just one joint and just one limb at a time, such as a dumbbell biceps curl), for the next 4 to 6 weeks you'll be doing lots of compound, bilateral movements that require your body to work as a functional unit rather than as a series of unrelated muscle groups. All that means is that you'll be doing exercises that require both limbs working at the same time and that involve more than one joint (squats, bench presses, etc.). Another difference is that the workouts in this chapter will offer more diversity and balance than the targeted stretching and strengthening of the corrective phase.

This phase isn't about increasing size or strength or even cardiovascular function to any significant degree. It's more inclusive of all aspects of fitness than the corrective phase, but it still prioritizes those qualities you need to work on the most. Say you're a 50-year-old ex-jock, for instance. As badly as you may want to just start pumping iron, the workouts in this phase will have you focusing on flexibility and cardiovascular efficiency first and foremost, leaving the weight training until near the end of your workout. On the other hand, if you're a younger, seasonal lifter, you may find that your workouts are comprised of near equal parts flexibility, strength, and cardiovascular training. Whatever the case, this is meant as a prep course for what's coming down the road, not as something you should stick with indefinitely.

I say this primarily because the lighter loads and higher reps you'll be using during this phase are something your body will quickly become accustomed to. They serve a great purpose for now: helping to bolster tendon and ligament strength and allowing you to familiarize yourself with the movement patterns of the exercises so you don't get hurt later on. Stick with them for too long, though, and they'll become staler than day-old bread. Their main purpose is to ease you into a structured training program by exposing you to the type of exercises, stretches, and cardio you'll be performing at a much more intensified pace later on.

UNDER CONSTRUCTION

BUILDING YOUR WORKOUT FROM THE GROUND UP

One of the things I think you'll like best about this phase is the relative simplicity of the workouts. I've divided the training into four major components: cardio, strength, flexibility, and core work. The first thing I'm going to ask you to do is rank these by level of importance, in accordance with the parameters that were set in Chapter 2. Say you're a total newbie under the age of 35. Your ranking system might look something like this:

1. Strength
2. Core
3. Flexibility
4. Cardio

This would differ significantly from an ex-jock over age 35, whose list might look more like this:

1. Flexibility
2. Cardio
3. Core
4. Strength

The next step is to figure out how much of your allotted workout time you plan to devote to each variable. I would suggest earmarking 60 to 70 percent of your time for your top two priorities. This strategy will help keep your workouts as time-efficient and individualized as possible.

As you may have noticed, the above model assumes that you'll be working on all aspects of fitness every time you train. This isn't an accident; it's how I recommend you proceed for the first 4 to 6 weeks. Because this workout is fairly basic, it's something you can and should do two or three times each week. This serves two purposes: (1) It makes exercise a habit, and (2) it allows you to become familiar with the exercises and stretches you'll be doing, in some cases with significantly more load, in the weeks ahead. However, I recommend doing this workout no more than three times per week. If you have the time and inclination to exercise a fourth day, throwing in some additional flexibility work and cardio should suffice. Outside of correcting specific imbalances, strength training four days per week is a bit much for someone who is just starting out, regardless of how simple the workout may be.

Okay, time to construct the actual workouts themselves. I'll provide you with a little synopsis of each training variable, as well as a couple of alternatives for how you can best implement the variables according to your needs. All you need to do is select the ones that work best for you and—with the exception of the warmup, which always goes first—arrange them in the appropriate order. Taking this kind of systematic approach to your workouts will make you feel much more organized and enable you to get more work done in your allotted time. You'll know you're going about things in a way that's appropriate for your current level of conditioning, and as result, you'll be able to progress much more rapidly. Okay, enough lecturing. Let's start putting together that workout.

A WARMING TREND

APPRECIATING THE IMPORTANCE OF A GOOD WARMUP

In order to get the most out of these workouts, you need to have your body properly prepared to train. The types of warmups I prefer to use are dynamic stretching warmups called mobility sequences, and they get your body used to moving lots of muscle mass through increasingly larger ranges of motion. They include lots of twisting and bending and other functional movements that mimic the way you move through the course of daily living.

Like any good warmup, they're designed to get your blood flowing and raise your body temperature. Movements like squatting, lunging, and pressing not only activate lots of muscle mass but also get your nervous system fired up to train. So once it's time to increase the intensity during your workout, you'll be more than ready. This isn't something you can accomplish by warming up for 5 minutes on a piece of cardio equipment. That kind of a "warmup" may increase bloodflow and body temperature, but there'll be little if any transfer to three-dimensional movements. This is why many people experience little aches and pains during the first couple of sets of strength training. They basically haven't given their bodies a chance to become familiar with the movement pattern of the exercise before loading on the weight.

So I've provided two different movement sequences, one for those of you under 35 (workout A) and one for us older guys (workout B). I've done this on the assumption that younger guys usually have slightly better flexibility. If, however, you're a younger guy who's inordinately tight or if you're a member of the over-35 set who's somewhat limber, feel free to mix and match them as you see fit.

These warmups are best done with a pair of light (5- to 10-pound) dumbbells or a medicine ball, but you can do them without weight as well. I count these dynamic warmups as part of your flexibility training due to the large ranges of motion you'll be moving through. You can also elect to include some additional static stretching at the end of your workout if you like.

Workout A

Rotational squat with dumbbells
Reaching lunge
Side lunge and touch
Spiderman
T-pushup

Workout B

Sumo deadlift
Reverse lunge with rotation
Woodchopper
Bootstrapper
Rotational shoulder press

Do 8 to 10 repetitions (4 to 5 per side, where applicable) of each exercise in succession, for two or three circuits. If you have poor flexibility, opt for three circuits. You may also find it helpful to do 3 to 5 minutes of low-intensity cardio exercises prior to beginning the mobility sequence, as a means of increasing bloodflow and lubricating your joints.

ROTATIONAL SQUAT WITH DUMBBELLS

Stand holding a pair of dumbbells at your sides with your feet shoulder-width apart and your knees slightly bent.

Descend into a squat by sitting your hips down and back and simultaneously rotate your torso so one arm ends up between your knees and the other one behind you. Then reverse this sequence and repeat to the other side.

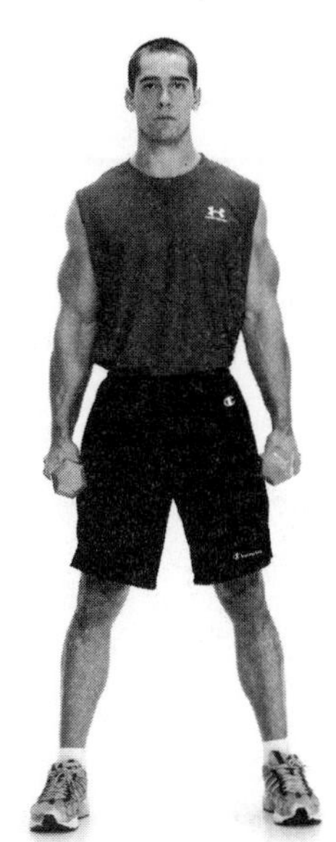

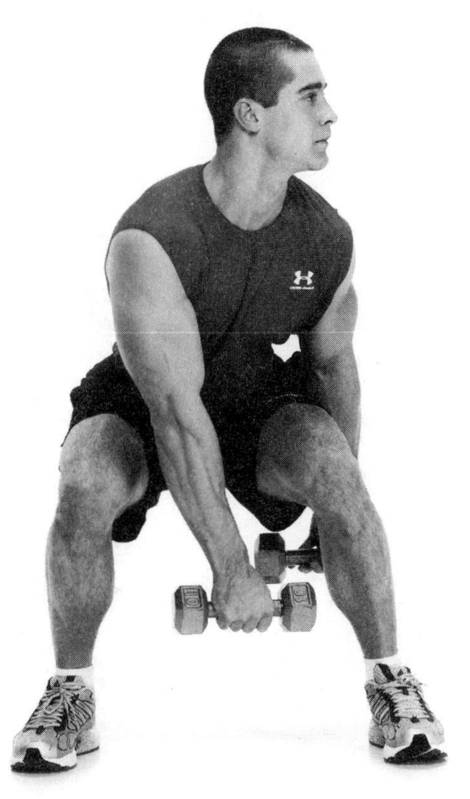

B

REACHING LUNGE

Stand holding a pair of light dumbbells at your sides.

Quickly lunge forward as you extend your arms in front of you and flex your spine while attempting to touch the dumbbells to the floor. Once there, brace your abs and explosively push back up to the starting position. Finish your set and do the same number of reps with your other leg lunging.

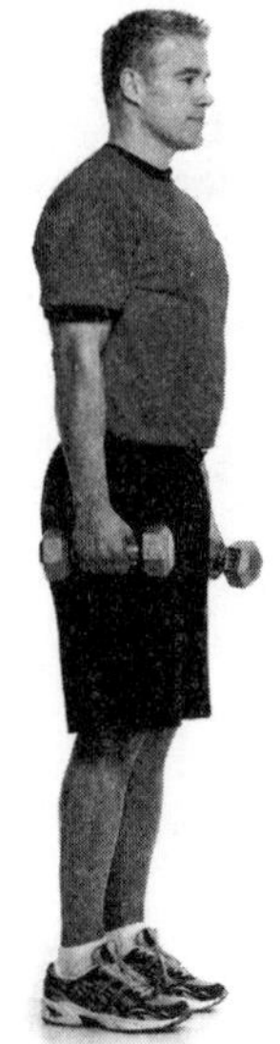

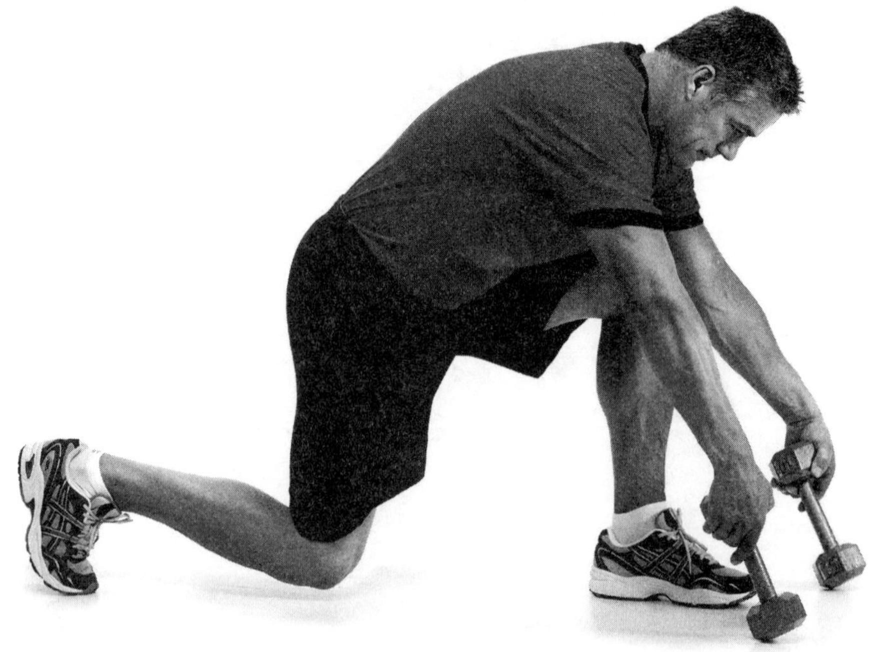

B

SIDE LUNGE AND TOUCH WITH MEDICINE BALL OR DUMBBELLS

Stand holding a medicine ball or dumbbells with your feet shoulder-width apart and your knees slightly bent. Step out to one side, making sure that your foot and knee continue to point straight forward as you lower yourself into the side lunge position. You'll need to lean slightly forward at the waist to reach your arms toward the floor—just be sure not to round your back excessively. In the bottom position, your working thigh should be parallel to the floor and your other leg should be completely straight as you extend the medicine ball or dumbbells toward the floor. Push back to the starting position and repeat to the other side.

SPIDERMAN

Get into a standard pushup position with your hands slightly wider than shoulder-width apart.

Raise one foot and bring it around until it plants softly right next to the corresponding hand. Simultaneously pick up that hand and drop that elbow toward the floor, with your forearm perpendicular to your shin. As you do so, drop your opposite hip and knee toward the floor. Return to a pushup position and repeat to the other side.

A

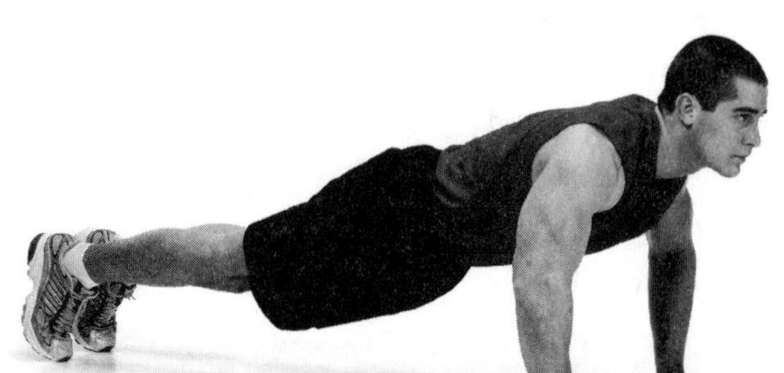

B

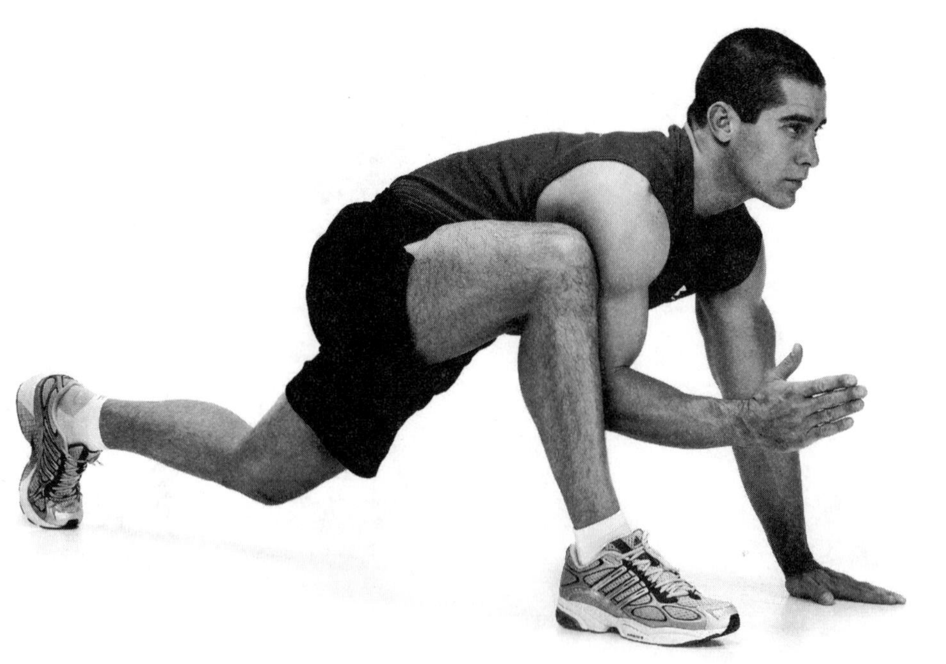

T-PUSHUP

Begin as you would a regular pushup, only with your feet spaced slightly wider apart, say just outside shoulder width.

Push up and, as you near the top of the pushup, immediately rotate one arm toward the ceiling as you simultaneously turn your hips and legs to the same side. At the top you should end up with your arms in a straight line, pointing from ceiling to floor, and your weight resting on the sides of your feet. Return to the starting position and execute another T-pushup before repeating to the other side.

A

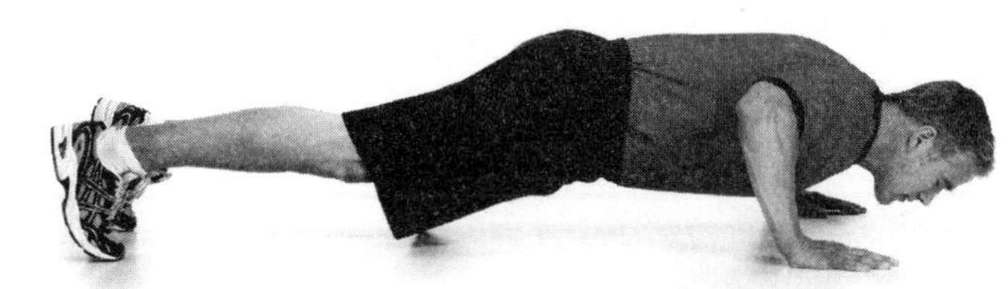

B

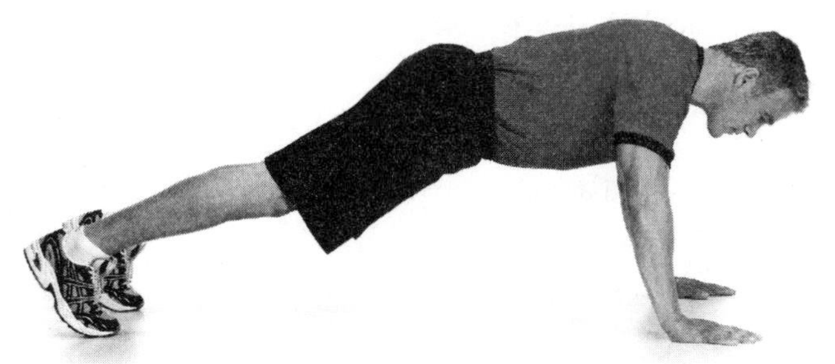

C

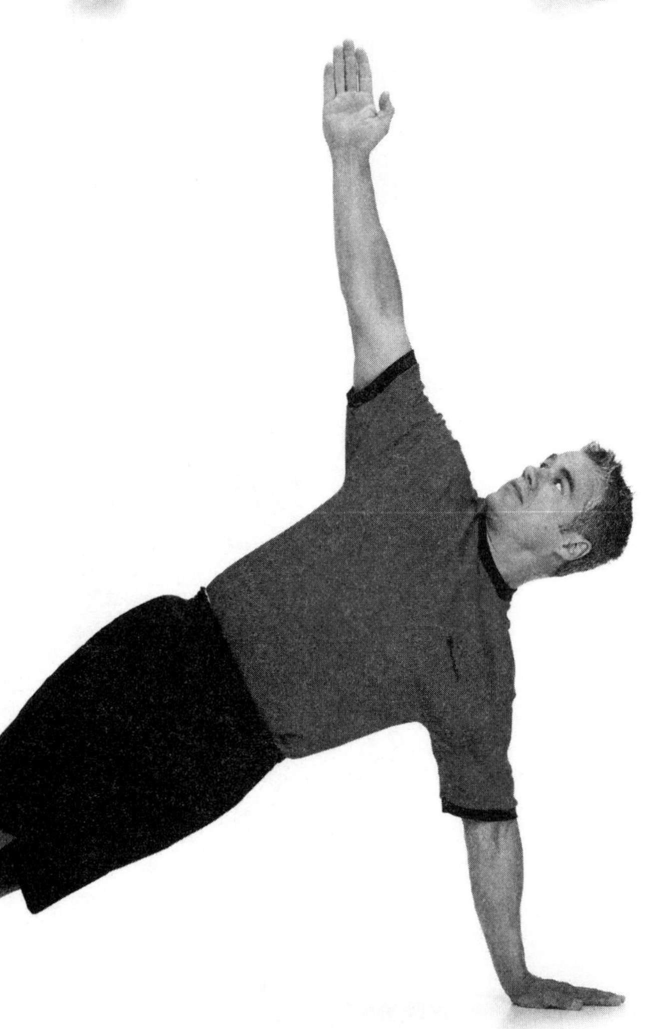

SUMO DEADLIFT WITH MEDICINE BALL OR DUMBBELLS

Standing with your feet spaced twice shoulder width and your toes turned out, hold a medicine ball or a pair of dumbbells at arm's length between your legs.

Keeping your back and arms straight, slowly descend until your thighs are parallel to the floor. Make sure your shoulder blades are still together at the bottom of the movement. Then press back up to the starting position.

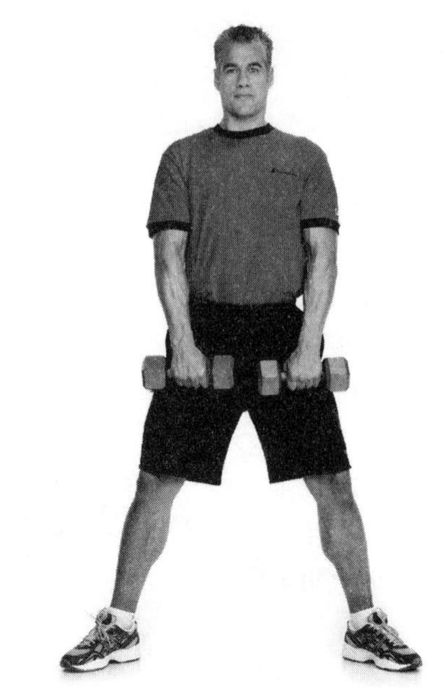

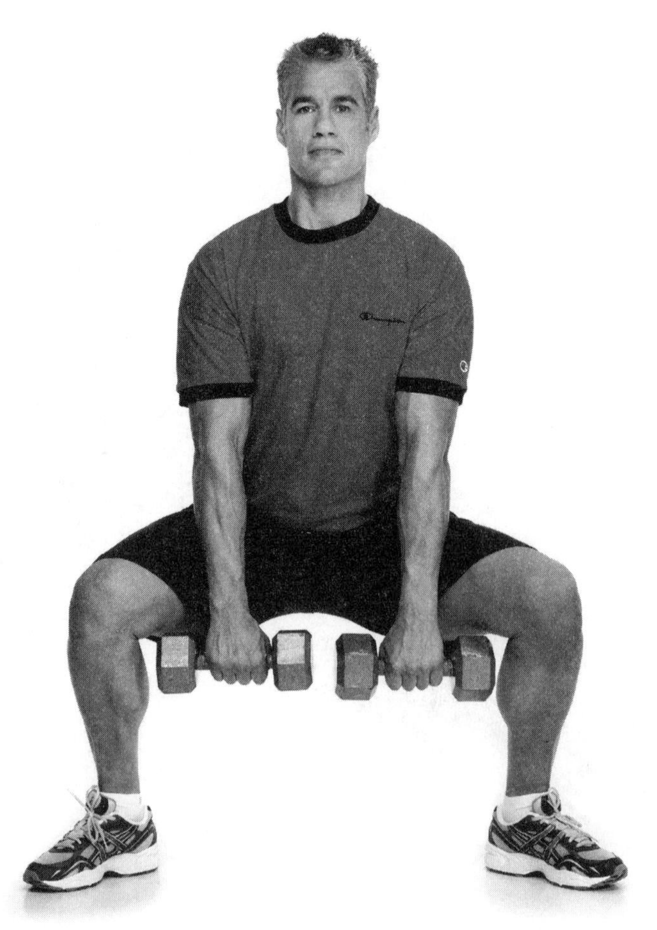

B

REVERSE LUNGE WITH ROTATION

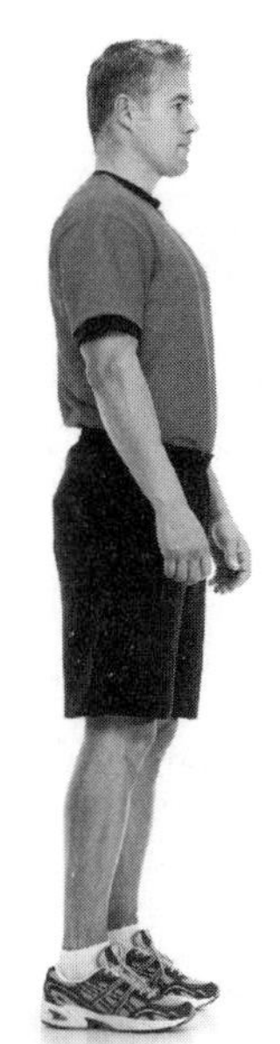

Stand with your feet shoulder-width apart.

With one leg, stride backward into a lunge position, allowing only the ball of that foot to contact the floor. As you do so, bend that knee until it almost touches the floor and allow your front knee to bend to a 90-degree angle. Once in this lunge position, rotate your torso and arms toward the same side as your forward leg (if you stepped back with your left, rotate your arms and torso to the right) and lean back slightly at the waist. Slowly reverse the process and repeat to the other side.

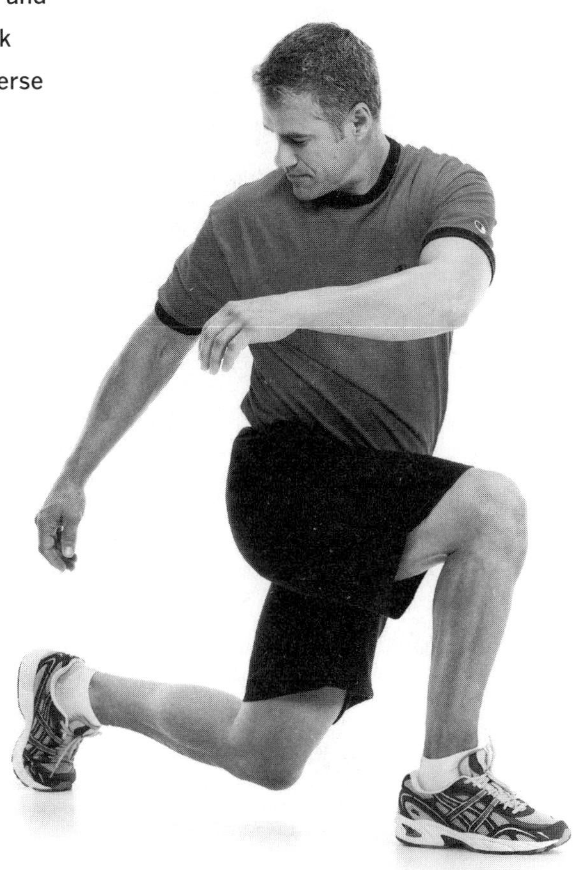

B

WOODCHOPPER WITH MEDICINE BALL OR DUMBBELLS

Standing with your feet shoulder-width apart and your knees slightly bent, hold a medicine ball or dumbbell with your arms outstretched over your left shoulder.

Using your core to initiate the movement, "chop" the weight down using a long, sweeping stroke so that you finish with the weight outside your right calf. Be sure to bend your knees and keep your back flat as you chop downward. Bring the ball back to the starting position and repeat. Finish your set and do the same number of reps with the weight starting above your right shoulder.

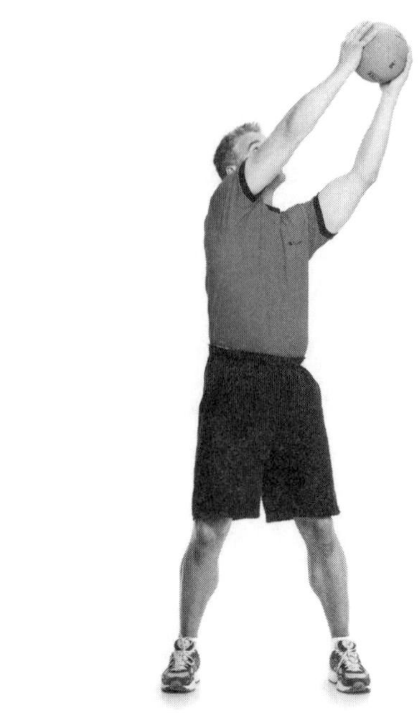

A

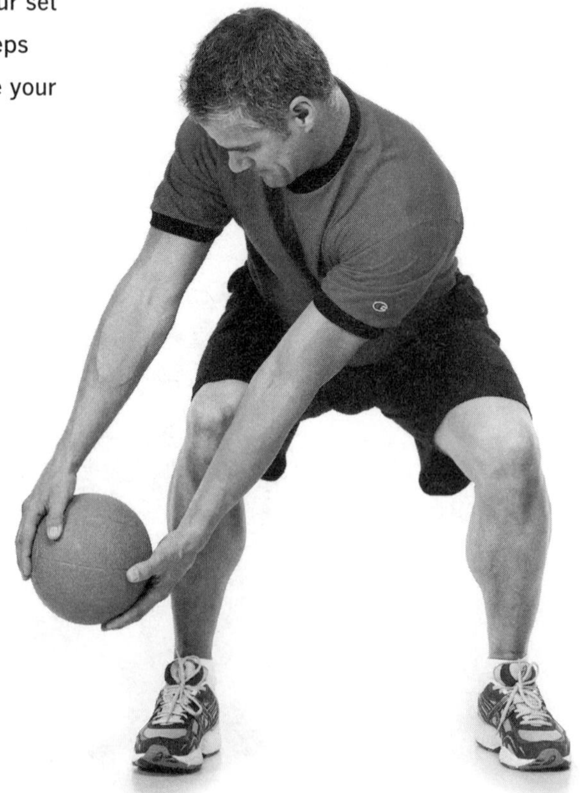

BOOTSTRAPPER

Standing with your feet spaced slightly wider than shoulder width, squat down so you can reach between your legs and grab the backs of your heels.

Holding your heels, straighten your legs as you slide your hands up your calves to just below your knees. Lower and repeat.

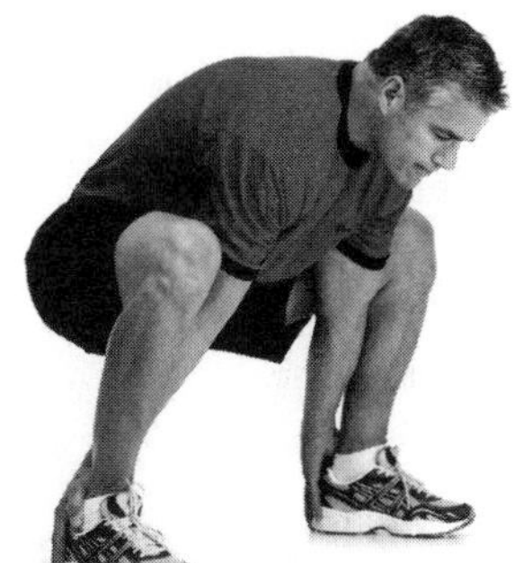

B

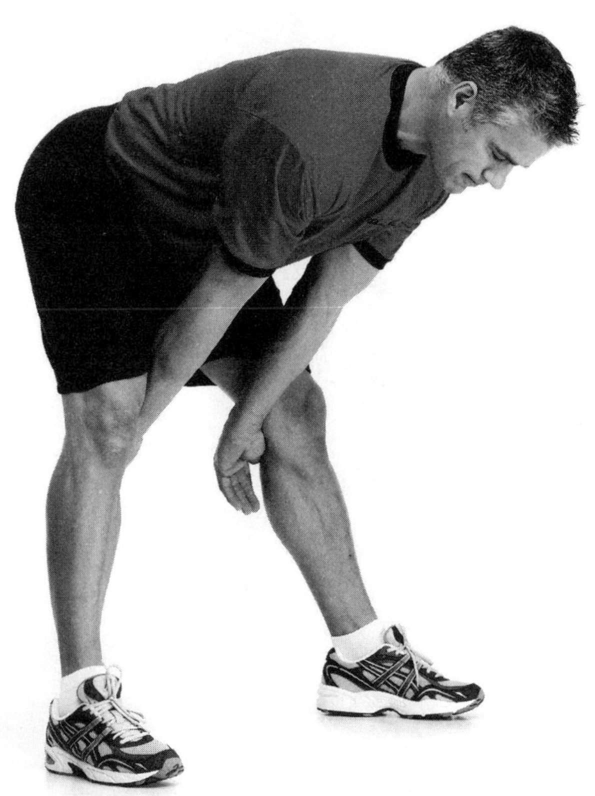

ROTATIONAL SHOULDER PRESS WITH DUMBBELLS

Stand holding a pair of dumbbells just outside your shoulders at jaw level, palms facing in.

Press the dumbbells overhead as you twist to your right. Lower the dumbbells as you twist back to the center, then twist to the left as you press the weights upward again.

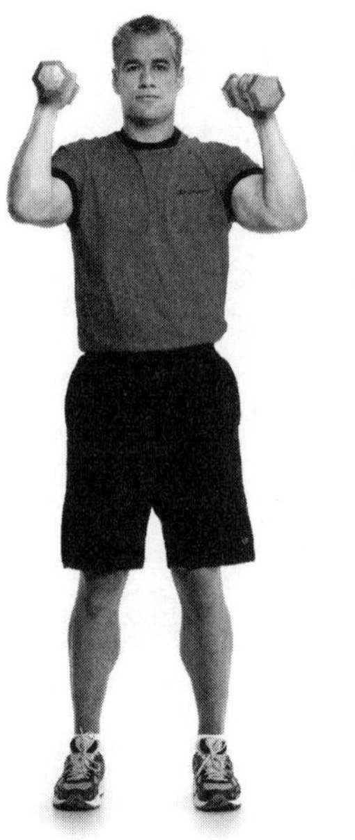

A

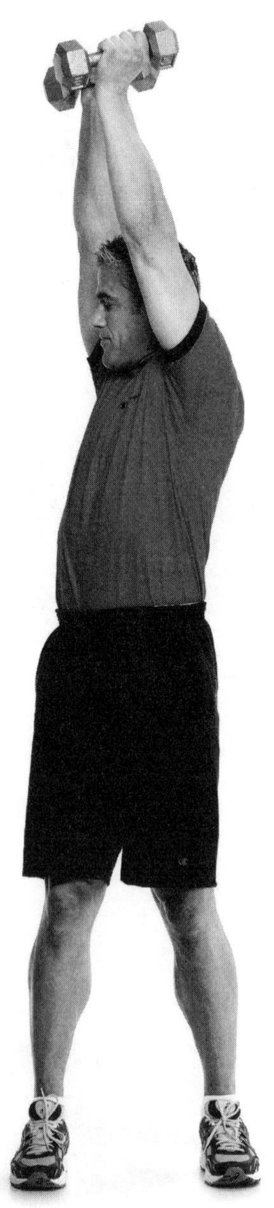

B

SPONTANEOUS COMBUSTION

REPLACING TRADITIONAL CARDIO WITH INTERVAL TRAINING

In the corrective phase, you just did light, unstructured cardio as a way to get into the flow of things. Now, it's time to up the ante a bit. You're about to enter the wonderful world of interval training. Get ready to forever change the way you think about cardio work.

With intervals, you work harder than you normally would for a brief time frame and then have an active recovery period. You then repeat this process for the desired number of intervals, allowing you to do more work at the higher-intensity level than you otherwise could. Training this way allows you to burn more calories in less time and offers a more potent stimulus than does traditional aerobic exercise, where you typically work at one set level of intensity.

Any mode of cardio training is fine. You can do intervals while running, riding a bike (road or stationary), jumping rope, or even swimming. They are a little tough to do on a treadmill, though, because changing the speed and grade makes it difficult to stick to the prescribed time intervals. I'll leave the mode of exercise up to you and concentrate on the workout format.

Workout option A is slightly more aggressive, so I recommend it mostly for ex-jocks and seasonal lifters under the age of 35. Its overall time frame is somewhat shorter since these guys don't need to focus as much on cardio work as some of us older guys do. Option B is a little kinder and gentler but still packs a decent punch in its own right. It's better suited to total newbies of any age and guys over the age of 35. As with the stretching programs, though, feel free to mix and match according to your current level of fitness.

	Workout A	**Workout B**
Work interval	15 seconds	30 seconds
Recovery interval	45 seconds	60 seconds
Number of intervals	12 to 15	14 to 16

In case you're unsure of what exactly this all means, relax—it's pretty simple. After a brief 3- to 5-minute lightly paced warmup, simply increase your intensity for the time frame listed as "work interval." Once you've completed that, decrease either your speed or the amount of resistance you're working against for the period of time listed as "recovery interval." Then repeat, alternating between these two different levels for the number of times listed as "number of intervals."

As for how hard you should be working during the work and recovery intervals, I want you to use a simple 1 to 10 scale where 1 would be taking a walk in the park and 10 would be sprinting to save your life. For workout A, since the intervals are shorter, you should work at a higher intensity—say, 8.5 to 9.5. You'll then want to be sure you're adequately recovered to repeat that kind of effort again, so lower your intensity to around 5 to 6.5 (for instance, go from a sprint to a light jog). For workout B, the longer intervals mean you won't be able to work quite as intensely, so shoot for 7.5 to 8. Since you won't be working as hard, you also won't need such a dramatic reduction in intensity during the recovery interval: 6 to 7 should work just fine.

GIVE YOURSELF A LIFT

FINDING A PLACE FOR STRENGTH TRAINING IN YOUR ROUTINE

The key to understanding the strength-training portion of this phase is to think movement, not muscles. During

(continued on page 146)

ADDED FLEXIBILITY

The following dynamic flexibility exercises can be done as either another warmup option prior to training or as a workout unto themselves. Be sure to use light weights and as full a range of motion as possible. Try 5 to 6 reps (per side, if applicable) of each for 1 or 2 sets as a warmup, or 2 or 3 sets as a workout.

OVERHEAD SPLIT SQUAT

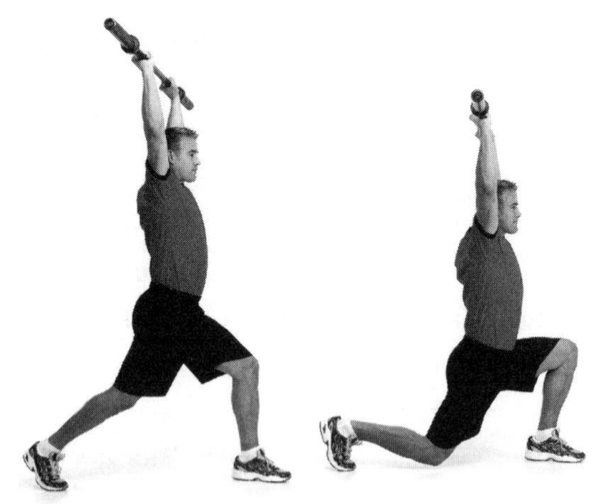

Stand with your feet spread front to back with 2½ to 3 feet between them. Using a grip that's approximately twice shoulder width, press an unloaded barbell up over your head until your arms are completely straight and you can't see them out of the corners of your eyes.

Balancing on the ball of your back foot, slowly begin to descend toward the floor, making sure to keep your torso as vertical as possible and not allowing your front knee to extend past a 90-degree angle. In the bottom position, be sure to keep your bottommost ribs as far away from your waist as possible. Pause, return to the starting position, and repeat. Finish your set and then do the same number of reps with your other leg.

ROTATIONAL SHOULDER PRESS

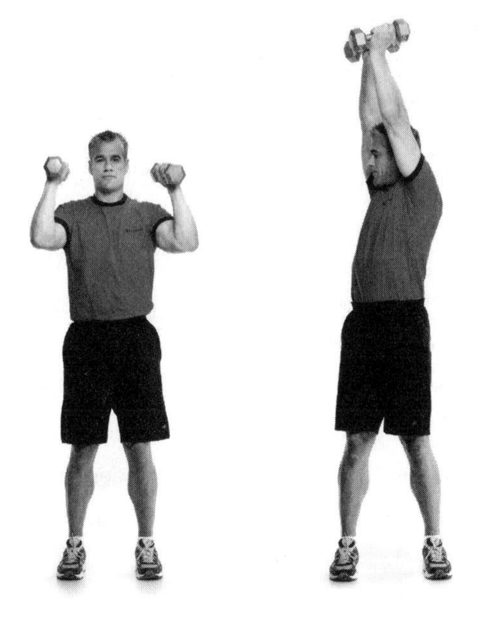

Stand holding a pair of dumbbells just outside your shoulders at jaw level, palms facing in.

Press the dumbbells overhead as you twist to your right. Lower the dumbbells as you twist back to the center, then twist to the left as you press the weights upward again.

ROMANIAN DEADLIFT

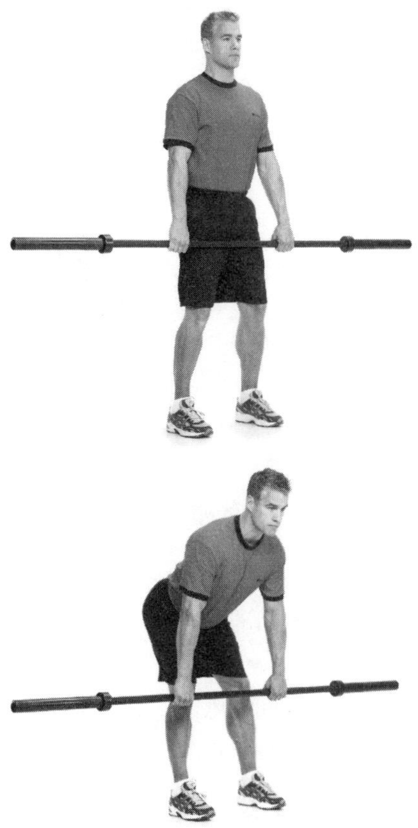

Grab an unloaded barbell (feel free to add weight to it as you get stronger) with an overhand grip that's just beyond shoulder width. Stand holding the bar at arm's length and resting on the fronts of your thighs. Your feet should be shoulder-width apart and your knees slightly bent. Focus your eyes straight ahead.

Slowly bend at the hips as you lower the bar to just below your knees. Don't change the angle of your knees. Keep your head and chest up and your lower back flat or slightly arched. Lift your torso back to the starting position, keeping the bar as close to your body as possible, and repeat.

DUMBBELL WOODCHOPPER

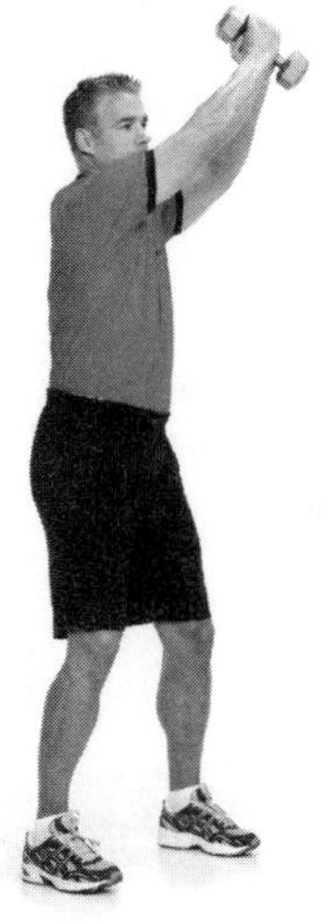

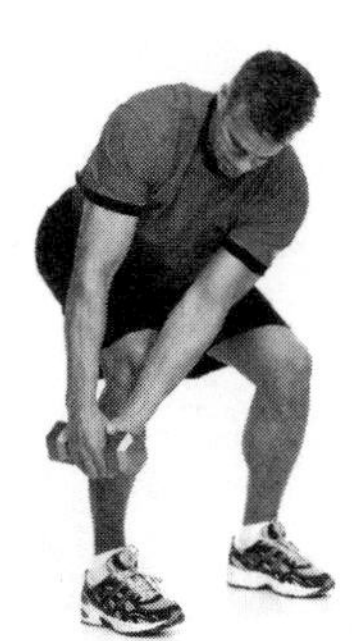

Stand holding a dumbbell with a hand-over-hand grip over one shoulder, with your arms straight and your knees slightly bent.

Chop the dumbbell down in a wide, sweeping motion so that your hands finish next to your opposite calf. Be sure to use your core muscles to initiate the movement and have your knees bent at the bottom of the movement. Return the dumbbell to the starting position and repeat.

(continued)

SUMO DEADLIFT

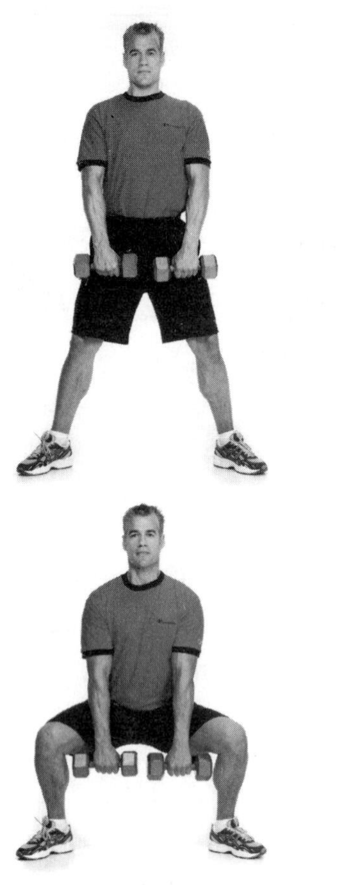

Using a wide stance that's twice shoulder width, with your toes turned out, hold a pair of dumbbells at arm's length, between your legs.

Keeping your back and arms straight, slowly descend until your thighs are parallel to the floor. Make sure your shoulder blades are still together at the bottom of the movement. Then press back up to the starting position and repeat.

SAXON SIDE BEND

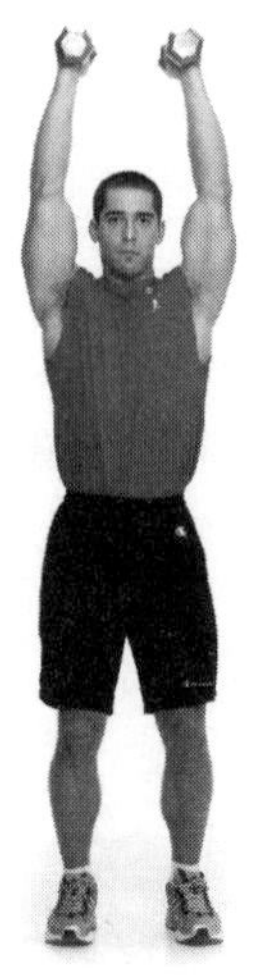

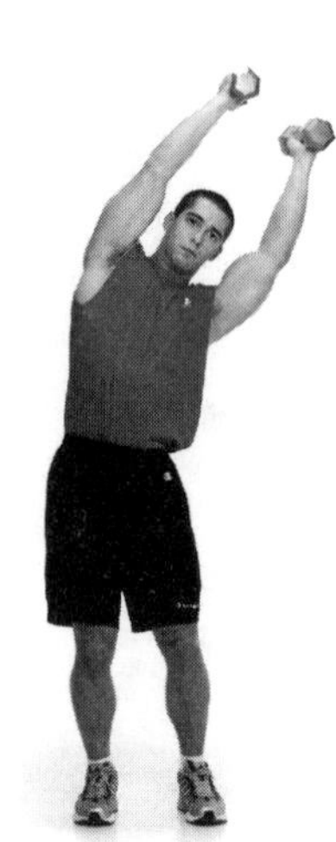

Stand holding a pair of light dumbbells directly overhead with your arms completely straight.

Keeping your knees slightly bent, lean over as far as you can to one side without allowing your arms to bend, your torso to twist, or the distance between the two dumbbells to change. When you've gone as far as you can, use your core muscles to bring yourself back to the starting position, and repeat. Finish your set, and then do the same number of reps on your other side.

REACHING LUNGE

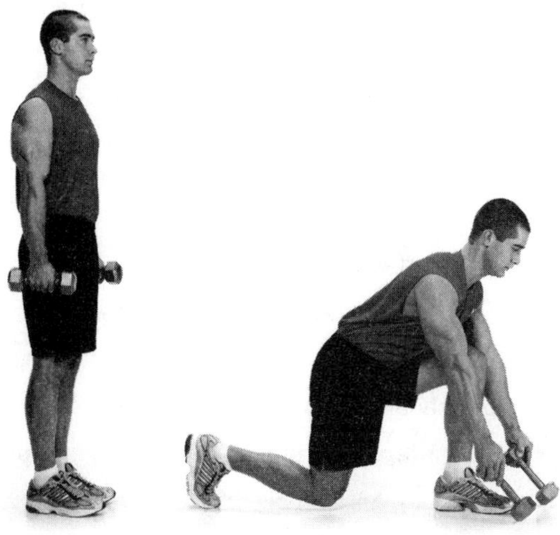

Stand holding a pair of light dumbbells with your arms hanging down at your sides. Quickly lunge forward as you extend your arms forward and flex your spine while attempting to touch the dumbbells to the floor. Once there, brace your abs and explosively push back up to the starting position, and repeat. Finish your set and then do the same number of reps with your other leg.

T-PUSHUP

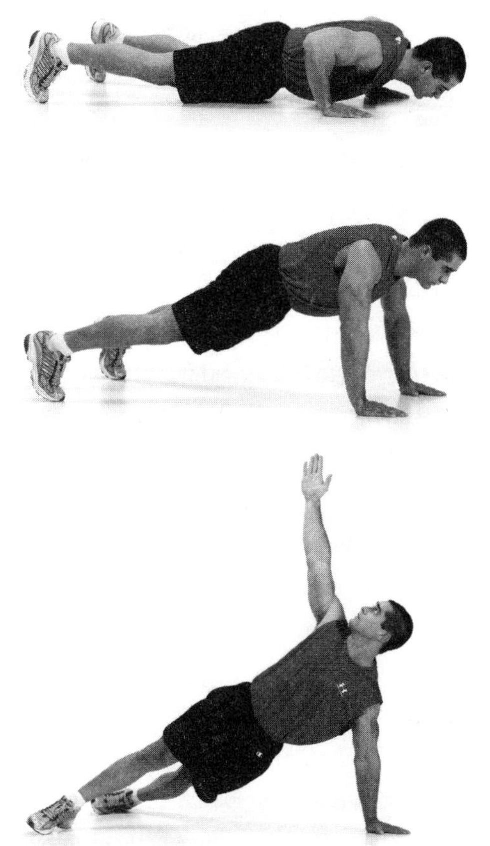

Begin as you would for a regular pushup, only with your feet spaced slightly wider apart.

Push up and, as you near the top of the pushup, immediately rotate one arm toward the ceiling as you simultaneously turn your hips and legs to the same side. At the top you should end up with your arms in a straight line, pointing from ceiling to floor, and your weight resting on the sides of your feet. Return to the starting position and execute another T-pushup before repeating to the other side.

(continued from page 141)

this phase you'll focus on four main movements: squatting, lunging, pushing, and pulling. That's it! The strength portion of your workout will contain a total of five or six exercises, at most. It will enable you to work lots of different muscle groups at once and get used to the idea of your body working as a functional unit—the way you use it outside of the gym.

In the interest of keeping things as basic as possible, I've provided you with two different workouts. Despite the fact that they're composed essentially of the same exercises, the way they're organized makes all the difference in the world. There are also slightly different set and rep schemes to further differentiate among the various types of beginners. Workout A is once again for the younger set, though those of you who are north of 35 can give it a go if you feel you're up to it. Workout B is somewhat simpler, to accommodate those who are completely inexperienced or have movement restrictions that could make more advanced exercises problematic.

Workout A

Dumbbell squat, hammer curl, and press/lat pulldown*: 2 or 3 sets × 10 reps

Alternating lunge: 2 or 3 sets × 10 reps (each leg)

Dumbbell bench press/one-arm row with elbow out*: 2 or 3 sets × 10 reps (each arm)

Workout B

Dumbbell squat: 1 or 2 sets × 15 reps

Lat pulldown: 1 or 2 sets × 15 reps

Reverse lunge: 1 or 2 sets × 15 (each leg)

Dumbbell bench press: 1 or 2 sets × 15

One-arm row with elbow out: 1 or 2 sets × 15

Neutral-grip dumbbell shoulder press: 1 or 2 sets × 15 reps

On the surface it might seem like workout B is more work. That's because workout A, for the most part, is arranged into supersets, where you do one exercise immediately after another without rest (the exception being the alternating lunge, which isn't grouped with anything else). Another big difference has to do with the training volume. While the prescribed repetition ranges are high (10 or 15 per set) for both workouts, workout A consists of 2 or 3 sets per exercise, as opposed to 1 or 2 sets in workout B. Finally, to help ensure adequate recovery between sets, be sure to take at least 30 seconds of rest after each set in workout B and a full 60 seconds of rest after each superset in workout A.

*These are supersets, pairs of exercises for which you perform a given number of repetitions of the first exercise and then take little or no rest before moving on to the second exercise (as indicated by the slash).

DUMBBELL SQUAT, HAMMER CURL, AND PRESS

Stand holding a pair of dumbbells at arm's length with a shoulder-width stance and your knees slightly bent. Begin by sitting down and back, descending into a squat until your thighs are parallel to the floor.

Reverse directions and stand back up. When your legs are almost completely straight, begin curling the weights up to your shoulders.

Once there, keep a slight bend in your knees as you press the weights overhead. Lower the dumbbells back down to your shoulders, then alongside your body, and repeat.

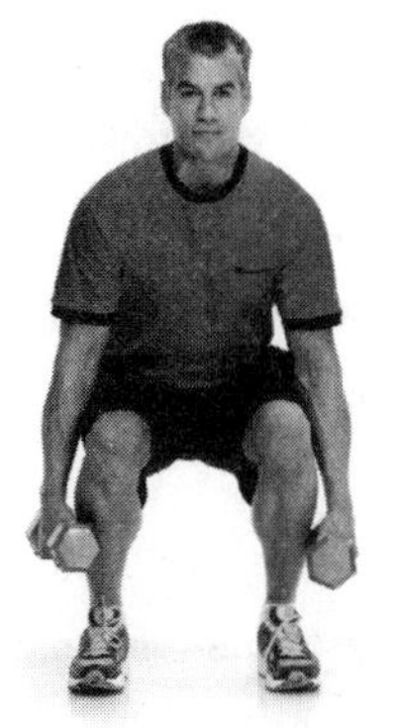

B

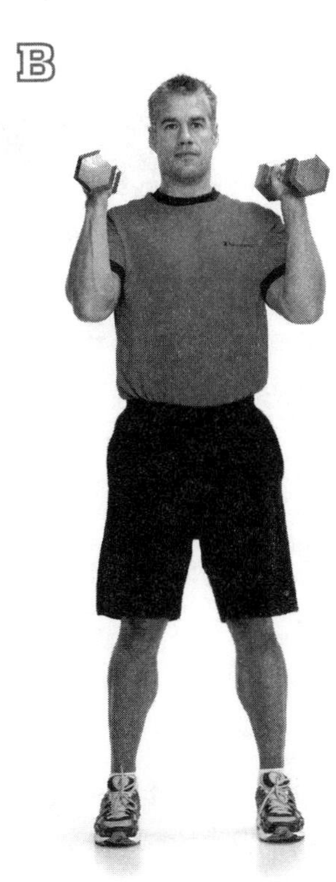

C

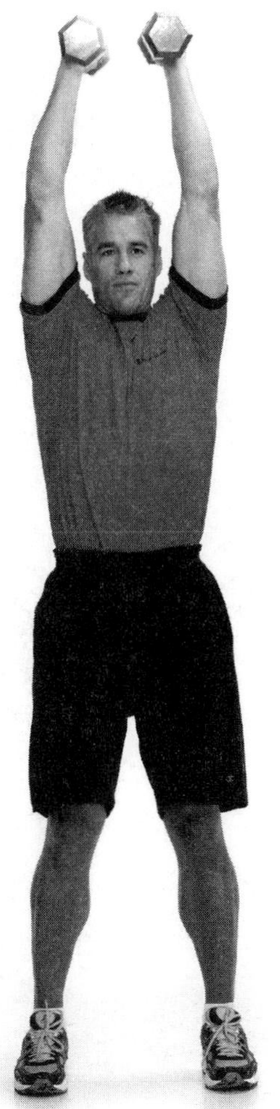

LAT PULLDOWN

Grab the bar of a lat pulldown machine (or a straight bar on the high pulley of a cable station) with a shoulder-width, overhand grip.

Moving only your arms, pull the bar down to your chest by squeezing your shoulder blades together. Hold for a second and then bring the bar back to the starting position.

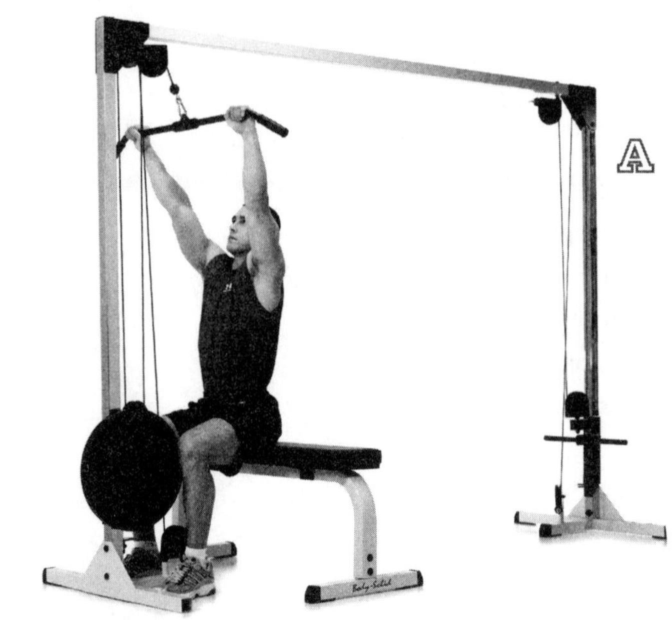
A

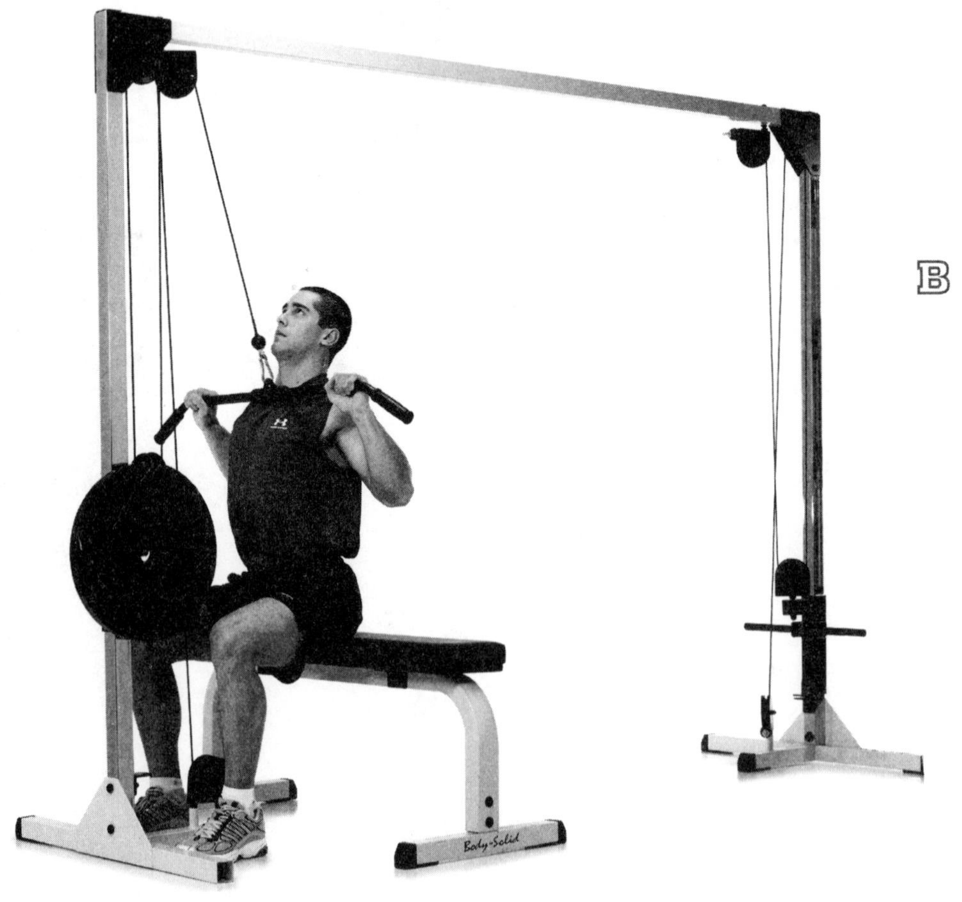
B

ALTERNATING LUNGE

Stand holding a pair of dumbbells at arm's length. Lunge forward until your front knee forms a 90-degree angle and your back knee almost touches the floor.

Immediately press back up to the starting position and lunge backward with the same leg. Be sure to allow only the ball of your back foot to contact the floor. In the bottom position your back knee should almost touch the floor and your front should once again form a right angle. Push back up to the starting position and repeat with your other leg.

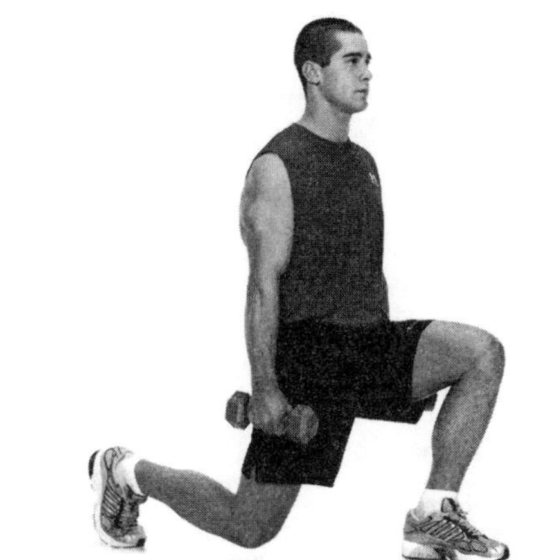

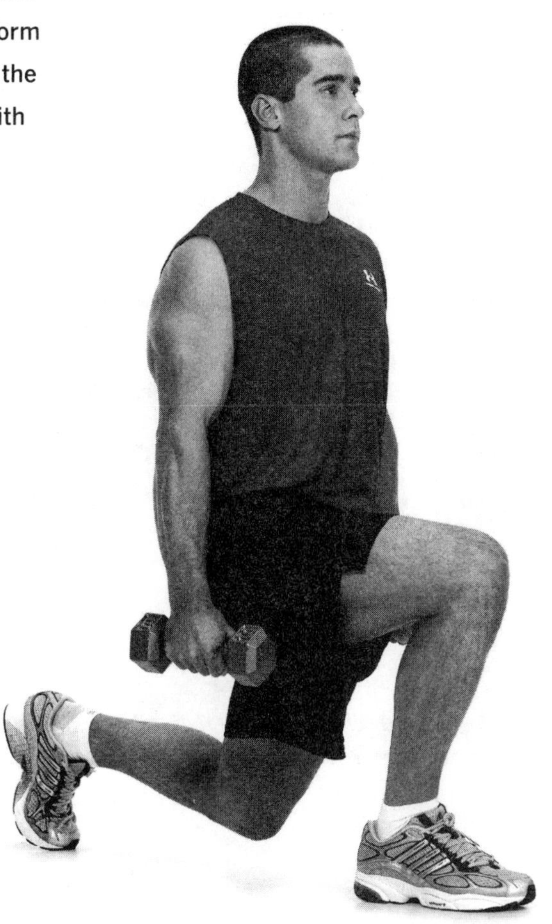

B

DUMBBELL BENCH PRESS

Grab a pair of dumbbells and lie faceup on a bench, holding the dumbbells over your chest with your palms facing forward.

Lower the dumbbells toward the floor, stopping when your elbows are even with, or just slightly below, your torso. Then reverse the motion and push the weights back up to the starting position.

You can make this exercise more shoulder friendly by using a neutral grip (palms facing each other) and keeping your elbows close to your body. If you suffer from lower-back pain, you might also want to place your feet up on the end of the bench instead of down on the floor.

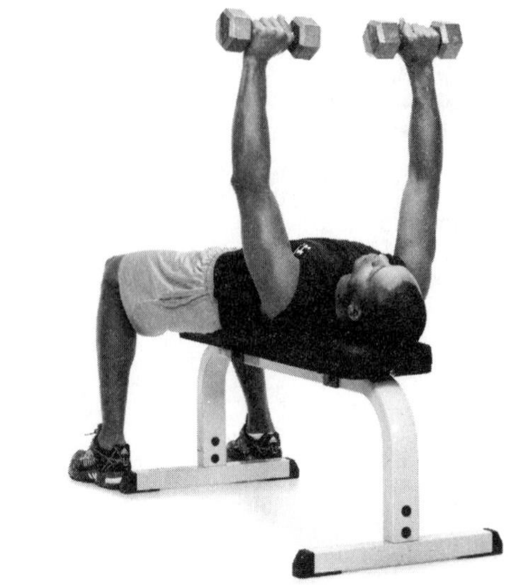

A

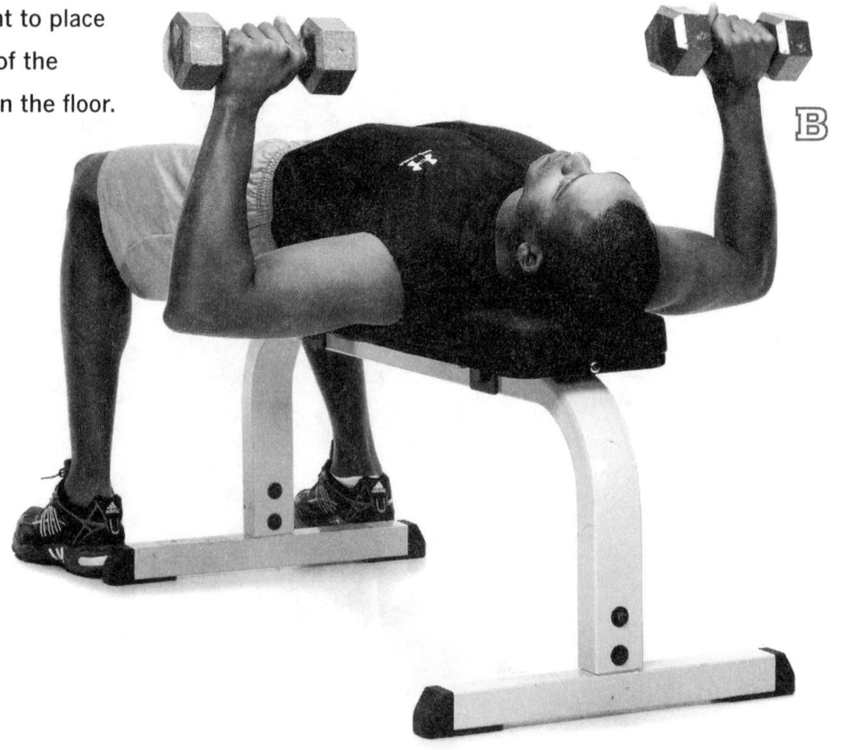

B

ONE-ARM ROW WITH ELBOW OUT

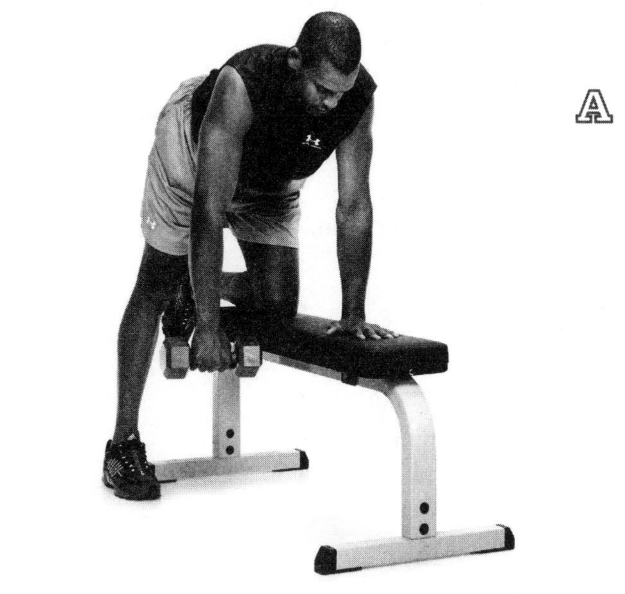

A

Support yourself on an exercise bench by placing one knee and the corresponding hand on the bench and keeping the other foot on the floor. Make sure your back is flat. With your free hand, grasp a dumbbell with a false, or hook grip (with your thumb wrapped around the same side of the bar as the rest of your fingers) and let it hang at arm's length beneath your shoulder, with your palm facing behind you.

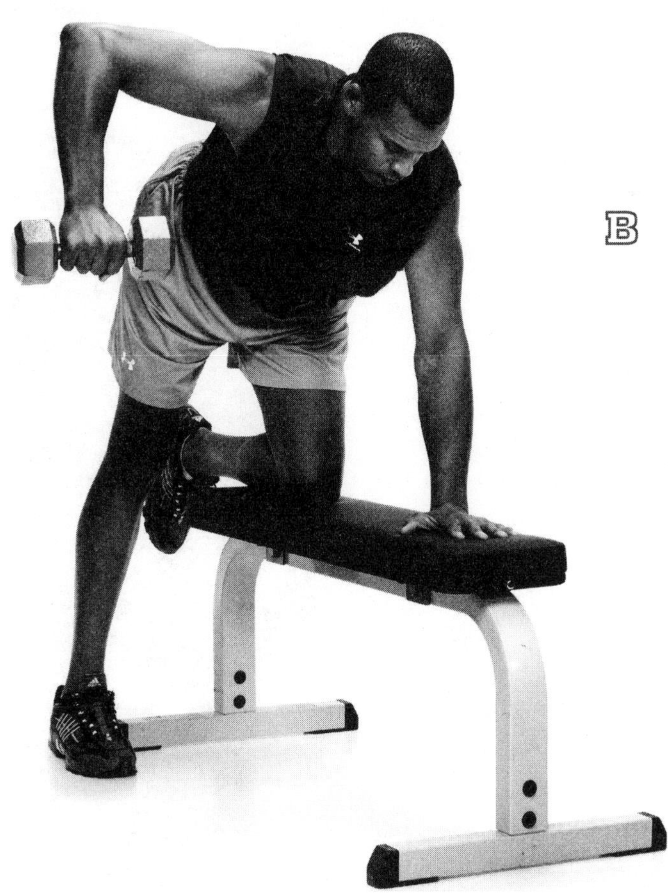

B

Draw your elbow up past your torso by pinching your shoulder blade in toward your spine. Avoid twisting or contorting your body to get the weight up. Hold for a second and then lower the weight back down to the starting position. Finish your set and then do the same number of reps with your other arm.

DUMBBELL SQUAT

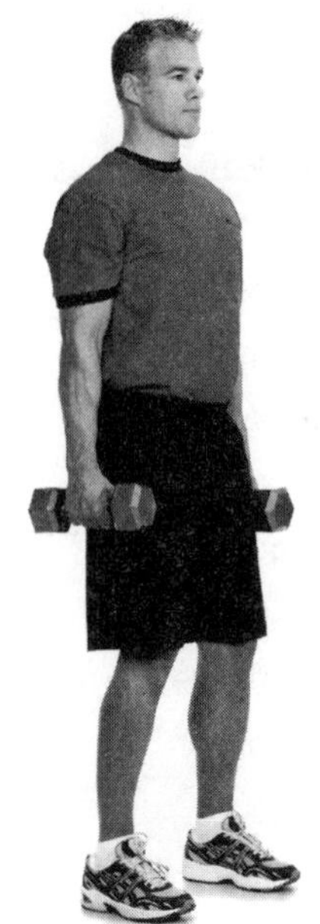

Stand holding a pair of dumbbells at arm's length with your palms facing each other and a stance slightly wider than shoulder width.

Sit down and back, keeping your back as straight as possible until your thighs are parallel to the floor. Pause for a second and then return to the starting position.

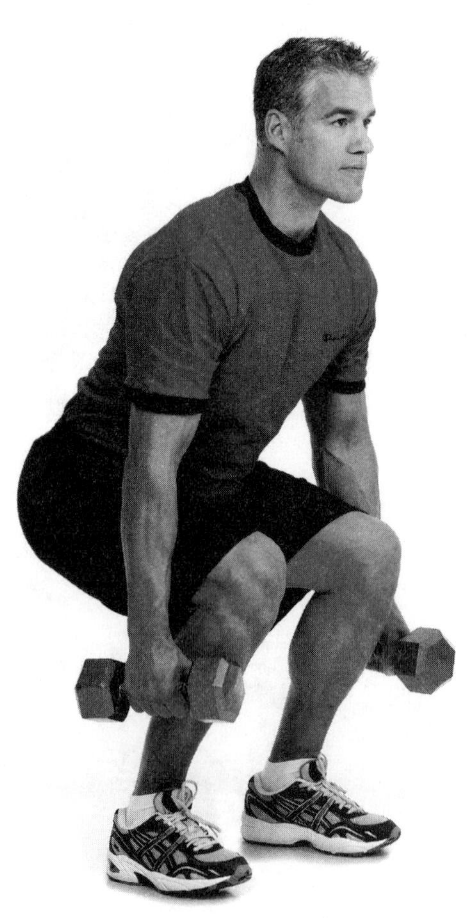

B

REVERSE LUNGE

Stand with your feet hip-width apart.

Step backward with one leg and lower your body until your front knee is bent 90 degrees and your rear knee nearly touches the floor. Your front lower leg should be perpendicular to the floor and your torso should remain upright. Push yourself back up to the starting position as quickly as you can and repeat with the other leg.

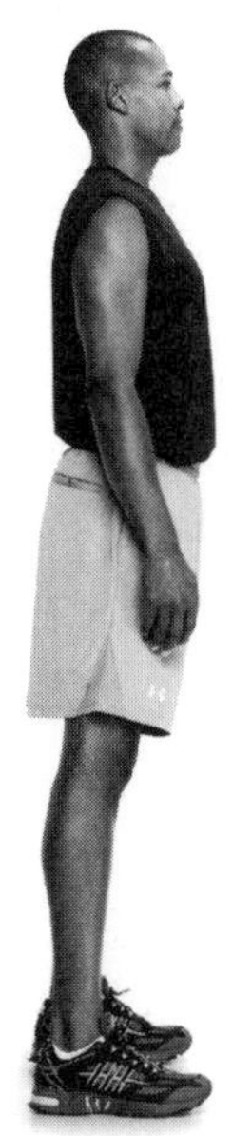

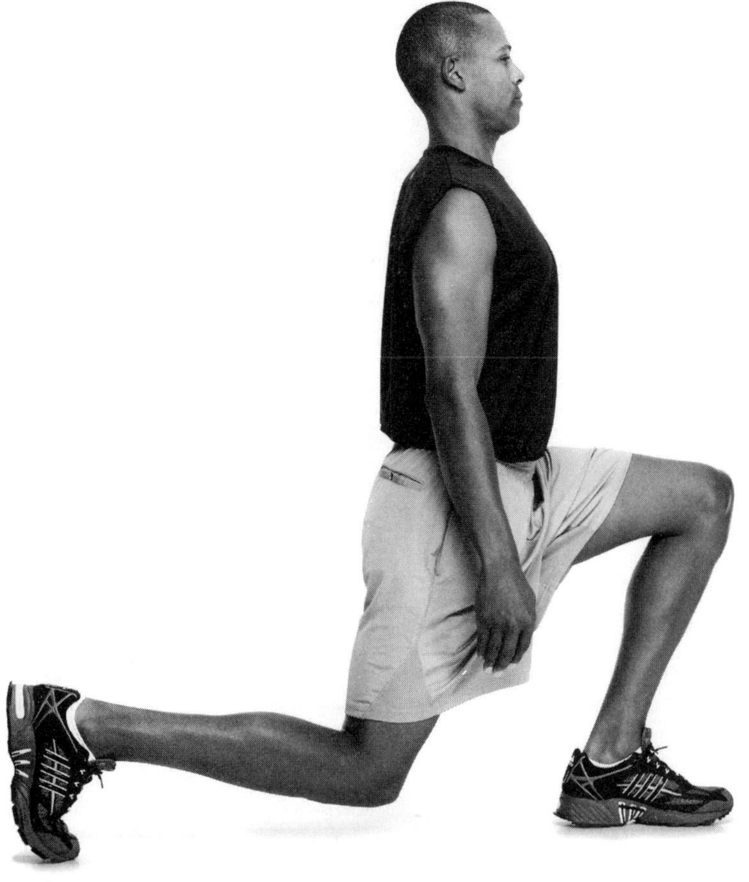

B

NEUTRAL-GRIP DUMBBELL SHOULDER PRESS

Stand holding a pair of dumbbells just outside your shoulders, with your arms bent and your palms facing each other.

Push the weights straight overhead (like a referee signaling a touchdown). Pause, then slowly lower them back to the starting position.

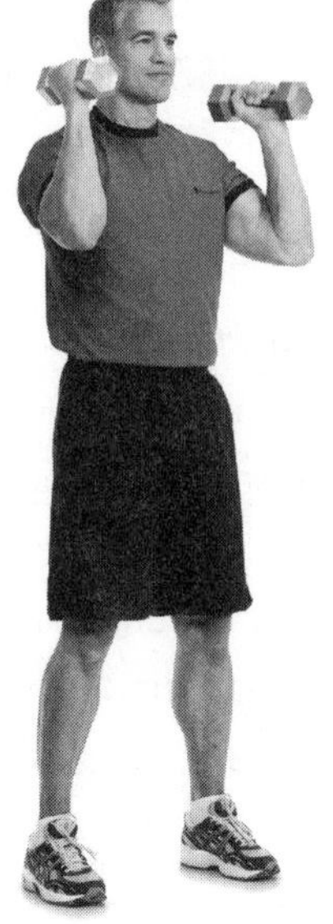

A

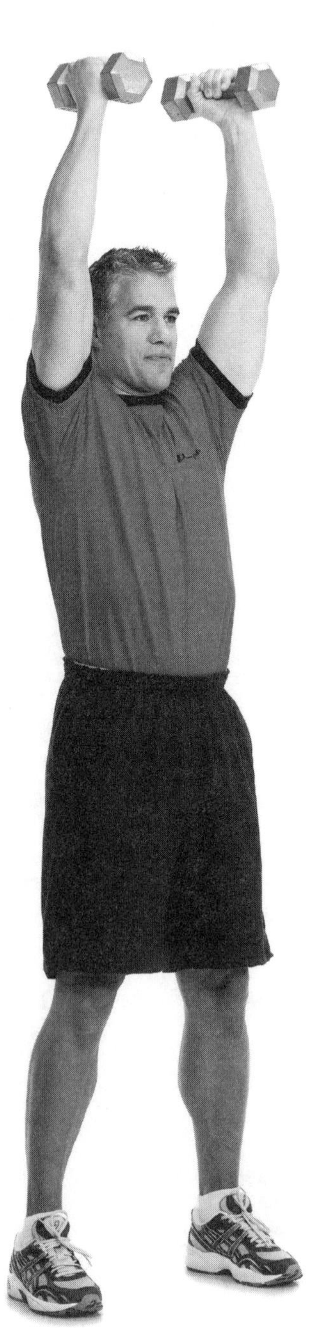

B

WEIGHTY ISSUES

Using free weights to burn fat

Despite what you may have heard, unless you're moving at a blistering pace, traditional cardiovascular exercise doesn't really cause long-term elevations in metabolism. Weight training, on the other hand, when done at the right pace causes significant elevations of your metabolism in two different ways. First off, it requires your body to consume extra oxygen for up to several hours after you've finished exercising, in order to restore itself to its pre-exercise condition. Second, the muscle you build as a result of this type of training helps increase your metabolic rate even when you're at rest.

The following two workouts can be done two or three times per week on a rotating basis. Use a weight that allows you to do between 10 and 15 reps per set, and limit your rest intervals to approximately 30 seconds between sets (which is just about enough time to set up for your next exercise). Upon completing the last exercise, take a 1-to-2-minute rest before repeating the sequence once or twice.

Workout A

Barbell squat or dumbell split squat
Prone row
Incline reverse crunch
Incline press
Side lunge

Workout B

Neutral-grip dumbbell shoulder press
Barbell deadlift or dumbbell deadlift
Situp
Dumbbell lunge
Reverse fly

Don't be fooled by their relative brevity; these two routines are pretty tough. They're going to get you winded, get your heart pumping through your chest, and give you a whole new appreciation for the versatility and power of free weights. Perhaps best of all, they're going to hammer home for you the notion that you don't need a bunch of specialized equipment to sculpt a lean, chiseled physique. All it takes is a little iron and a lot of effort.

BARBELL SQUAT

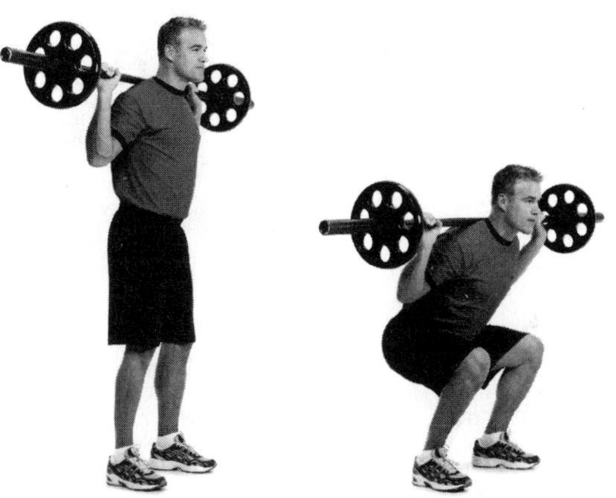

Hold a barbell with an overhand grip so that it rests comfortably on your upper back (not on your neck). Set your feet shoulder-width apart, with your knees slightly bent, your back straight, and your eyes focused straight ahead.

Slowly lower your body as if you were sitting back into a chair, keeping your back in its natural alignment and your lower legs nearly perpendicular to the floor. When your thighs are parallel to the floor, pause, and then return to the starting position.

(continued)

DUMBBELL SPLIT SQUAT

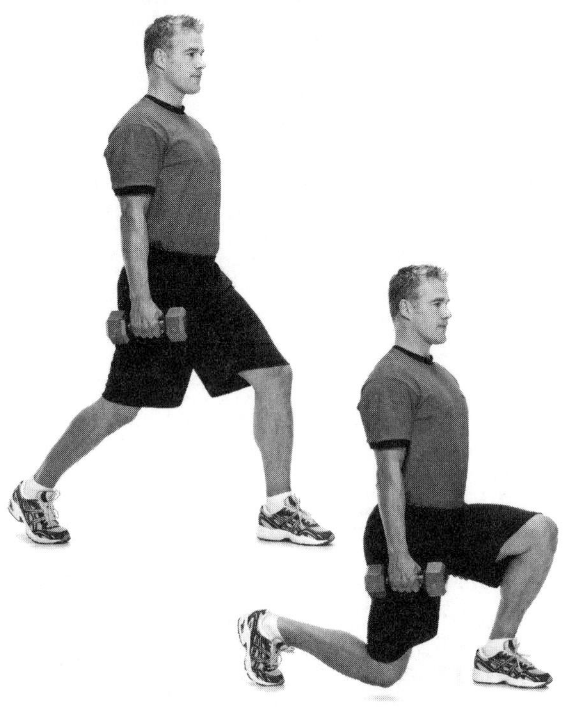

Grab a pair of dumbbells and hold them at your sides. Stand in a staggered stance with your left foot 2½ to 3 feet in front of your right.

Lower your body until your front knee is bent 90 degrees and your rear knee nearly touches the floor. Your front lower leg should be perpendicular to the floor and your torso should remain upright. Push yourself back up to the starting position as quickly as you can. Finish your set, then do the same number of reps with your right foot in front of your left.

PRONE DUMBBELL ROW WITH ELBOWS OUT

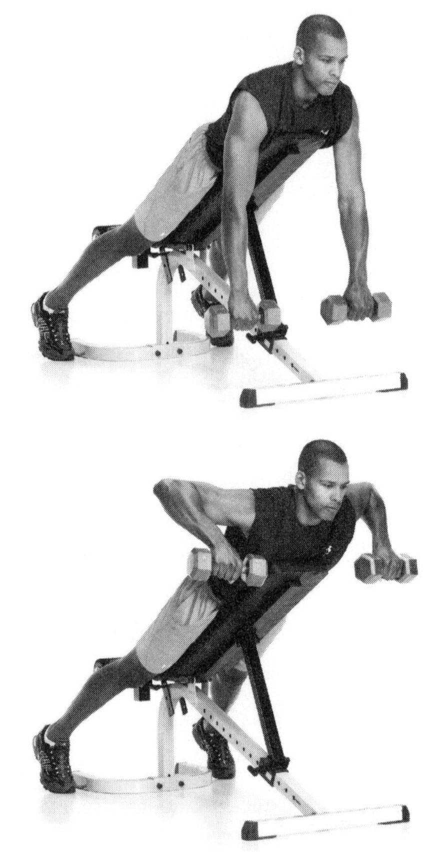

Set an incline bench to a 30-degree angle. Grab a pair of dumbbells and lie with your chest against the pad. Let your arms hang straight down from your shoulders and turn your palms so that your thumbs are facing each other.

Lift your upper arms as high as you can by bending your elbows and squeezing your shoulder blades together. Your upper arms should be perpendicular to your body at the top of the move. Your lower arms should be pointing toward the floor. Pause, then slowly lower the weights to the starting position.

INCLINE REVERSE CRUNCH

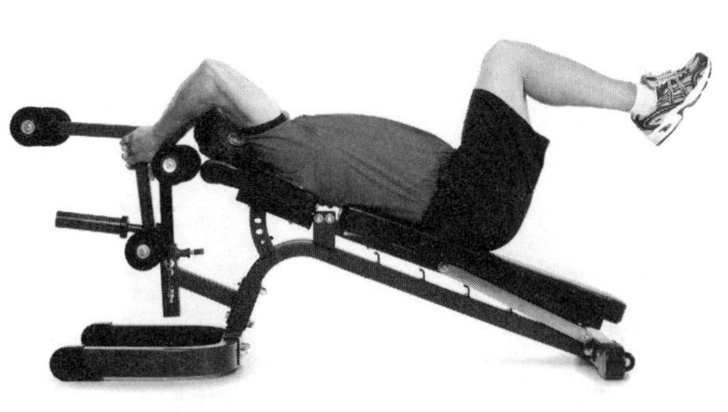

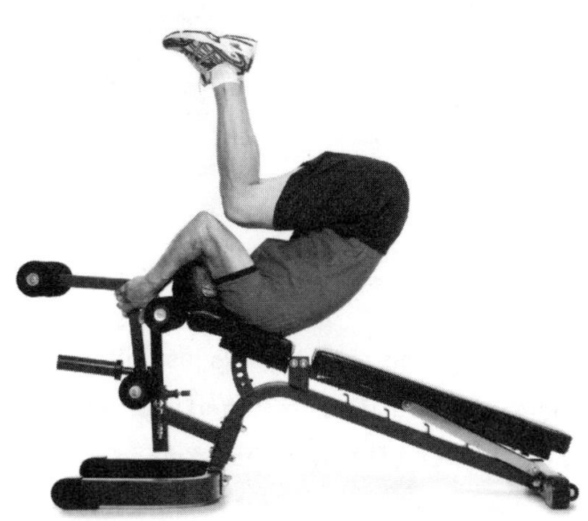

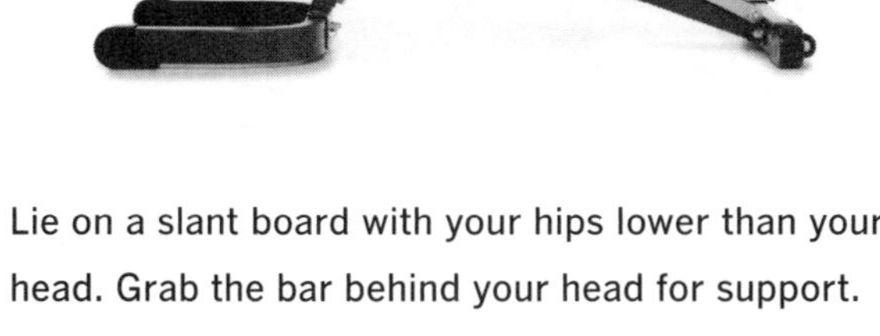

Lie on a slant board with your hips lower than your head. Grab the bar behind your head for support. Bend your hips and knees 90 degrees.

Pull your hips upward and crunch them inward, as if you were emptying a bucket of water that was resting on your pelvis. Keep your hips and knees at 90-degree angles throughout the exercise. Pause and then slowly lower your hips to the starting position.

INCLINE DUMBBELL BENCH PRESS

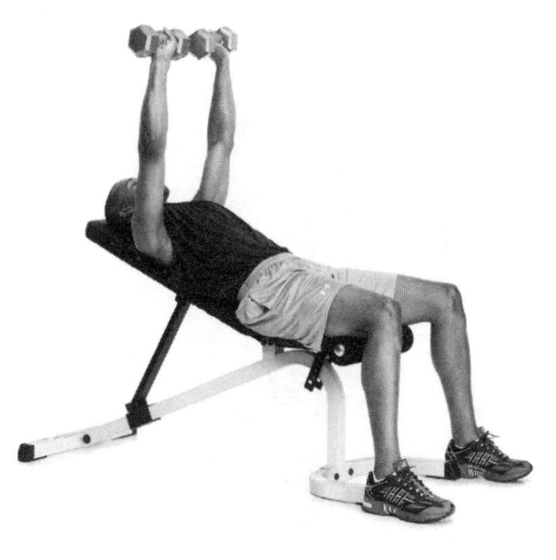

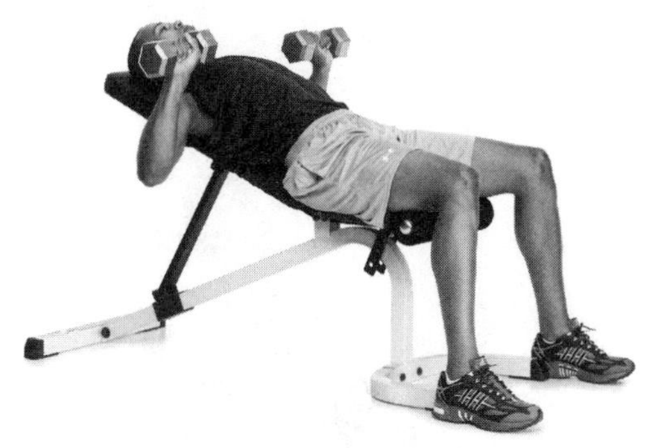

Grab a pair of dumbbells and lie faceup on a bench set to a low incline (15 to 30 degrees). Lift the dumbbells so they're over your chin and hold them with your palms turned out (thumbs facing each other).

Slowly lower the weights to your upper chest, pause, and then push them back up over your chin.

(continued)

SIDE LUNGE

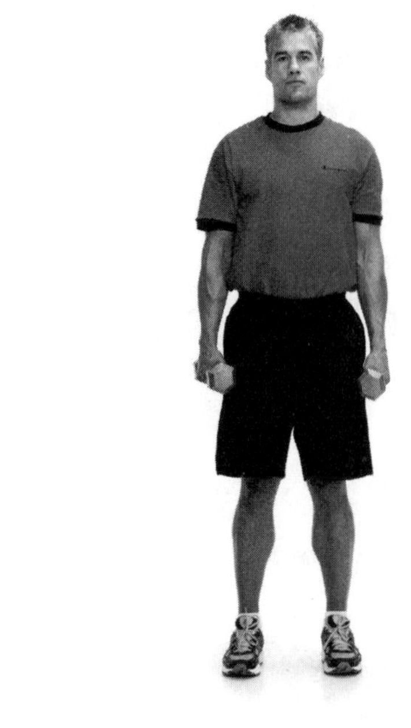

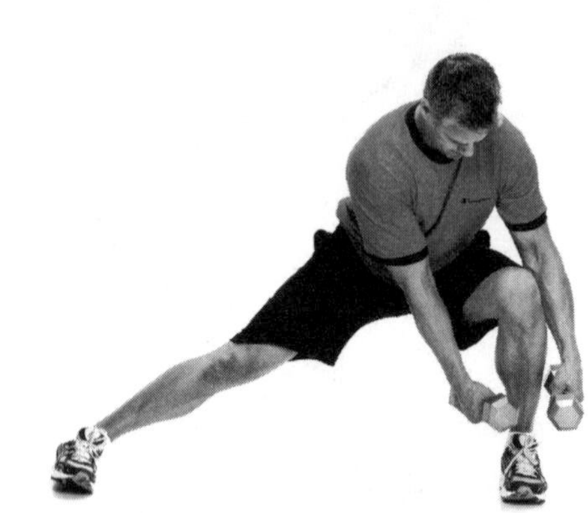

Stand holding a pair of dumbbells at arm's length, and step out to the side so that the knee and toe of the leg you're stepping with continue to point straight ahead as you lower yourself into a squat. As you're doing this be sure that the other leg is completely straight. Pause for a second and push back up to the starting position. Finish your set, then do the same number of reps with your other leg lunging.

NEUTRAL-GRIP DUMBBELL SHOULDER PRESS

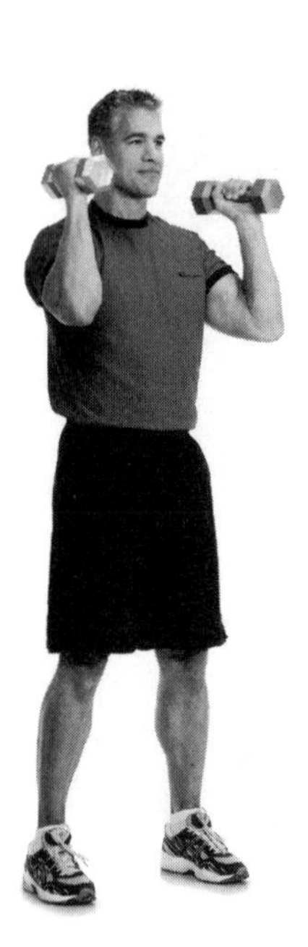

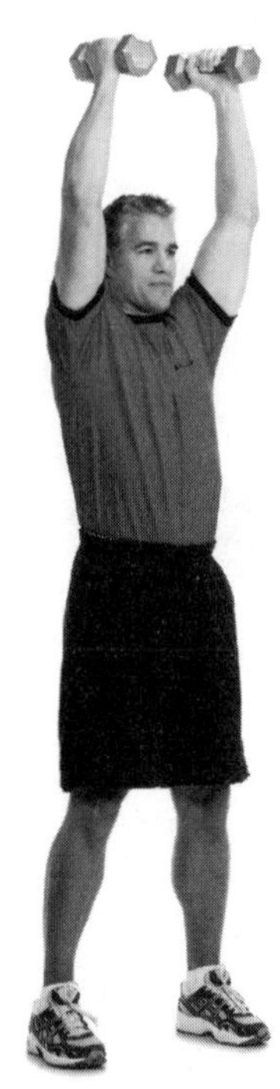

Stand holding a pair of dumbbells just outside your shoulders, with your arms bent and your palms facing each other. (This will free up some space within the shoulder joint making it less problematic for guys with previous shoulder injuries.)

Push the weights straight overhead (like a referee signaling a touchdown). Pause, and then slowly lower them back to the starting position.

BARBELL DEADLIFT

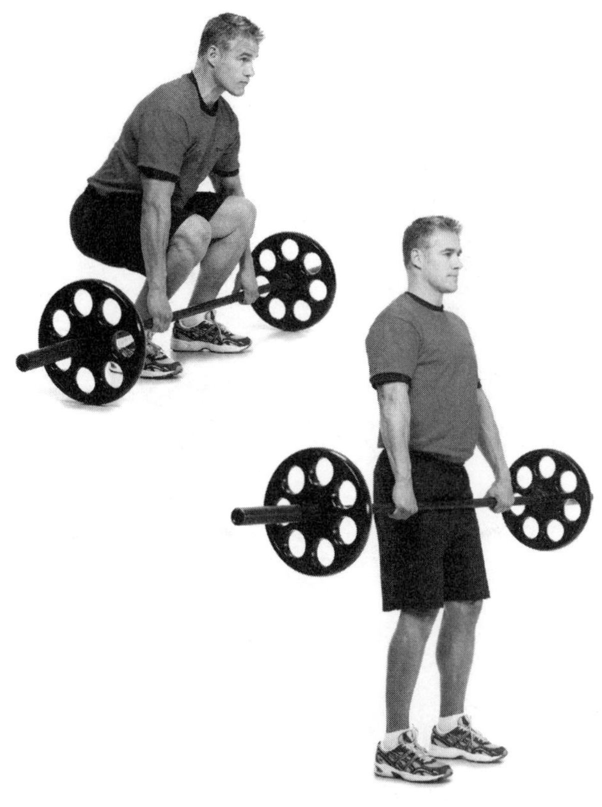

Set a barbell on the floor and stand facing it. Squat down and grab it with an overhand grip (palms facing you), your hands just outside your legs.

With your back flat and your head up, stand up with the barbell, pulling your shoulder blades back. Slowly lower the bar to the starting position.

DUMBBELL DEADLIFT

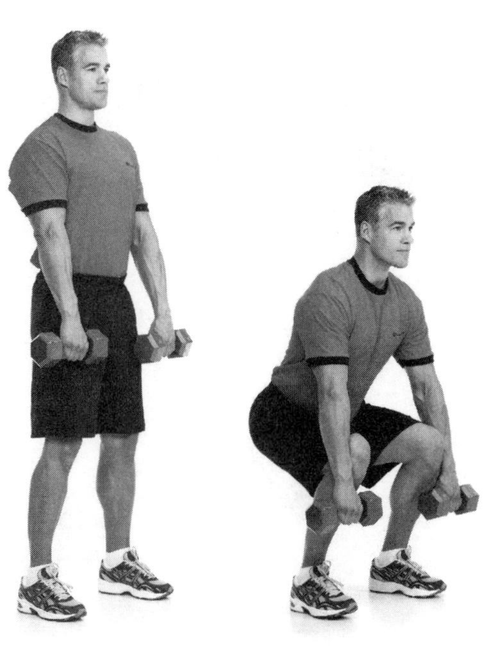

Stand holding a pair of dumbbells at arm's length with your palms facing your thighs and a stance that's slightly wider than shoulder width. (The position of the weight here allows you to remain more upright and reduces lower-back strain as compared to the barbell deadlift.)

Keeping a slight arch in your back and your shoulders pinched together, begin to sit down and back until your thighs are parallel to the floor. Pause there for a second and then press back up to the starting position.

(continued)

SITUP

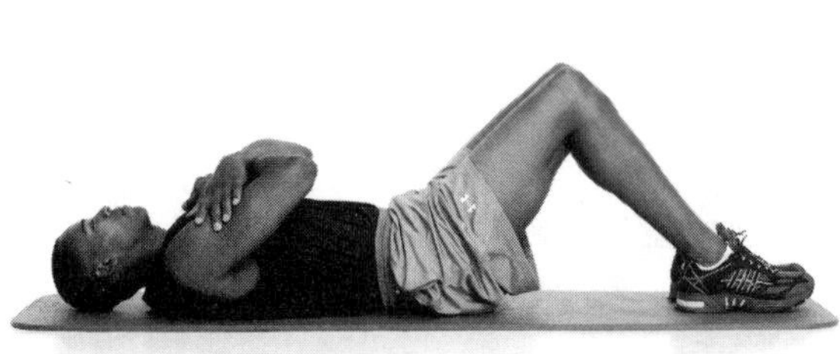

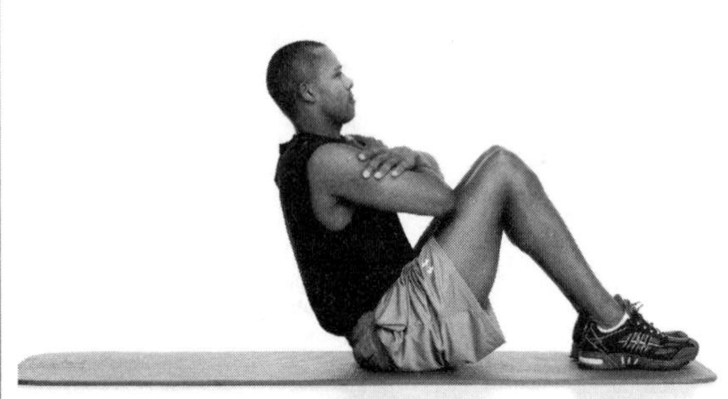

Lie faceup on the floor with your knees bent about 90 degrees and your arms folded across your chest.

Without anchoring your feet or using momentum, sit up by contracting your abdominals until your arms make contact with your thighs. Pause for a second and then slowly lower yourself.

DUMBBELL LUNGE

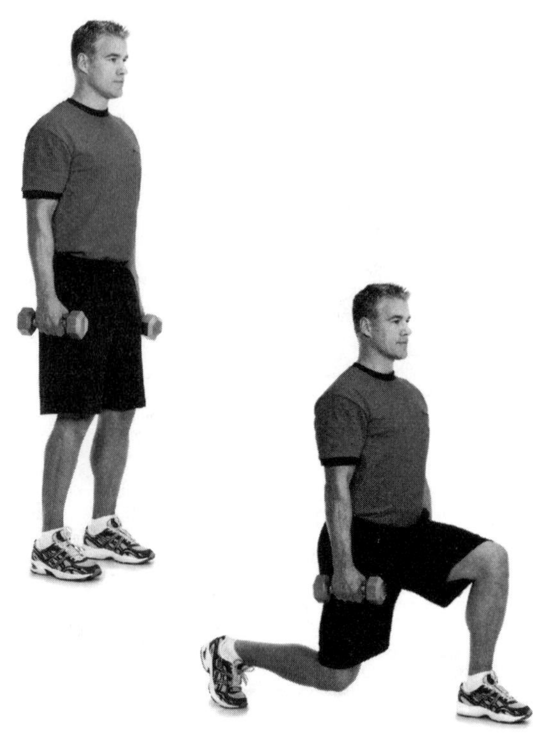

Grab a pair of dumbbells and hold them at your sides. Stand with your feet hip-width apart.

Step forward with one leg and lower your body until your front knee is bent 90 degrees and your rear knee nearly touches the floor. Your front lower leg should be perpendicular to the floor and your torso should remain upright. Push yourself back up to the starting position as quickly as you can and repeat with your other leg.

REVERSE FLY

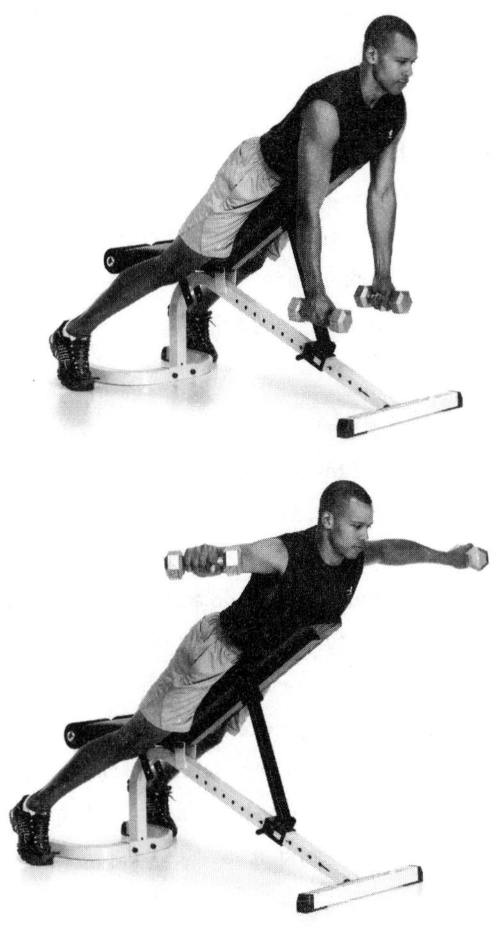

Lie facedown on a 45-degree exercise bench holding a pair of dumbbells at arm's length.

Keeping a slight bend in your elbows, pinch your shoulder blades together and work your arms up in a wide, arcing motion. At the top of the movement your elbows should remain slightly bent and you should see the weights out of the corners of your eyes.

MIDDLE MANAGEMENT

YOU'RE NOTHING WITHOUT A STRONG CORE

Believe it or not, there's more to working your core than throwing in a few sets of crunches at the end of your workout. A good, well-rounded core workout not only includes exercises that target the main muscle group of the abs—the rectus abdominis, which flexes, or bends, your spine—but also involves bending your spine laterally (side to side), as well as some form of rotation. And seeing as how the core musculature also includes the lower back, you need at least one exercise that extends the spine as well. Building on the foundation you created during the corrective phase, the following workouts should provide you with a nice challenge.

This time, rather than just using age and experience as the parameters for which of the two workouts you should do, I'm going to recommend that anyone who scored low on their core test during the self-assessment and/or suffers from lower-back pain opt for workout B. Those with higher self-assessment scores should be fine with workout A. Either way, you'll be getting a very inclusive core workout that's a far cry from just doing crunches.

Workout A

Unanchored situp: 2 or 3 sets × 6 to 10 reps
Russian twist: 2 or 3 sets × 4 to 6 reps per side
Lateral crunch: 2 or 3 sets × 4 to 6 reps per side
Swiss ball back extension: 2 or 3 sets × 10 to 12 reps

Workout B

Swiss ball pass-off: 2 or 3 sets × 6 to 8 reps
Bicycle: 2 or 3 sets × 8 to 10 reps per side
Oblique jackknife: 2 or 3 sets × 6 to 8 reps per side
Unilateral bird dog: 2 or 3 sets × 10 to 12 reps per side

As with the strength training, we'll once again keep the reps high and the rest intervals relatively brief (30 seconds max between sets) due to the postural component and the high resistance to fatigue displayed by these muscle groups. You could also opt to perform the exercises circuit-style, where you bang them out one after another, without rest in between, and then take a brief rest only before going around again. Whether you choose to do them as straight sets or as circuits, two or three sets of each exercise should be more than enough, regardless of which workout you choose.

UNANCHORED SITUP

Lie faceup on the floor with your arms at your sides or folded across your chest, your knees slightly bent, and your feet flat. (The more bend you have in your knees, the harder the exercise will be.)

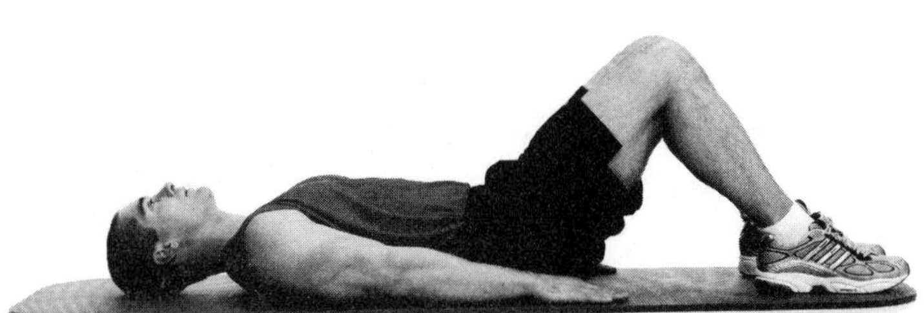

Use your abdominals to slowly pull yourself up to a seated position; avoid using any momentum to lift yourself off the floor. Hold for a second and lower back down under control.

B

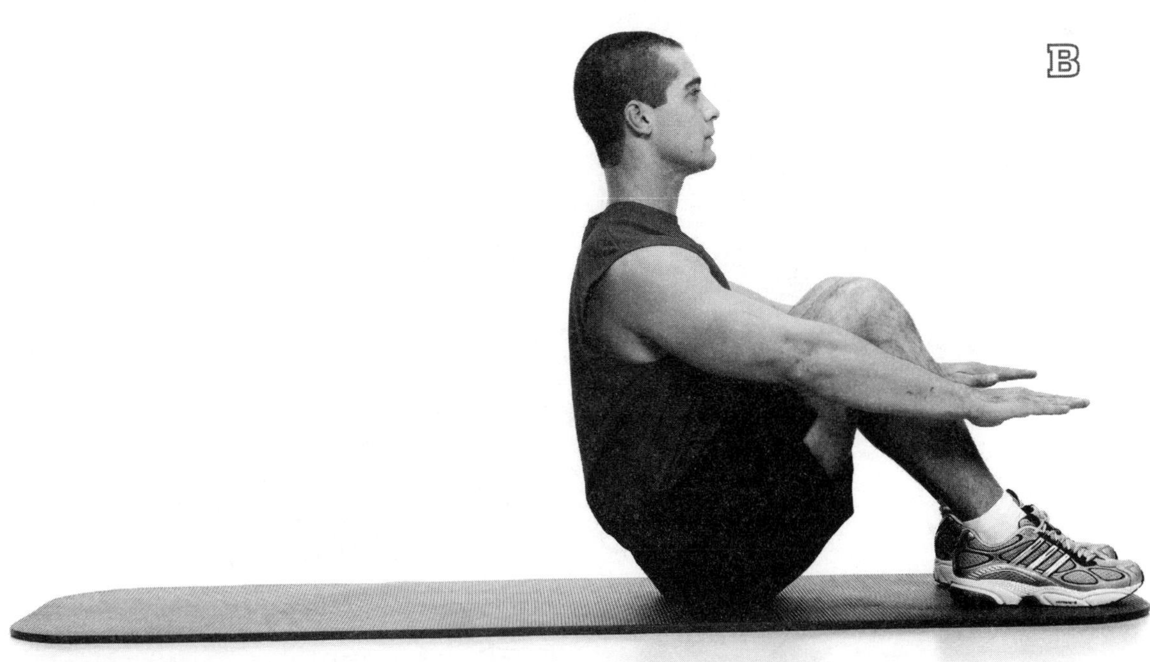

RUSSIAN TWIST

Sit on the floor with your knees bent about 90 degrees and your feet flat on the floor. Next, extend your arms and lean back until your wrists line up over your knees.

Hold this same trunk angle as you twist as far as possible to one side and then the other.

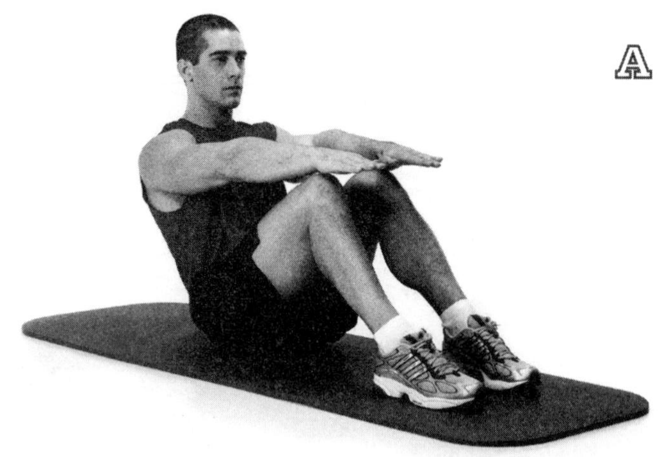

A

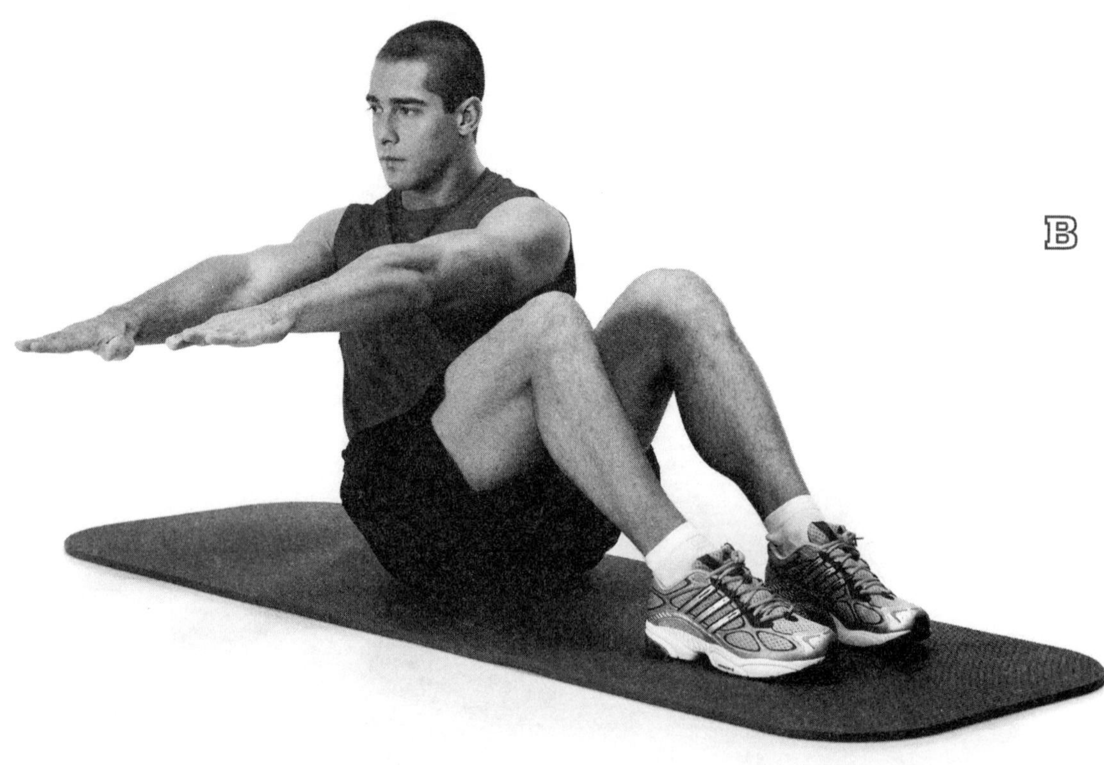

B

LATERAL CRUNCH

Lie faceup on the floor with your knees bent, your feet flat, and your hands placed lightly on the sides of your head. Crunch up until your shoulder blades are a few inches off the floor.

Hold that position as you attempt to bring your left armpit towards your right hip. Reverse the motion and slowly go to the other side without allowing your shoulder blades to touch the floor. Continue for the desired number of repetitions.

A

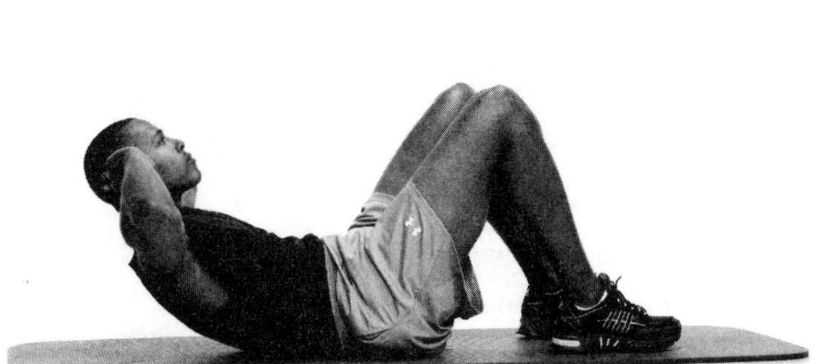

B

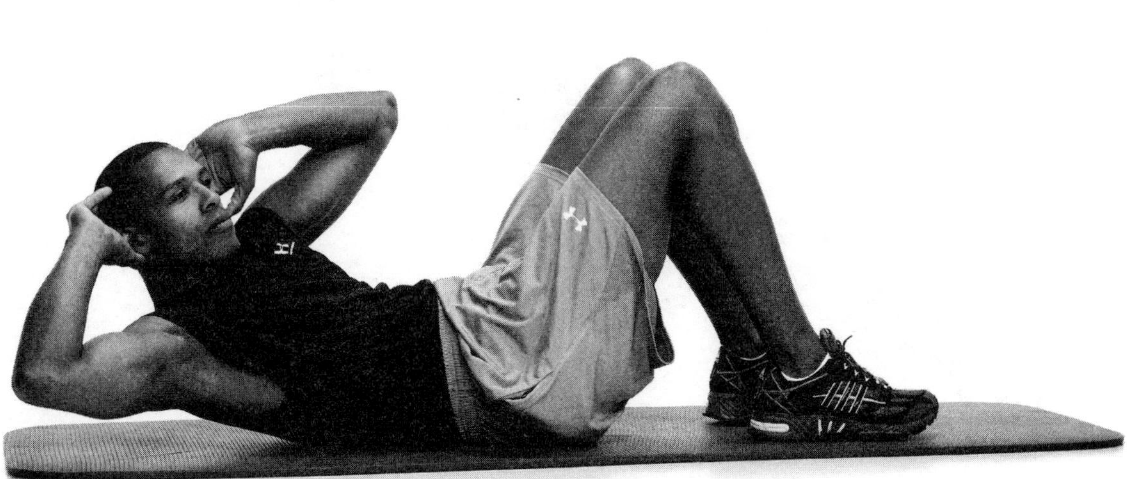

SWISS BALL BACK EXTENSION

Lie facedown with your torso rounded over a Swiss ball, your legs straight and your hands folded behind your back.

A

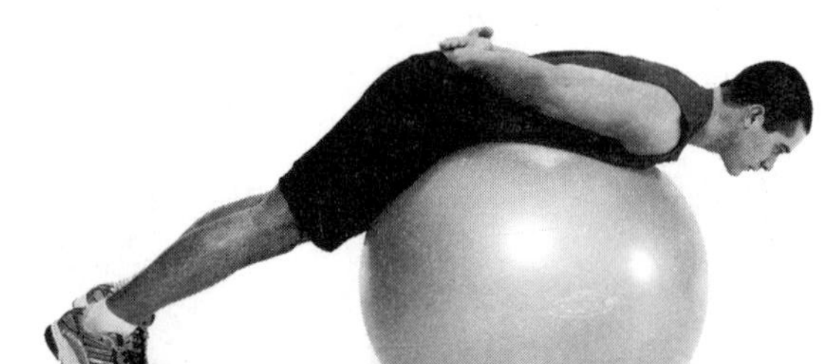

Using the muscles that run up and down along your spine, extend your spine and lift your chest completely off the ball. Hold for 20 to 30 seconds and then release.

B

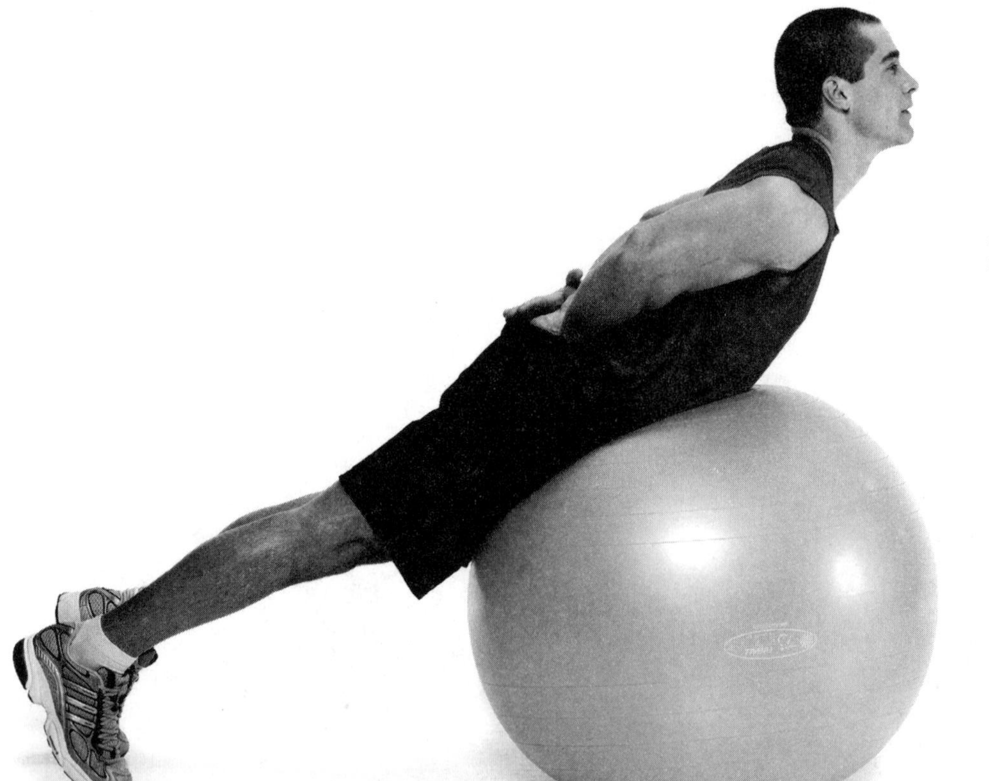

SWISS BALL PASS-OFF

Lie faceup on the floor with your arms over your head, holding a Swiss ball, and your legs extended straight up over your hips.

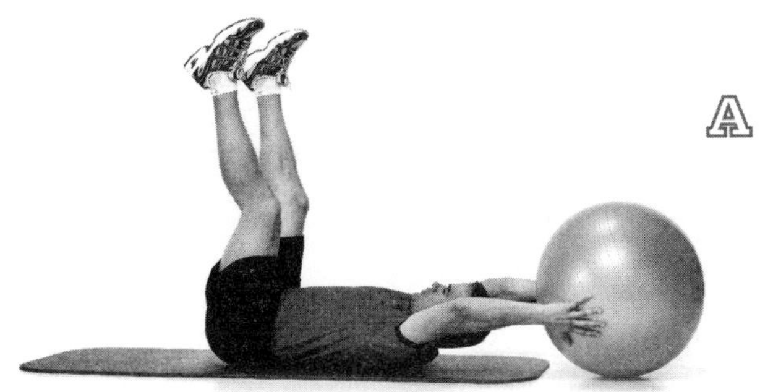

A

Lift your torso up off the floor and place the ball between your feet.

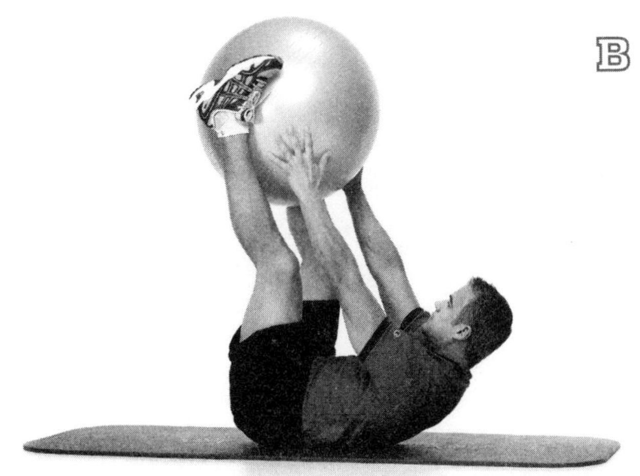

B

Keeping your torso off the floor and your arms extended, lower your legs as far toward the floor as you can without allowing your lower back to arch. Once you reach this point, use your abdominals and hip flexors (the muscles at the very tops of your thighs) to bring the ball back up to your hands and then lower yourself back to the starting position.

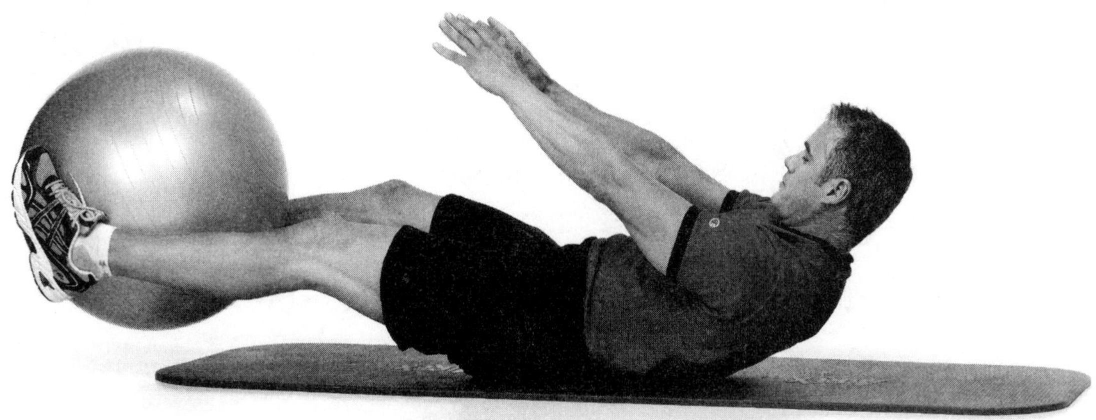

BICYCLE

Lie faceup on the floor with your hands on the sides of your head and your legs bent at 90 degrees up over your hips. Cycle one leg after the other in toward your chest as you simultaneously bring the opposite armpit toward each knee as it comes up. Be sure to keep your back flat and your elbows back out of sight.

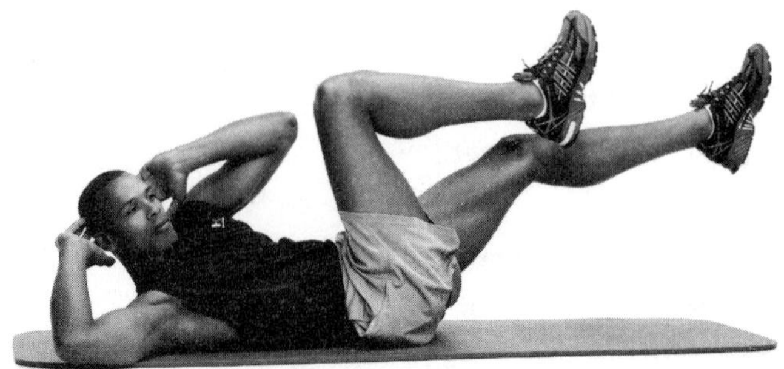

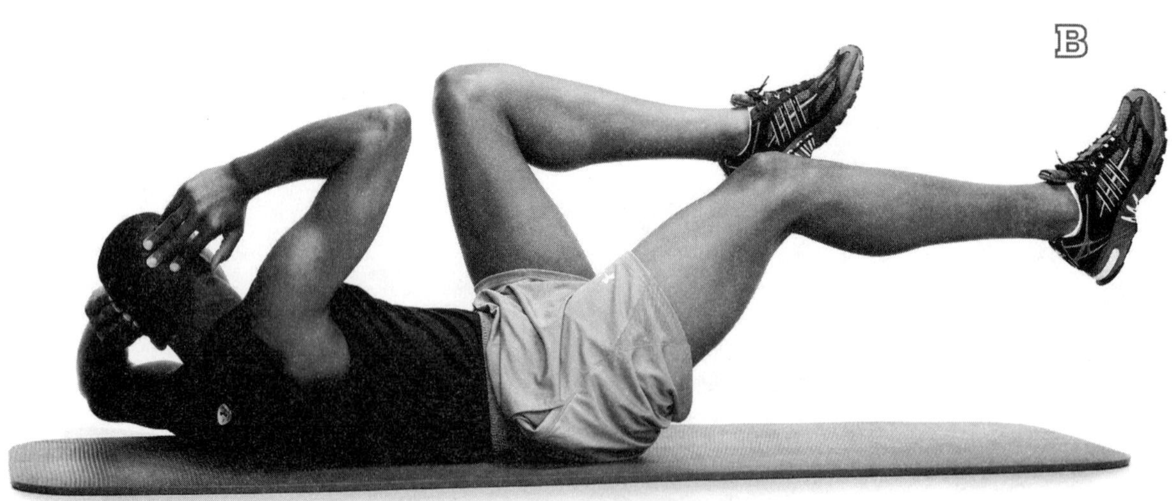

OBLIQUE JACKKNIFE

Lie on your side on the floor so that your shoulders, hips, knees and feet are stacked over each other. Fold your arms across your chest.

Balance on your bottom arm as you lift your legs off the floor and attempt to bring your top elbow toward your top hip. Hold and then slowly lower back to the starting position. Finish your set and then do the same number of reps on your other side.

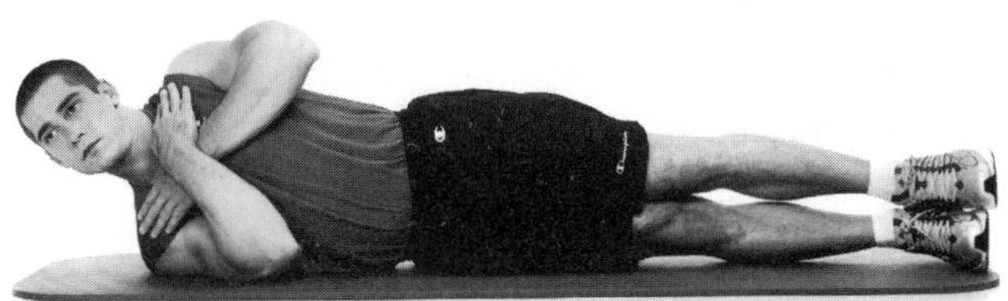

B

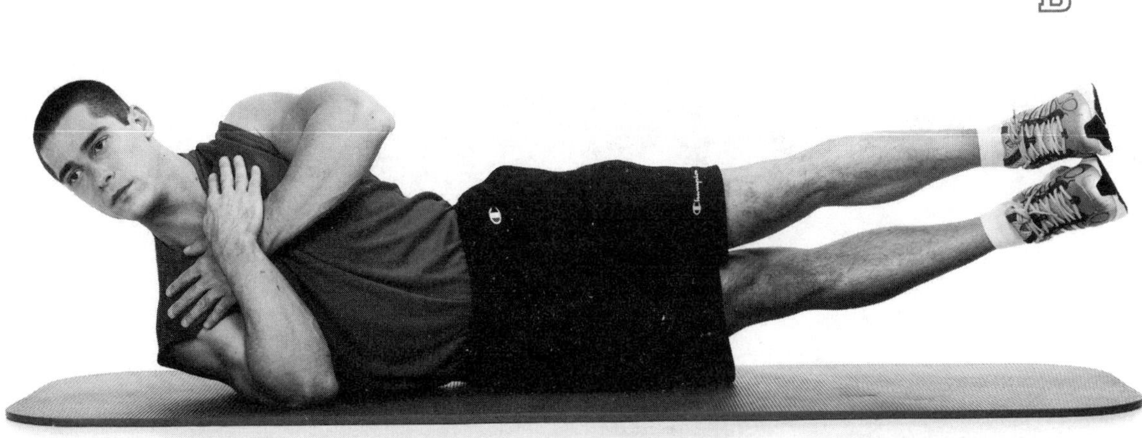

UNILATERAL BIRD DOG

Get down on all fours with your knees bent 90 degrees and your arms directly beneath your shoulders.

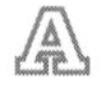

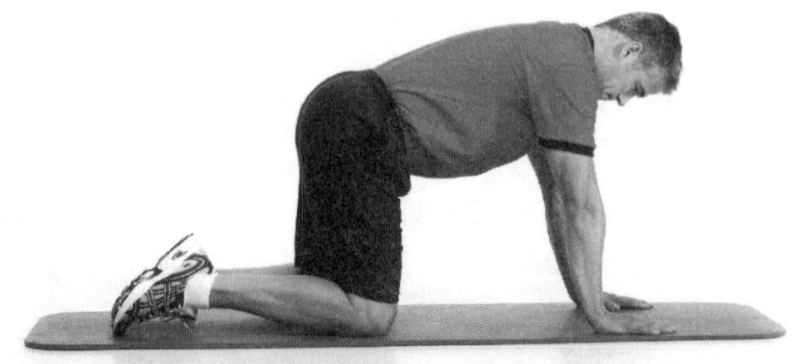

Brace your core muscles as you simultaneously attempt to lift up your right arm and leg until they're parallel to the floor, allowing as little rotation in your hips and torso as possible. Lower and repeat with your left side.

B

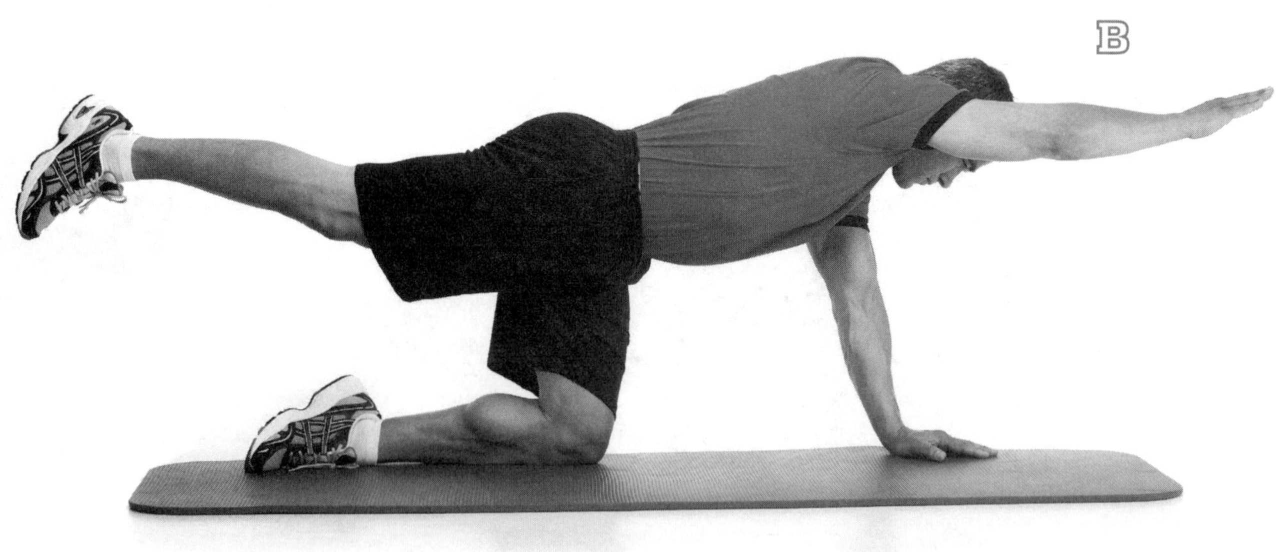

A MODEL FOR SUCCESS

EXAMPLES OF HOW TO PUT YOUR PLAN INTO ACTION

Having now established a thorough understanding of just what these workouts entail, let's look at examples of how two different types of beginners might put them into action. Let's start with an 18-year-old newbie who's never even walked into a gym before and wants to build a little muscle mass. The workout prescription for this person, according to his current physical status and goals, would be as follows:

Flexibility: Workout A

Strength: Workout B

Core: Workout A

Cardio: Workout A

Based on this model, he would determine his allotted workout time and make it fit his specifications. How can he do this, seeing as how the workout guidelines seem to have specific time requirements? Simple: He just chooses the appropriate number of repetitions for each component of the training. For instance, the cardio workout he selected calls for 12 to 15 intervals. Since cardio work isn't a big priority to him, he could opt to stay closer to the shorter time frame.

Compare this to the approach of a 55-year-old ex-jock who'd like to improve his golf game and drop a few pounds. His priority list might look more like this:

Flexibility: Workout B, plus additional static stretching at the end of the workout

Cardio: Workout B

Strength: Workout B

Core: Workout B

Given his age and low level of fitness, I would advise him to stay near the lower end of the scale when it comes to the volume recommendations. This means doing fewer cardio intervals and fewer sets of strength and core training. However, since his training volume will be so low, he should be able to work out more frequently without fear of overtraining. So doing a routine like this as often as three times per week would not be unreasonable.

A *NEW* BEGINNING

CHOOSING A DIFFERENT PATH CAN BE TOUGH

I know what you're thinking: "If this is basic, what are the workouts going to be like in the latter phases of the program?" Not everyone has the wherewithal and the patience to take the path you've chosen. You have put in a lot of work so far and should be commended for the tremendous strides you've already made. Just don't go resting on your laurels, because this is far from the end of the road. You've got a lot more work to do in the pages ahead.

Take solace in the fact that you've given yourself an excellent chance to succeed. If you implement everything you've learned up until this point, your body will not only look better but actually *work* better. You'll be stronger, able to endure more, and, perhaps best of all, able to move more freely and efficiently. Rather than just treating fitness as some completely vanity-driven pursuit, you're well on your way to building yourself a body that can actually be useful outside of the gym. That's more than most beginners can say. In fact, it's more than many of the guys pumping up in front of the mirrors at the local sweat palace can lay claim to. Stick around, though. If you think the changes you've made so far are inspiring, you ain't seen nothing yet.

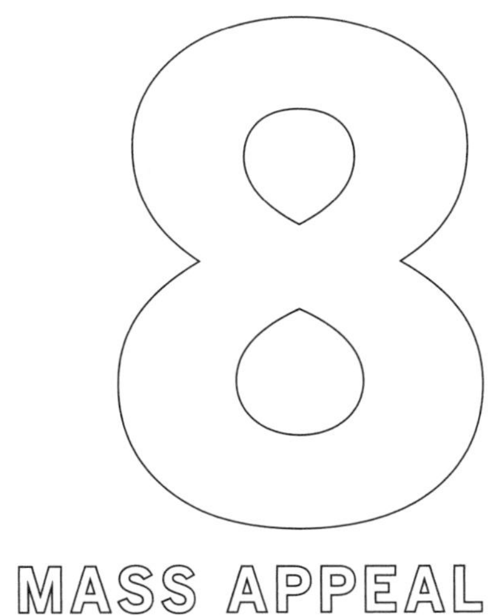

MASS APPEAL

PHASE 4: EVEN BEGINNERS CAN BENEFIT FROM ADDING A LITTLE MUSCLE

When it comes to strength training, one of the most common complaints I hear from beginners is that they don't want to get "too big." Newbies constantly look at the biggest, buffest guys at the gym and start listing all the reasons why they don't want to look like them. As if having a body like that were easy. The truth is, it takes months if not years of hard work and determination to sport the kind of physique that will turn heads. Granted, some guys take the shortcut and use steroids, but most rely on nothing more than gut-busting effort and meticulous attention to their training and nutritional habits. To think you could look like them by merely picking up a loaded barbell is ludicrous.

I can't help but laugh when I overhear a novice trainee telling his personal trainer that he doesn't want to increase the weight on the bar because he's worried about getting "too bulky." I mean, sure, if he's struggling with a certain amount of weight or using improper technique, I can understand his point. But when he's just cranked out 12 to 15 reps without breaking a sweat, it's time to increase the load a bit!

If you want to increase your muscle mass, you must present your body with enough of a training stimulus to create an overload (gym-speak for challenging your muscles to do more than they have before). And believe me, you *do* want to increase the amount of muscle you're carrying on your frame. Consider the effect that a few extra pounds of muscle will have on your metabolism. Because it's so much more metabolically active than fat, muscle tissue burns calories when you're just sitting around doing nothing, let alone when you're working out. That's a big help in keeping body fat in check. Then there's the whole aesthetic angle. A little added muscle might result in some extra attention. By the way, you're kidding yourself if you think adding a few extra pounds is going to make you look too bulky. It would take a lot more than the workouts you'll find in this book to make you look like the guys on the cover of the muscle magazines, so quit worrying about that.

I realize that for some of you this requires a radical shift in the way you perceive strength training. There are legions of runners and other endurance athletes who feel that adding too much muscle mass will somehow impede their performance. Believe me, it's not going to happen, for a couple of reasons. First, with all the endurance exercise you do, it's going to be extremely difficult to add the amount of muscle mass that would negatively impact your performance. Consuming enough calories is imperative to supporting muscle growth, and considering the number of calories you burn through endurance exercise, making huge increases in muscle mass will be next to impossible. And second, any muscle mass you do add will likely prove beneficial, adding more strength and support to the muscles and joints that you use for your sport.

On the other hand, there are those to whom this whole notion of picking up a little extra muscle mass will be more than welcome. Just don't be surprised if you, too, need to change your current mind-set when it comes to pumping iron. I say this because most of the information about strength training circulated by the mainstream media is extremely misguided. It relies too heavily on machines (more on why this is a problem shortly), often warns of the "dangers" of exercises like squats and deadlifts (lifts that when done properly are some of the most effective), and perpetuates the archaic bodybuilding mentality that should have died out years ago.

TIME FOR A CHANGE

A NEW APPROACH TO MUSCLE BUILDING

To build muscle, there are basically two things you need to do. One is eating enough calories to support muscle growth (more on this shortly) and the other is overloading your muscles with enough resistance to spur growth. In order to accomplish the latter, your best bet is to lift as much weight as you can through the use of big, compound lifts such as squats, chinups, and overhead presses. When done with proper form, such movements not only activate large amounts of muscle mass but in doing so also trigger a greater release of muscle-building hormones like growth hormone and testosterone, compared to isolation exercises like biceps curls or calf raises.

It's important to keep in mind that your objective should be overload, not overkill. A few good, intense sets of a couple of different compound movements are more than adequate to bring about noticeable changes in your physique over the course of several weeks. You don't have to spend 2 hours a day "blasting your muscles from every conceivable angle" as you would read about in the muscle mags. You also don't have to worry about dividing your body into little individualized segments and then devoting an entire workout to each of those segments just to gain a little extra size. In fact, unless you have superior genetics or an awfully good pharmacist, that kind of approach just doesn't work for us "regular guys."

And yet, in weight rooms far and wide, marathon workouts rife with isolation exercises seem to be the rule rather than the exception. Why? One word: bodybuilding. Somewhere along the line, the idea of lifting weights to get bigger muscles became synonymous with a bunch of guys with bad tans and Day-Glo spandex tank tops admiring themselves in the mirror while they

BETTER SAFE THAN SORRY

Safety tips for free-weight training

Always use collars. These handy little clamps that secure the weights to the bar can be a real godsend if you somehow lose your balance during a lift. In addition to keeping you from getting hurt, they can also save you tons of embarrassment by preventing weights from crashing to the floor.

Ask for a spot when working with heavy weights. Do yourself a favor and can the macho attitude. There's no shame in having someone keep an eye on you when you're lifting the heavy iron. A spotter is simply someone who stands by from a position where he or she can offer just enough assistance to help you if you get stuck. Most of your fellow gym members will be more than happy to comply with your request for a spot; just be sure to return the favor when asked.

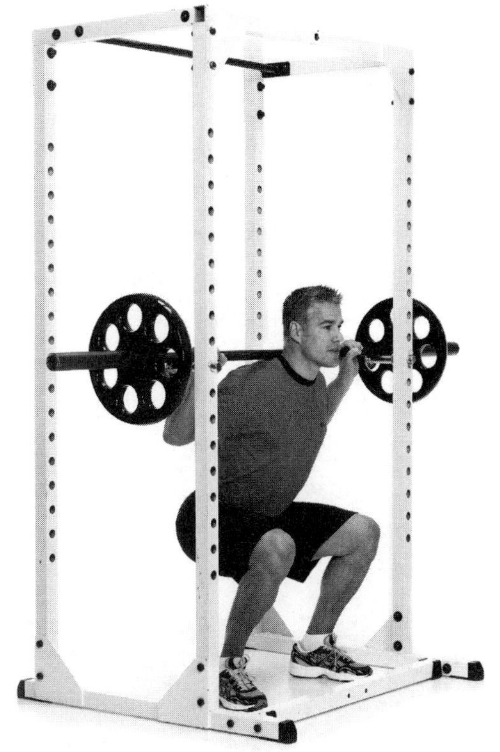

Never attempt a repetition you're not sure you can get. In case you don't have access to a spotter, always be sure you can complete that last rep. If there's even the slightest bit of hesitation in your mind, take a pass. The only exception to this rule is if you perform the exercise inside a squat rack or power cage with safety supports on each side as in the photo at right. In the event that you can't get the bar back up, you can simply lower it down until it rests on the supports.

Use light weights when trying out a new exercise. Free weights can be tricky, especially for the uninitiated. There's a lot more to them than simply raising and lowering the weights. Things like balance and coordination come into play in a big way. If you've never tried an exercise before, be sure to go slowly at first and resist the urge to impress others. There'll be plenty of time down the road to add more weight once you get the form down right.

Use good form at all times. Yeah, yeah, I know you've heard it before. Apparently it bears repeating, though, because so many people fail to heed this seemingly simple advice. It is never a good idea to sacrifice form in the quest to bang out another rep or two. When your technique starts to suffer, it's your body's way of telling you the target muscles have given it all they've got. You don't get extra points for pushing beyond the limits of what your body can endure. In fact, you might end up seriously hurting yourself.

pumped up. Believe it or not, the overwhelming majority of guys who lift have no aspirations of getting up on stage in front of a bunch of strangers, clad only in a Speedo. So why, then, is this style of training still considered by many to be the preferred method?

If you ask me, it really all boils down to blind tradition and a fear of deviating from the norm. After all, if the average guy walks into a gym and all he sees is people doing bench presses and biceps curls, chances are, he's going to follow suit, especially if he has no training experience of his own from which to draw. Not to mention the fact that, as I alluded to earlier, whatever training advice he's able to glean from muscle mags will feature this same, tired approach. So what is he supposed to do? Rock the boat by training in a manner considered to be foreign by "those in the know"?

In a word, yes!

Remember a few chapters ago when I kidded you about getting strange looks from other gym members because of some of the exercises you'll be doing? Well, as you're now well aware, I wasn't kidding. And I've got news for you: Those strange looks aren't going to stop anytime soon. I speak from experience here. About a decade ago, when I first started buying into this more individualized approach and doing some innovative exercises I learned from some of the best strength coaches in the world, I got my share of funny looks. But I stayed the course because I knew I was onto something. And I'm urging you to do the same.

Even when you start doing some more "traditional" types of exercises, like the ones contained in this chapter, you're bound to raise an eyebrow or two because of the way the exercises are grouped or the seemingly low volume of the programs. Case in point: I once had this huge guy tell me that I shouldn't superset squats with chinups. When I asked him why, he got all agitated and finally blurted out, "Because you just shouldn't." What he really meant to say was that it was because he had never seen it done before in any of the bodybuilding magazines, and it must therefore be a useless way to train. Then again, maybe he actually did say that, and I just couldn't hear him over his clown pants and neon tank top.

The cynicism of others aside for a moment, even those of you who train at home alone may find yourself questioning the relative brevity of the routines contained in this chapter. Keep in mind that you're a beginner. One of the biggest mistakes most beginners make is that they do too much, too soon and end up turning themselves off to the whole idea of exercise for months, if not years, to come. By starting out with what I like to call the "real guy's" approach to muscle building, you'll not only see results but also avoid the type of burnout and fatigue that will prevent you from building on those results. It doesn't take endless hours in the gym or a fortune spent on supplements. It does, however, require an open mind.

HEAVY METAL

ADDING MORE WEIGHT TO YOUR WORKOUTS

In this 4-to-6-week muscle-building phase, you'll probably notice quite a bit of carryover from the exercises in the Basic Training phase. The biggest difference between these workouts and the ones you did in that previous phase will undoubtedly be the amount of weight that you're using. That's because loading is the variable that your body most quickly adapts to. Meaning that there's no need to change all of the exercises just for variety's sake. As a beginner, you're much better off sticking with exercises longer to help build familiarization. Periodically altering the amount of weight you're using will be enough to bring about increases in size and strength.

There'll be plenty of time to change the exercises later on, when you become more advanced.

One of the things that makes heavier loads so effective in terms of building muscle is that they cause a greater release of muscle-building hormones. However, in order to take full advantage of this hormonal surge, you need adequate recovery time between sets. String your sets together too closely and you'll compromise your ability to handle weights heavy enough to produce muscle growth. So, where you might have taken only 30 to 60 seconds between sets in the previous phase, this time around count on more like 90 seconds to 2 minutes. That may sound like a lot, but you're going to need it. If it feels like too much, you can always use the opportunity to sneak in some extra flexibility work between sets.

FREESTYLING

BUILDING THE CASE FOR FREE WEIGHTS

Another thing you're bound to notice is the continued emphasis on free weights over machine training. Now, I realize that many experts deem machines safer for beginners than free weights. These folks usually cite the fact that free weights require balance and coordination, whereas machines for the most part offer a set path of resistance that's much easier to control. If you ask me, though, one of the real benefits of free-weight training *is* the stability and control issue. Life requires balance and coordination, so what sense does it make to avoid developing the very attributes your body needs to perform optimally?

Free weights place a far greater demand on all the little stabilizer muscles that assist what are known as the prime movers in taking a weight through the range of motion. An example of these small muscles are those of the rotator cuff, which help stabilize the shoulder joint during upper-body lifts like bench presses and rows. These muscles need strengthening because they help protect and support your shoulder during activities like throwing a ball or loading something up on a high shelf. When you use only machines for upper-body strengthening, these muscles go largely unchallenged because they work through only one set path of motion. This ends up leaving you at a distinct disadvantage when it comes to "real world" activities outside of the gym. Sure, you can increase your muscle mass by using mostly machines, but it'll be the kind of nonfunctional muscle that's good for little other than admiring in the mirror.

Another great thing about free weights is that you can make alterations to the way certain exercises are done in order to both increase their effectiveness and alleviate unnecessary strain on joints, tendons, and ligaments. Take a machine versus a dumbbell chest press, for instance. With the machine you're locked into one set range of motion, but with dumbbells, you can alter the path of the weight, by say using a neutral grip (palms facing each other) and keeping your elbows in closer to your sides.

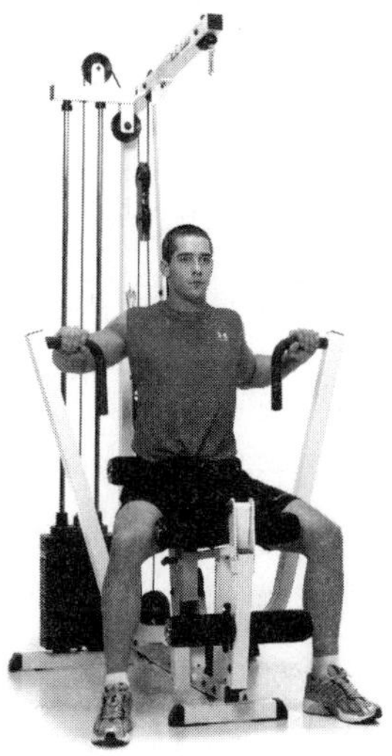

MACHINE CHEST PRESS WITH PRONATED (OVERHAND) GRIP

(continued on page 182)

Sometimes you're all the gym you need

A bodyweight-only muscle-building workout can help kick-start you on your way to more advanced forms of training later on. The following routine can be done two or three times per week and is appropriate for all beginners of all levels. The exercises in this workout have all been arranged into supersets, pairs of exercises for which you perform a given number of repetitions of the first exercise and then take little or no rest before moving on to the second exercise (as indicated by the slash). You then rest for 60 seconds before repeated pairings. Once you've completed the desired number of sets for that pairing, move on to the next. Do each exercise for 2 or 3 sets of 6 to 12 repetitions each. After 6 to 8 weeks, you'll need to start adding some additional weight to your exercises.

Incline pushup/Reverse pushup

Unilateral touch/Unilateral supine bridge

Bird dog/Situp

Lunge/Chair dip

INCLINE PUSHUP

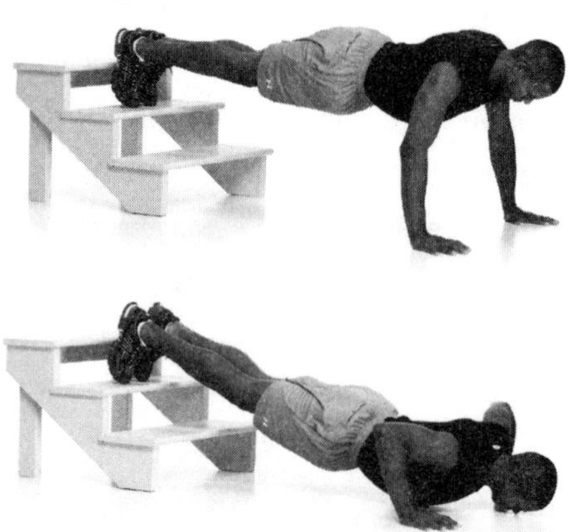

Get into a pushup position with your feet propped up on a step or crate.

Keeping your back completely straight, slowly bend your elbows and lower your body until your face is just a couple of inches from the floor. Pause and then push back up to the starting position.

REVERSE PUSHUP

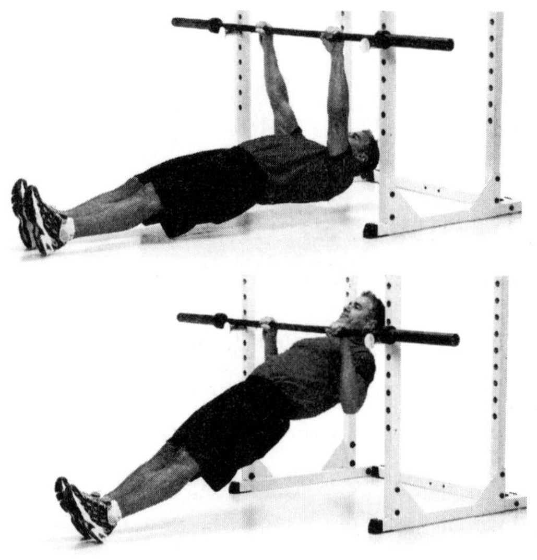

Lie under a heavy, sturdy table or secure a chinup bar in a doorway, 3 to 4 feet above the floor. Lie under the table or the bar and grab it with a shoulder-width, overhand grip. Hang at arm's length with your body in a straight line from your ankles to your shoulders.

Keeping your body rigid, pull your chest up as far as possible. Pause, then lower yourself back to the starting position.

UNILATERAL TOUCH

Set a water bottle or other handy object on the floor about $1\frac{1}{2}$ feet in front of you. Next, stand upright and lift one leg off the floor and hold it bent behind you at a 90-degree angle.

Begin by sitting back into your hips as you squat down and simultaneously reach forward to touch the bottle. Reach with the arm on the same side as your bent leg. Once you touch it, pause for a second before pushing back up to the starting position. Finish your set and then do the same number of reps with your other leg bent.

UNILATERAL SUPINE BRIDGE

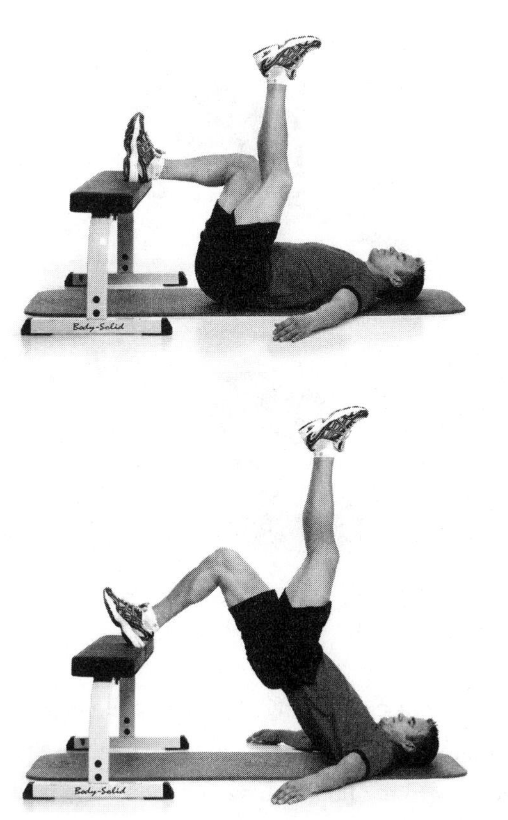

Lie faceup on the floor in front of an exercise bench or sturdy step. Bend one knee at a 90-degree angle and place it on the bench or step as you lift the other leg up so it lines up over your hip.

Begin by pressing the heel of the leg with the bent knee into the bench or step and lifting your hips off the floor until your body forms a diagonal line from your head to your knees. Pause, lower, and repeat. Once you finish the desired number of repetitions, switch to the other leg.

(continued)

BIRD DOG

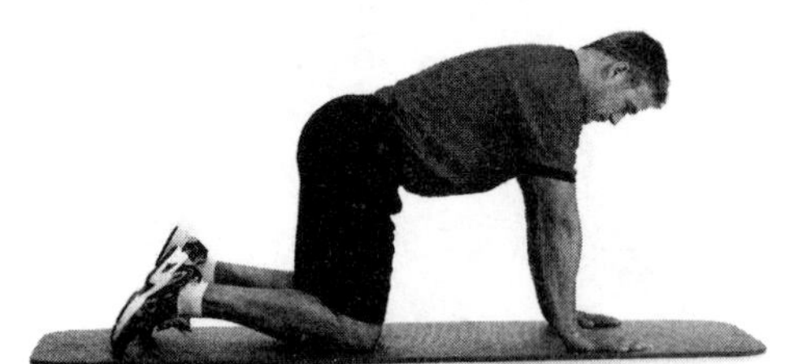

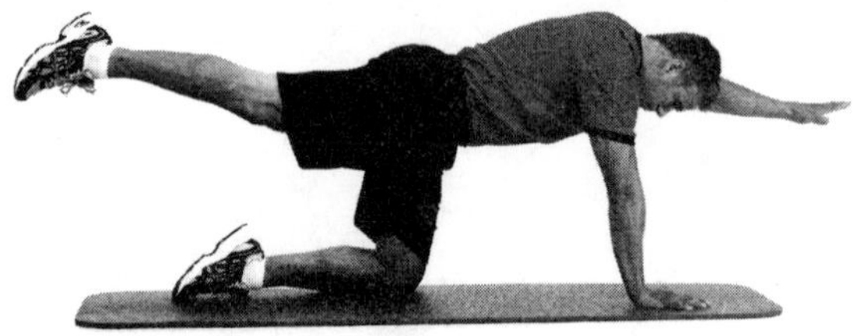

Get down on the floor on all fours.

Brace your core tightly and simultaneously straighten your left arm and right leg until they're parallel to the floor. Pause and then lower and repeat on the other side, lifting your right arm and left leg. That's one rep. Continue this pattern until you've completed the desired number of repetitions.

SITUP

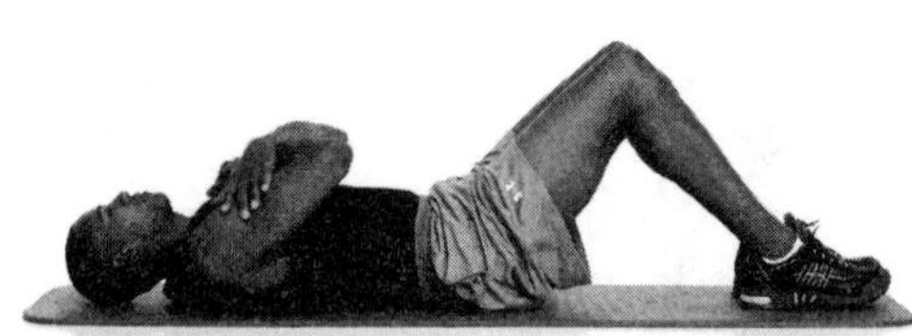

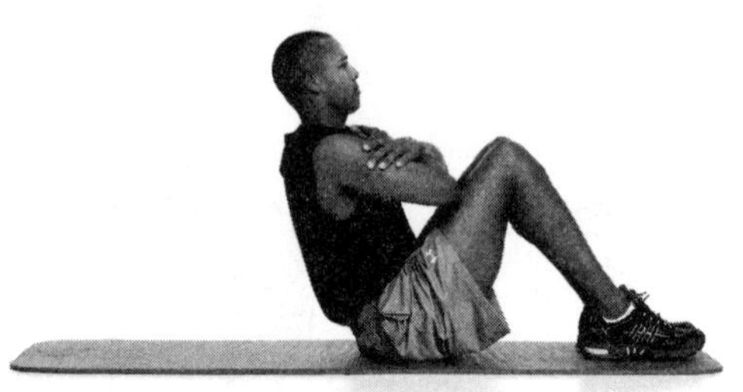

Lie faceup on the floor with your knees bent about 90 degrees and your feet flat.

Keeping your arms at your sides, or folded across your chest, use your abdominals to pull yourself up to a seated position. Hold for a second and lower back down with control.

LUNGE

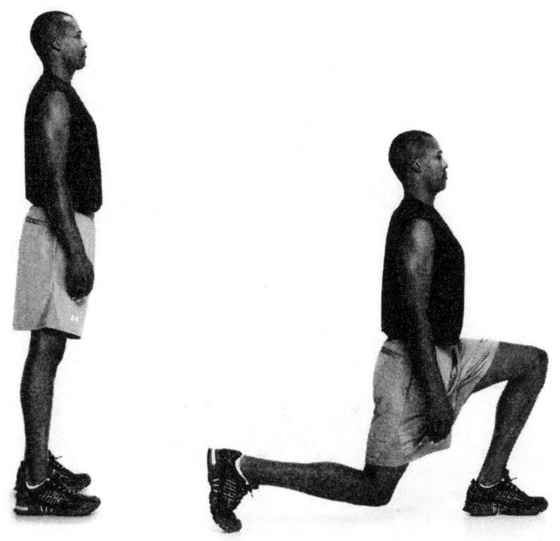

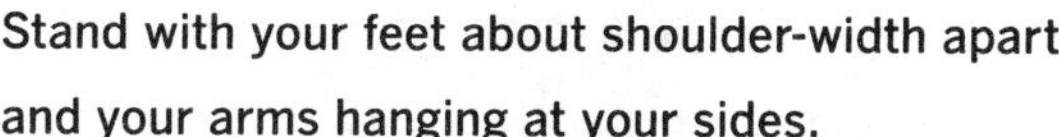

Stand with your feet about shoulder-width apart and your arms hanging at your sides.

Begin by stepping forward and bending both knees until the front knee reaches a 90-degree angle and the back one almost touches the floor. Once there, immediately press back up to the starting position and repeat on the other side. That's one rep. Continue this pattern until you complete the desired number of repetitions.

CHAIR DIP

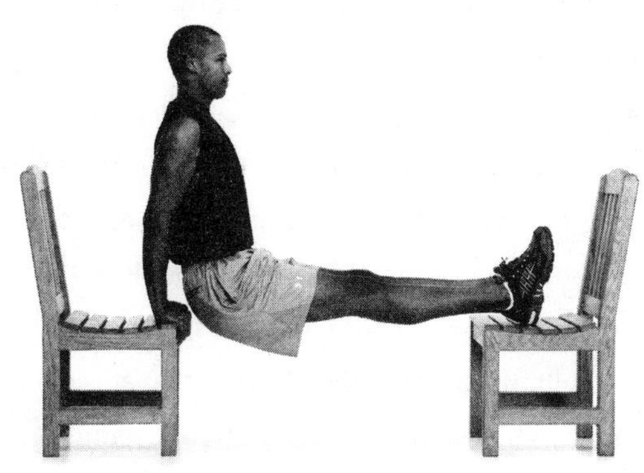

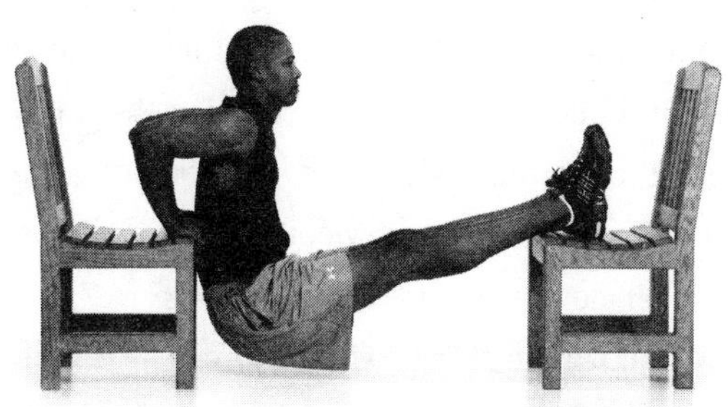

Set up a couple of chairs or sturdy benches several feet apart. Begin by placing both hands on the seat of one chair or bench and your outstretched legs on the other one.

Keeping your torso as straight as possible, bend at the elbows and lower yourself until your upper arms are parallel to the floor. Pause for a second and push yourself back up to the starting position.

Such a dumbbell press technique can reduce the likelihood of developing a shoulder impingement, a painful condition that often results from doing too many pressing movements (both overhead and lying) with your elbows flared out away from your body.

Let's assume that shoulder pain isn't a concern. You can also intensify the contraction you get in your chest by doing dumbbell presses this same way but rotating the dumbbells at the top. Using a neutral grip at the bottom of the movement (photo A), press the dumbbells up while simultaneously rotating them so that at the top of the movement the thumb sides of your hands come together in a pronated grip (photo B).

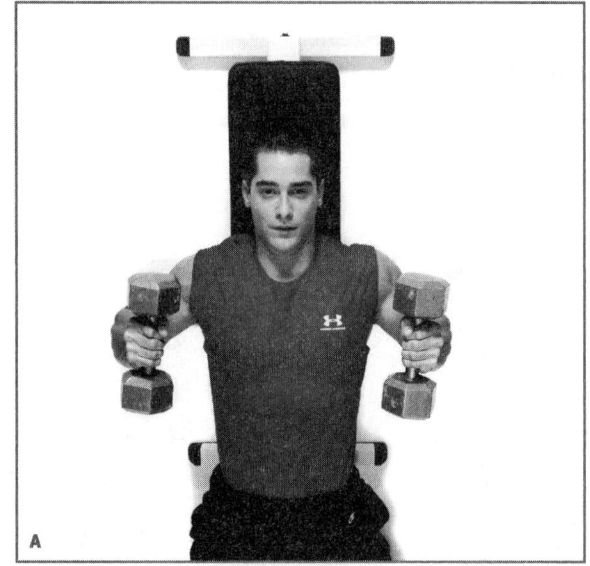
A

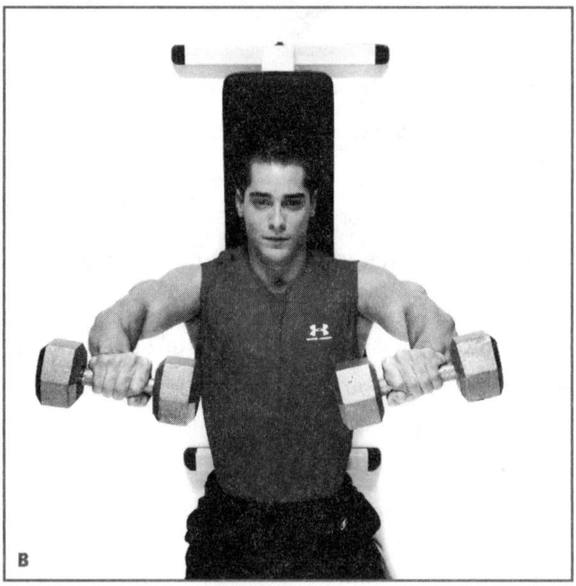
B

DUMBBELL BENCH PRESS WITH GRIP ROTATION

This combines the two primary functions of the chest, or pectoral, muscles in one motion. You're not only bringing your arms across the front of your body (known as horizontal adduction) but also rotating them inward (internal rotation). This produces a much more forceful contraction of the pecs than would a standard dumbbell press—let alone a machine press.

You can achieve a similar effect with overhead presses, rows, and a whole slew of other free-weight exercises. Several times throughout the book, I'll provide more effective and/or joint friendly alternatives to staple lifts. This way, regardless of your age, previous injury history, or current level of conditioning, you'll still be able to reap plenty of benefits from the programs. It might be as simple as changing the width of your stance or grip, or maybe altering the path in which you lift or lower the bar. Whatever the case, it's a feature unique to free weights.

Finally, I'd like to examine the issue of safety. As I mentioned earlier, one of the biggest reasons that beginners often avoid free weights is because they think they're somehow dangerous. The only things that make a free-weight exercise dangerous are using too much weight, sloppy technique, or both. Granted, preexisting injuries may preclude doing particular exercises like squats and deadlifts. But when you're healthy, there is nothing inherently dangerous about free-weight training. Oh sure, do something stupid like bench press alone in a basement and get pinned, or forget to use collars and dump all your weights on the floor, and you might get hurt. Nothing bad will happen, though, as long as you lift with your head instead of your ego and always take proper safety precautions (see "Better Safe Than Sorry on page 175").

Having said all that, I'm certainly not against the use of machines altogether. There are times when machines can prove useful. So, if all you have access to are machines, you're still going to learn how to use them, because I will include some in the workouts that follow. I'll even go so far as to offer machine alternatives to certain free-weight lifts that I think some might find too challenging, like chinups and squats, for instance. For the most part, though, it's going to be all free weights, all the time.

APPETITE FOR CONSTRUCTION

MUSCLE-BUILDING NUTRITION

By now you're probably thinking that this whole muscle-building phase is stacking up to be quite a bit different than what you did during the first 8 weeks. Well, you ain't seen nothing yet. I'm about to go into detail about the nutritional changes you're going to have to make to add more muscle to your frame. Building on the good habits you've already established in the first two phases, we're going to examine the impact of things like increasing your caloric intake, adding more protein to your diet, adjusting what you eat before and after your workouts, and considering what types of nutritional supplements may prove beneficial.

Feeding Frenzy

You've Got to Eat If You Want to Grow

If you're not eating enough to build muscle, it doesn't matter what workout program you're doing. So the first thing you'll need to do is increase your caloric intake above your total daily energy requirement (TDEE) that you calculated in Chapter 3. As mentioned previously, just how much of an increase you need depends on both the amount of muscle you want to build and how quickly you're looking to build it. Keeping within a manageable 10 to 20 percent above your TDEE should help ensure that the bulk of the weight you gain will be in the form of muscle mass and not body fat.

Of course, these excess calories can't come from just any old source. It's not like scoffing down a couple of Twinkies and a quart of chocolate milk is going to give you bulging biceps. You'll want to try to ensure that these extra calories come in the form of quality food choices like the ones I'm about to discuss.

As you'll notice, I've tried to keep things as realistic as possible here. I'm not telling you that you should never eat the foods in the "Avoid or Eat Less of These" category on page 187. All I ask is that you limit their consumption and, instead, more often opt for some of the suggested foods in the "Eat More of These" section on that page. In fact, here's a nice little trick I learned from my colleague John Berardi, who co-authored *Scrawny to Brawny*: Try to be good 85 to 90 percent of the time, and you'll be way ahead of the game. Say you figure out that it's going to take you five meals per day to take in all the calories you need for muscle growth. Five meals multiplied by seven days per week add up to 35 meals a week. That means that anywhere between 27 and 32 of those meals need to be made up of the foods from the "Eat More of These" list. That leaves anywhere from three to eight meals of "Avoid or Eat Less of These" foods, depending on just how good you want to be.

One way to get some of your additional calories, especially immediately after your workout, is through

(continued on page 186)

JOHNNY-ON-THE-SPOT

Spotting techniques for staple lifts

A spotter is someone who keeps a watchful eye over you as you perform an exercise. He or she is usually positioned in close proximity to you to help you keep the bar moving if you get stuck. A spotter can also help you unrack and rerack your weights during heavy squats and bench presses, assisting you in guiding the bar off of and then back onto the supports at the end of the set.

Being a good spotter requires focus as well as a thorough understanding of how to best position yourself to assist the lifter should he or she experience any difficulty. Here's a quick spotting guide for several key exercises.

BARBELL BENCH PRESS

Stand behind the bench press rack so that you are positioned directly over the bar. Once the lifter sets his grip, ask if he needs a "lift off" (this would entail your helping lift the bar off the supports and guiding it directly over his chest). As the lifter begins to lower the bar, bend your knees and lean over him slightly with your hands positioned close to the bar in a pronated (palms facing downward) position. Continue to stay close to the bar as the lifter presses it up and lowers it back down again.

Touch the bar only if you notice it start to slow down appreciably. If it does slow, do not wait for it to come to a dead stop so that the lifter struggles! Grasp the bar, gently guide it back up to the top position, and help the lifter rerack the weight onto the supports.

DUMBBELL BENCH OR SHOULDER PRESS

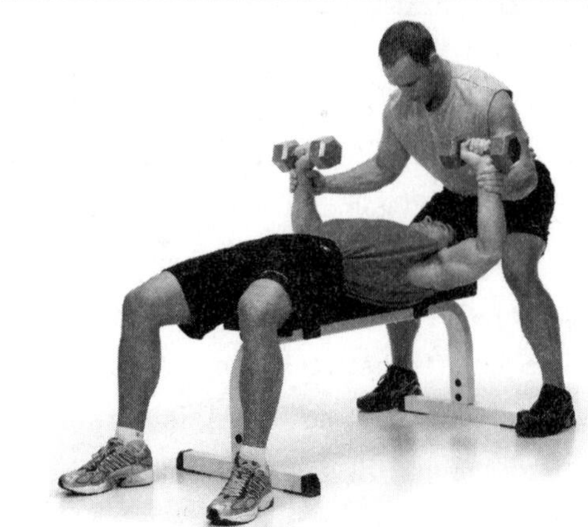

DUMBBELL BENCH PRESS, HANDS ON WRISTS

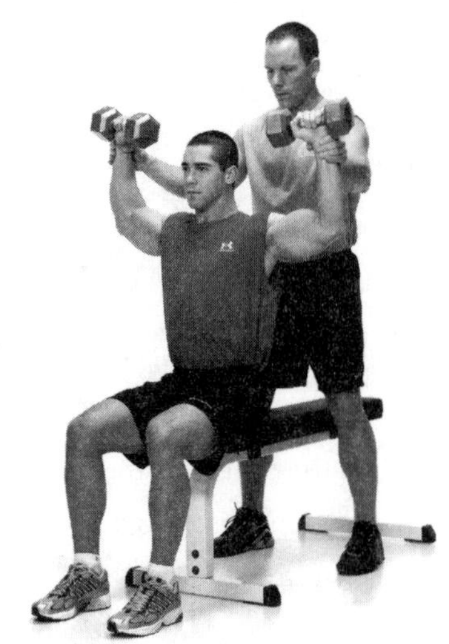

DUMBBELL SHOULDER PRESS, HANDS ON WRISTS

Spotting dumbbell exercises is a little bit tougher because the weight is more concentrated in each hand. Some feel that the spotter pushing on the lifter's elbows is the best way to get the weight up, while others are more inclined to grasp the wrists. I personally opt for the wrists and here's why: When pushing on someone's elbows, it's easy to give too much of an inward, rather than an upward, push. If the lifter is somewhat inexperienced, this could result in the weights collapsing inward onto his chest (during bench presses) or head (during shoulder presses). Obviously, this presents a potentially disastrous situation. If, however, you grasp a person's wrists during these lifts, you can more easily guide the weights upward.

The only knock on spotting in this fashion comes from those who argue that the spotter will not be able to offer much assistance from this position. True enough. But a spotter is supposed to offer just enough of an assist to get the lifter through the sticking point. If the lifter requires a big push from under his elbows, it could be argued that the weight he's using is too heavy for him to use for the desired number of reps.

To spot people during either of these exercises, keep your hands just outside their wrists or upper forearms and, once they get into trouble, grasp them around this area and guide the weight up. When spotting a shoulder press, you can do this from a standing position just behind the person, whereas a bench press might require you to squat, or to kneel down behind him to avoid potential strain on your lower back.

BARBELL SQUAT

This is without question one of the toughest exercises to spot properly. Once the lifter unracks the bar and walks back into position, your job as the spotter is to get in right behind him and position your arms underneath his armpits. Once he begins his descent, you then proceed to squat up and down with him, keeping those arms extended beneath his armpits so you can grab and steady his torso should he begin to lean forward. Your primary objectives as a spotter during this exercise are to keep his torso as upright as possible and keep the weight moving. If you wait until he gets stuck and the weight is heavy enough, it is unlikely you'll be able to get him back up, and you could both get seriously hurt.

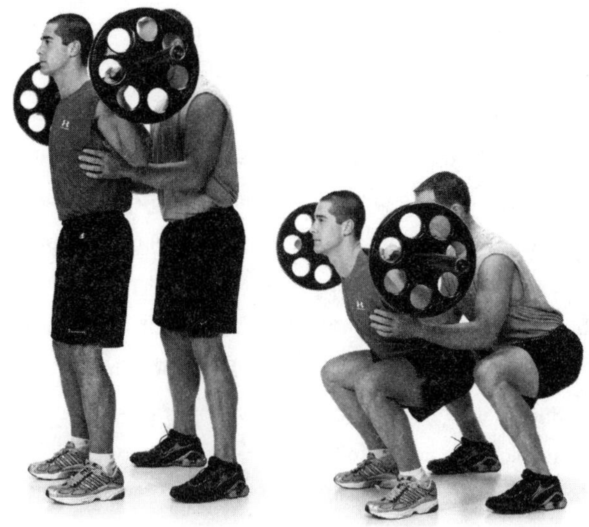

CHINUP/PULLUP

Begin by positioning yourself directly behind the lifter. As soon as he begins to pull himself up, fan out your hands and place them just above the curvature of his lower back, at the base of his rib cage. Once he starts to struggle, gently push him up toward the bar. While most people opt to spot pullups from the ankles, I prefer this position because it stresses proper form. When you spot someone from the ankles, it's easy for him to cave in his chest at the top of the movement. This takes away from the contraction of the upper-back musculature. By pushing him up from his middle back, you essentially make it impossible for him to cave in his chest and, as a result, you increase the effectiveness of the exercise.

(continued from page 183)

the use of liquid meals. When it comes to muscle growth, nutrition experts refer to the first 30 minutes following resistance exercise as the "window of opportunity." That's because this is the time when your muscles are looking to replenish some of the energy you used and repair the damage caused by your workout. Drinking a mixture of whey protein and fast-acting carbohydrates like fruit juices or maltodextrin after your workout has been shown to accelerate the muscle-building process more rapidly than not eating or consuming a solid meal. You can find whey protein at most vitamin/ nutritional supplement suppliers, and maltodextrin can be bought either online or, believe it or not, from liquor stores.

Why such specific ingredients? It's all about the absorption rate. Whey protein is more rapidly absorbed than other protein sources, and the fast-acting carbs are sucked up by hungry muscles looking for a quick fix for the energy deficit caused by your workout. As effective as these ingredients are, though, you can't just combine them haphazardly. The conventional wisdom holds that a 2:1 ratio of fast-acting carbs to protein seems to work best. So if you use a typical one-scoop serving (approximately 24 grams) of whey protein, count on combining that with at least 48 grams of carbs, or about the amount contained in one large, single-serving fruit juice.

As long as we're on the topic of carbs, I would like you to pay attention to the type of carbs you're eating. Simple carbs, like those in your post-workout drink and in fruits and sugary drinks, are very rapidly absorbed by your bloodstream. This causes an initial burst of energy followed by a quick drop once the hormone insulin is released to help bring your blood sugar levels back to normal. Why should you care about that? Besides making you feel lethargic once the insulin does kick in, it also has the nasty little habit of promoting fat storage. So the more times per day you trigger insulin's release, the more apt you are to store the calories you're consuming as fat.

You'd be much better off eating more complex, or slow-acting, carbs like yams, oatmeal, brown rice, whole grain breads and cereals, and vegetables. These types of carbs take longer for your body to break down, and they create a more sustained energy release, rather than the quick blood sugar spike of simple carbs. Beware, though: All complex carbs are not created equal. There are actually a few so-called complex carbs that really act like simple carbs, as evidenced by the effect they have on your blood sugar levels. White potatoes and white breads are perfect examples of this, since both raise your blood sugar levels about as fast as will eating a tablespoon of pure sugar.

It's all got to do with something called the glycemic index (GI), a measure of how quickly a food breaks down into blood sugar (see the table on the page 189). The higher the number, the faster the breakdown and the less desirable the food. Familiarize yourself with this index and focus on eating mainly low-GI foods throughout the day, saving high-GI choices for the period leading up to and immediately following your workout. This way, as long as you keep their intake within reason, you'll be able to enjoy carbohydrates without having to worry about storing them as excess body fat.

SUPPLEMENTAL FOCUS

A BEGINNER'S GUIDE TO SUPPLEMENT USAGE

I know that a lot of beginners, especially those past their early twenties, are wary about using nutritional supplements. I'm not talking about creatine or weight

Eat More of These	Avoid or Eat Less of These
Breakfast	
Slow-cooked oatmeal	Instant hot cereals
Yogurt (plain, with added fruit)	Cold cereals
Eggs (one yolk to every three whites)	Doughnuts
Whole grain breads	White breads and bagels
Fruits	Pop Tarts, etc.
Unsalted nuts	Cookies and crackers
Granola bars	Bacon and sausage
Peanut butter	Cream cheese and margarine
Juices	Butter (use sparingly)
Lunch and Dinner	
Turkey, fish, and lean red meat	Cold cuts
Pasta (especially whole wheat, cooked al dente)	White breads and bagels
Rice (brown)	White rice and potatoes
Yams and sweet potatoes	Fried foods
Steamed vegetables	Instant microwave meals
Pizza (occasionally)	Hot dogs
Whole grain breads	Soda
Yogurt (plain, with added fruit)	Whole milk
Nuts	
Granola bars	
Water and sports drinks (after or during physical activity)	
Milk (skim, 1, and 2 percent)	
Snacks	
Fresh fruit	Cookies
Trail mix	Chips
Nuts and seeds (lightly salted or unsalted)	
Cottage cheese	
Yogurt (plain, with added fruit)	
Granola and energy bars (watch sugar content)	

gainer drinks. Think more along the lines of a good multivitamin/mineral formula, some essential fatty acids, and meal-replacing protein drinks that can provide a quick, convenient source of that most precious of nutrients. These supplements act as an insurance policy of sorts to help you cover all your bases and make sure you provide everything your body needs to support muscle growth. Here are a few details about each type, plus some advice on how you can best fit them into your daily diet.

Multivitamin/mineral formula. It's difficult to provide your body with all of the nutrients it needs from food sources alone, so a good multivitamin/mineral helps cover all of your nutritional bases. Look for a brand that offers sustained release or that allows you to split up your dosage over the course of the day. Your body uses vitamins at different times throughout the day, so taking them all at once may not allow you to derive the maximum benefit. Also, look for minerals that come in "chelated" form, as this is the way they're most rapidly absorbed by your body.

There's currently a lot of confusion surrounding what to look for in a multivitamin/mineral. Here are a few tips most experts seem to agree on.

- Always choose natural and not synthetic brands of multis.
- Make sure the multivitamin possesses 100 percent of the Recommended Daily Allowance (RDA) for *most* of the nutrients listed on the label.
- Look for a copper to zinc ratio of 1:1.
- Make sure it has adequate amounts of key nutrients such as calcium (at least 45 percent RDA), magnesium (at least 50 percent RDA), and phosphorus (at least 35 percent RDA).

Meal replacement drinks (MRDs). With today's hectic schedules, meal replacement drinks offer a convenient way to ensure you get high-quality protein to build muscle, slow-acting carbs to give you more long-lasting energy, and essential fats to help keep your hunger in check. Most MRDs have fewer than 300 calories per serving and mix well in water with a simple shaker bottle. Some even come in ready-to-drink containers for the ultimate in convenience. Among the best are Myoplex, Met-RX, and Prolab's Lean Mass Matrix.

Protein powders. These are different from meal replacement drinks in that they are straight protein. Sometimes you may not want all the carbs and essential fats that come in MRDs. Whether you are cutting carbs and want a quick snack before bed or you're just looking for ways to add more protein to your diet, protein powder offers the perfect solution. For a healthy, muscle-building breakfast, you can blend it into a shake or just sprinkle some on your oatmeal in the morning. Just be sure that the kind you get is a mixture of several different proteins (like whey, casein, and egg albumin) and not just straight whey. A protein mix will give you a more sustained protein release, instead of the quick absorption of whey, which is only desirable immediately post workout (more on this shortly). Pro Blend 55 made by Human Development Technologies is one of the best of this type.

Essential fatty acids. Not all fats are created equal. Essential fatty acids, or EFAs, are naturally occurring unsaturated fats that are considered essential because they are not produced by the human body. There are two essential fatty acids: linoleic, sometimes referred to as omega-6 fatty acid, and alpha-linolenic, referred to as omega-3 fatty acid. EFAs help support the cardiovascular, reproductive, immune,

GLYCEMIC INDEX

Cereals

Food	GI
All Bran	51
Bran Flakes	74
Cheerios	74
Corn Chex	83
Cornflakes	83
Cream of Wheat	66
Frosted Flakes	55
Grape-Nuts	67
Life	66
Muesli, natural	54
Nutri-grain	66
Oatmeal, old fashioned	48
Puffed Wheat	67
Raisin Bran	73
Rice Chex	89
Shredded Wheat	67
Special K	54
Total	76

Fruit

Food	GI
Apple	38
Apricots	57
Banana	56
Cantaloupe	65
Cherries	22
Dates	103
Grapefruit	25
Grapes	46
Kiwi	52
Mango	55
Orange	43
Papaya	58
Peach	42
Pear	58
Pineapple	66
Plums	39
Prunes	15
Raisins	64
Watermelon	72

Snacks

Food	GI
Chocolate bar	49
Corn chips	72
Croissant	67
Doughnut	76
Jelly beans	80
Life Savers	70
Oatmeal cookie	57
Pizza, cheese & tomato	60
Pizza Hut, supreme	33
Popcorn, light micro	55
Potato chips	56
Pound cake	54
Power bars	58
Pretzels	83
Rice cakes	80
Saltine crackers	74
Shortbread cookies	64
Snickers bar	41
Strawberry jam	51
Vanilla wafers	77

Crackers

Food	GI
Graham	74
Rye	68
Soda	72
Wheat Thins	67

Cereal Grains

Food	GI
Barley	25
Basmati white rice	58
Bulgur	48
Couscous	65
Cornmeal	68
Millet	71

Sugars

Food	GI
Fructose	22
Honey	62
Maltose	105
Table sugar	64

Pasta

Food	GI
Cheese tortellini	50
Fettuccini	32
Linguini	50
Macaroni	46
Spaghetti, 5 min boiled	33
Spaghetti, 15 min boiled	44
Spaghetti, protein enrich	28
Vermicelli	35

Soups/Vegetables

Food	GI
Beets, canned	64
Black bean soup	64
Carrots, fresh, boiled	49
Corn, sweet	56
Green pea soup	66
Green peas, frozen	47
Parsnips	97
Peas, fresh, boiled	48
Split pea soup w/ham	66
Tomato soup	38

Drinks

Food	GI
Apple juice	40
Colas	65
Gatorade	78
Grapefruit juice	48
Orange juice	46
Pineapple juice	46

Milk Products

Food	GI
Chocolate milk	35
Custard	43
Ice cream, vanilla	60
Ice milk, vanilla	50
Skim milk	32
Soy milk	31
Tofu frozen dessert	115
Whole milk	30
Yogurt, fruit	36
Yogurt, plain	14

Beans

Food	GI
Baked	44
Black beans, boiled	30
Butter, boiled	33
Cannellini beans	31
Garbanzo, boiled	34
Kidney, boiled	29
Kidney, canned	52
Lentils, green, brown	30
Lima, boiled	32
Lima beans, frozen	32
Navy beans	38
Pinto, boiled	39
Red lentils, boiled	27
Soy, boiled	16

Breads

Food	GI
Bagel, plain	72
Baguette, French	95
Croissant	67
Dark rye	76
Hamburger bun	61
Pita	57
Pizza, cheese	60
Pumpernickel	49
Sourdough	54
Rye	64
White	70
Wheat	68

Muffins

Food	GI
Apple, cinnamon	44
Blueberry	59
Oat & raisin	54

Root Crops

Food	GI
French fries	75
Potato, new, boiled	59
Potato, red, baked	93
Potato, sweet	52
Potato, white, boiled	63
Potato, white, mashed	70
Yam	54

and nervous systems and are also involved in the manufacturing and repair of cell membranes, enabling the cells to obtain optimum nutrition and expel harmful waste products. EFA deficiency is a big problem in this country—especially omega-3 deficiency, with the average American falling well short of the optimal intake for this vital nutrient. This imbalance in omega 6/3 intake can be linked to such conditions as heart attacks, cancer, high cholesterol, obesity, and even accelerated aging.

Most nutritionists recommend supplementing with 1,000 milligrams of fish oil (in capsule form), which is rich in omega 3s, and 125 milligrams of omega-6s from sources such as borage oil.

To review, the basics of muscle-building nutrition are as follows:

- Increase your caloric intake by anywhere from 10 to 20 percent over your TDER for a reasonable 1-pound muscle gain per week. If that seems like too much for you to eat, or if you're not interested in gaining that much, you can scale back and consume slightly less. Just know that if your goal is to build muscle, you will have to eat above your daily TDER.

- Start supplementing with a good multivitamin/mineral formula, essential fatty acids, and easy-to-mix or ready-made protein drinks.

- Immediately following your workout, down a post-workout drink of simple carbs and whey protein at a 2:1 ratio.

- Stick mainly with low-GI carbohydrate sources throughout the day, reserving faster-acting carbs for immediately after your workout.

THE WORKOUTS

TIME TO START MUSCLE CONSTRUCTION

Finally, after all that buildup, it's time to get down to the actual workouts. Here are three different workout scenarios based on whether you can commit to a 2-, 3-, or 4-day weekly training routine. I've even gone so far as to recommend what workouts work best for different types of beginners based on age and level of previous training experience. Keep in mind that if the recommended workout plan doesn't fit your schedule, you can always select one of the others. These are just general guidelines, so feel free to tailor them to your individual requirements. And in keeping with the true spirit of periodization, you should stick with each of these workouts for 4 to 6 weeks at a time.

Workout Plan	Suggested For
2 days per week total-body plan	Newbies and ex-jocks, 35 and over
3 days per week total-body rotating schedule	Newbies and ex-jocks, under 35
4 days per week upper-and-lower-body split routine	Seasonals of any age and ex-jocks, under 35

To help keep things as simple as possible, all of the workouts in this chapter were put together using a template of just 25 exercises. This will show you how it's possible to vary little more than the sequence of the exercises or the training volume to make three distinctly different workout plans with one set of common exercises. As usual, detailed descriptions and pictures of these lifts are provided, starting on page 195.

It Takes Two

2 Days per Week Total-Body Plan

Do each of the following two workouts once a week, with anywhere from 48 to 72 hours between them. Complete all the sets of a given exercise before moving on to the next one, and keep your rest intervals between 90 seconds and 2 minutes.

Workout A

Barbell squat or leg press: 2 sets × 8 to 10 reps
Lying leg curl: 2 sets × 8 to 10 reps
Barbell bench press: 2 sets × 8 to 10 reps
Prone dumbbell row with elbows out: 2 sets × 8 to 10 reps
Dumbbell calf raise: 2 sets × 8 to 10 reps
Cable external rotation: 2 sets × 10 to 12 reps
Incline reverse crunch: 2 sets × 8 to 10 reps
Weighted Russian twist: 2 sets × 10 to 12 reps (5 to 6 per side)

Workout B

Barbell deadlift or dumbbell deadlift: 2 sets × 8 to 10 reps
Dumbbell lunge: 2 sets × 8 to 10 reps (each leg)
Chinup or lat pulldown: 2 sets × max reps (if more than 5)
Standing barbell shoulder press: 2 sets × 8 to 10 reps
One-arm row with elbow out: 2 sets × 8 to 10 reps
Back extension: 2 sets × 10 to 12 reps
Lateral bridge: 2 sets × 8 to 10 reps (4 or 5 per side)
Swiss ball crunch: 2 sets × 8 to 10 reps

Yes, this is a beginner's workout and, yes, you read correctly when you saw exercises like squats, deadlifts, and chinups included in the program. Bear in mind that you don't have to—and, in fact, shouldn't—lift weights you can't handle. As I mentioned earlier, squats and deadlifts are among the best lifts you can perform. There's no reason for you to steer clear of them just because you're a beginner. Besides, what do you think the corrective phase was for? The whole purpose of doing all of those weird exercises was to get you ready to do exercises like these without fear of injuring yourself.

Of course, if you suffer from lower-back pain of any sort, these lifts might actually do more harm than good. You can try substituting the leg press for the squat; just be careful not to go any lower than parallel (see "Parallel Universe" on page 192). And substitute either a dumbbell deadlift or a trap bar deadlift for the barbell deadlift, since each allows for a more upright posture and less lower-back strain. As for the chinups, maybe I'm just being stubborn, but by the time you finish all the programs in this book, I expect you to be able to do a complete set of them. For now, if you can't muster more than 5 per set, lat pulldowns can be substituted as an acceptable alternative. Try 2 to 3 sets of 6 to 8 reps.

Lower-body exercises are given priority on both days because they activate the largest amount of muscle mass and require the most energy, so you might as well hit them while you're fresh. They also stimulate the biggest release of those aforementioned anabolic hormones that are so important to the muscle-building process. Besides which, if I put them first in the workout, I know they'll get done. Since most guys tend to skimp on leg training anyway, putting them later in the workout is practically guaranteeing they'll get a lousy effort, if not be left out entirely.

Finally, if you're looking for any direct biceps and triceps work, you're out of luck. This phase is about building muscle, plain and simple. The best way to do that is to move the most weight you can handle. If you're doing that, believe me when I tell you that your arms will get all the work they need simply by assisting with your compound lifts. Your triceps will get pounded during bench presses and shoulder presses, and your biceps will get all they can handle on chinups and rows. So resist the urge to improvise by adding in a few sets of biceps and triceps work at the end of your workout.

Triple Play

3 Days per Week Total-Body Rotating Schedule

These two workouts are to be performed on a 3-day-per-week rotating schedule so that each week you do one of the workouts twice and the other just once. That order will then be reversed the following week. So in week one, you do workout A on Monday, B on Wednesday, and A again on Friday. The following Monday then kicks off with workout B, followed by workout A on Wednesday, and then B again on Friday.

In addition, both workouts are series of supersets, meaning that two exercises will be grouped together, with one performed immediately after the other without rest in between. Once you've done both, you then rest for 90 seconds to 2 minutes before repeating the same grouping again (since you're doing 2 sets of each pair) and moving on to the next one.

PARALLEL UNIVERSE

How low should you go during lower-body compound lifts?

The question of how far one should descend during various forms of squats, deadlifts, and leg presses is one of the most hotly debated in the entire fitness industry. For years, physical therapists and personal trainers have advised their clients to stop the lowering portions of these exercises when the thighs have reached a position parallel to the floor (or, in the case of the leg press, the thighs should be parallel to the force plate your feet are planted on). They chose this position because it is supposed to protect the knees against the dangerous shearing forces they might be subjected to if one were to descend lower than parallel. The lower back has also been identified as an area prone to additional stress when the thighs drop below the desired depth.

In recent years, however, more and more experts are advising that people descend lower than parallel (primarily because of increased glute and inner-thigh involvement), maintaining that the shearing forces to the knees are actually lower in a deep squat position than they are in the vaunted 90-degree position. To be able to descend into a deep squat position without compromising proper technique, one must be free of preexisting injuries to the knees and lower back and must display adequate flexibility.

Not being able to personally assess your flexibility, I feel it best to stick with the parallel recommendation in this instance, particularly in the case of the leg press, as dropping lower has been known to subject the lower back to injury. If, however, you're comfortable with the form and you feel you have the flexibility necessary to properly descend below parallel, feel free. Just be sure to avoid bouncing out of the bottom position, "sitting" on the backs of your calves in the bottom position, or raising your hips faster than your shoulders as you ascend.

If you're worried about going directly from one exercise to the next without rest, don't be. I purposely selected unrelated muscle groups so fatigue wouldn't pose much of a problem. After you've done your set of squats, you get to lie back on a bench and hit your chest. Once you've finished taxing your upper body with shoulder presses, you then go after your legs with some lunges. True, your whole body is still working in some manner regardless of what pairings you do, but the fatigue should be more manageable than if I had you supersetting two exercises for the same muscle group (like bench presses followed by flies). That's a little ways down the road yet.

The complete reliance on supersets will really help make your workouts more time efficient. That's a good thing. Keep your training sessions short and sweet. Work hard, not long, and live to fight another day. Don't be one of these guys who thinks that a workout has to last for a certain amount of time to be effective. You're just starting out, and your body has only a limited capacity for recovering from intensive training. Don't try to exceed that capacity, or else your results will be few and far between.

Workout A

Barbell squat/incline dumbbell bench press: 2 sets × 6 to 10 reps

Lying leg curl/one-arm row with elbow out: 2 sets × 8 to 10 reps (each arm)

Dumbbell calf raise/cable external rotation: 2 sets × 10 to 12 reps

Lateral bridge/Swiss ball crunch: 2 sets × 10 to 12 reps

Workout B

Chinup/barbell deadlift: 2 sets × 6 to 10 reps

Standing barbell shoulder press/dumbbell lunge: 2 sets × 8 to 10 reps

Prone dumbbell row with elbows out/reverse fly: 2 sets × 10 to 12 reps

Back extension/weighted Russian twist: 2 sets × 10 to 12 reps

Fourth and Goal

4 Days per Week Upper-and-Lower-Body Split Routine

This plan is by far the most difficult one in this phase. It's divided into two upper- and two lower-body workouts that will each be done once a week. All of the exercises in the upper-body workout are grouped into supersets, whereby you do both exercises in each pairing one after the other before resting for 90 seconds to 2 minutes. You then repeat that pairing for the desired number of sets before moving on to the next pair. In most instances you'll be supersetting muscle groups that work in direct opposition to each other (for instance, biceps and triceps), which is a terrific way to promote more balanced development. It also enables you to train with weights that are just a little bit heavier since the muscles on one side of a given joint will be forced to relax while the others are working. When the former are called into action, that previous relaxation actually allows them to contract with more force. It's a cool little trick and one that I've used many times both with my clients and myself.

Because of the amount of muscular overlap with the lower-body exercises, I felt that fatigue might become a problem if I used supersets. For instance, a squat hits the quadriceps, hamstrings, and glutes, which are themselves opposing muscle groups. There's just no way to superset a squat and lunge without trashing someone's legs. And while a squat and a leg curl might work better, it's still a little too much local muscular fatigue for a beginner, in my opinion. So I elected to stay with straight sets. With those, you'll simply rest for 60 to 90 seconds after each exercise. You'll just do more sets per exercise during your lower-body workouts to make up for the disparity in training volume. There'll be plenty of time down the line, after you've built a good conditioning base, to experiment by combining some of the more challenging lower-body exercises. For now, this'll be plenty.

Workout A

Barbell bench press/prone dumbbell row with elbows out: 2 sets × 6 to 10 reps

Standing barbell shoulder press/chinup: 2 sets × 8 to 10 reps

Cable external rotation/incline reverse crunch: 2 sets × 10 to 12 reps

Modified V-up: 2 sets × 6 to 8 reps

Workout B

Barbell squat: 3 sets × 6 to 10 reps

Dumbbell lunge: 3 sets × 8 to 10 reps

Dumbbell calf raise: 3 sets × 10 to 12 reps

Romanian deadlift: 2 sets × 8 to 10 reps

Workout C

Incline dumbbell bench press/one-arm row with elbow out: 2 sets × 6 to 10 reps (each arm, for row)

Chair dip/prone dumbbell row with elbows out: 2 sets × 8 to 10 reps

Lateral bridge/reverse fly: 2 sets × 8 to 10 reps

Weighted situp: 2 sets × 8 to 10 reps

Workout D

Barbell deadlift or dumbbell deadlift: 3 sets × 6 to 10 reps

Lying leg curl: 3 sets × 8 to 10 reps

Dumbbell calf raise: 3 sets × 10 to 12 reps

Back extension: 2 sets × 10 to 12 reps

BARBELL SQUAT

Hold a barbell with an overhand grip so that it rests comfortably on your upper back, just below the base of your neck. Set your feet shoulder-width apart, knees slightly bent, back straight, eyes focused straight ahead.

Next, slowly lower your body as if you were sitting back into a chair, keeping your back in its natural alignment and lower legs nearly perpendicular to the floor. When your thighs are parallel to the floor, pause, and then return to the starting position.

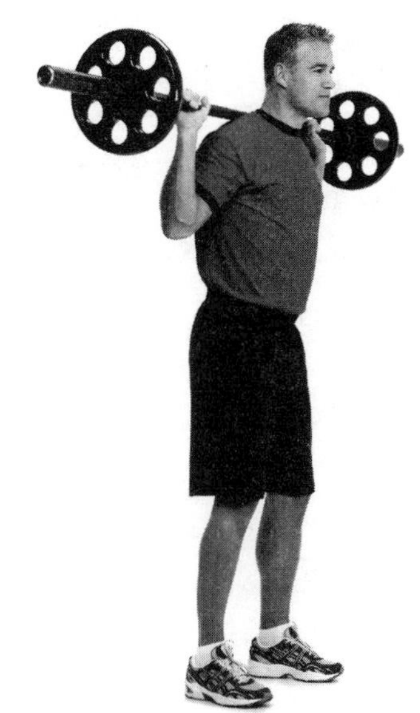

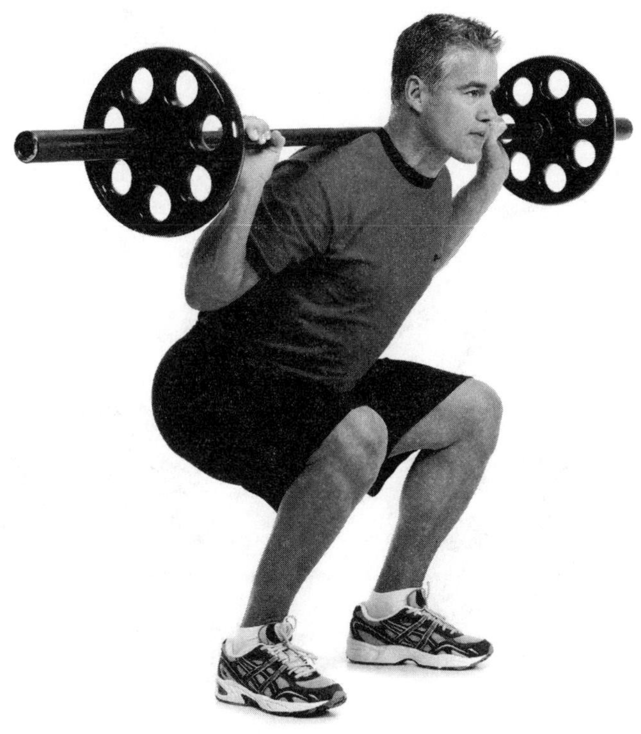

B

LEG PRESS

Position yourself in a 45-degree plate-loaded leg press sled with your feet about shoulder-width apart and your lower back pressed into the pad.

Unlock the sled and slowly lower the weight down toward your chest. Once your thighs are parallel to the force plate, pause for a second, then push back up to the starting position.

A

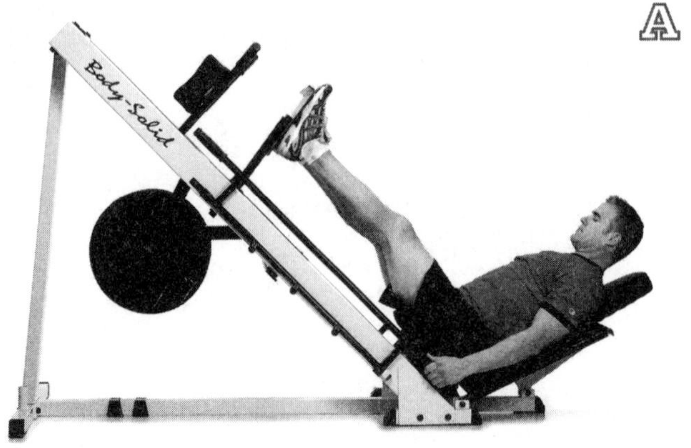

B

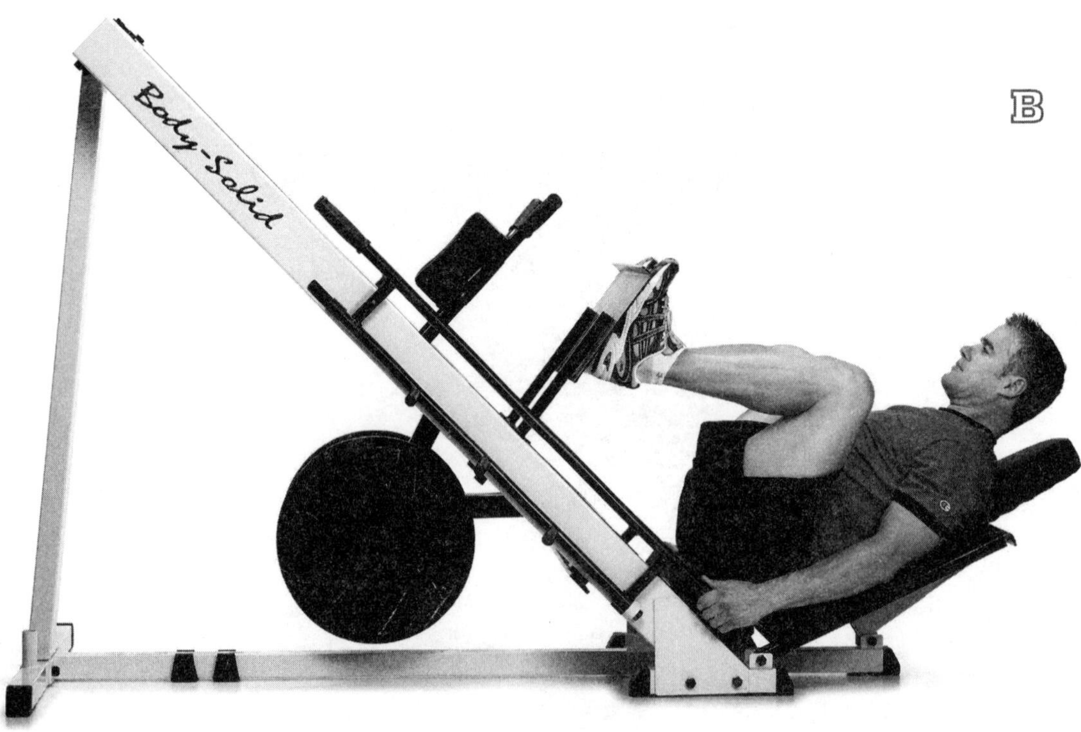

LYING LEG CURL

Lie facedown on a leg curl machine so that your knees are just off the bench and the ankle pad lines up just above your Achilles tendons.

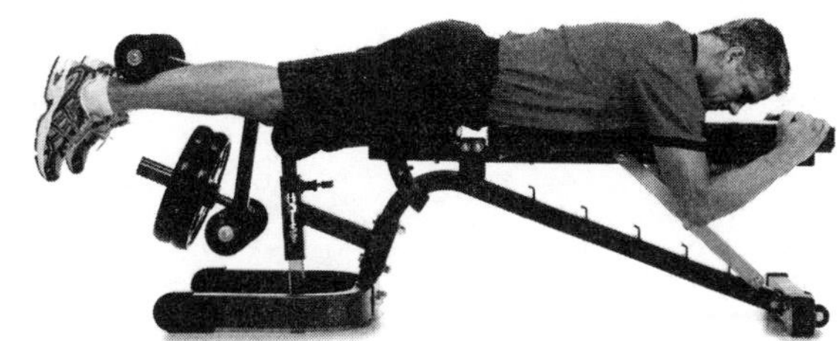

Keeping your feet relaxed (toes not pulled toward your shins or pointed away from them), use your hamstrings to pull the weights toward your rear end. Pause at the top just short of touching the backs of your thighs with the pad before lowering the weight back down.

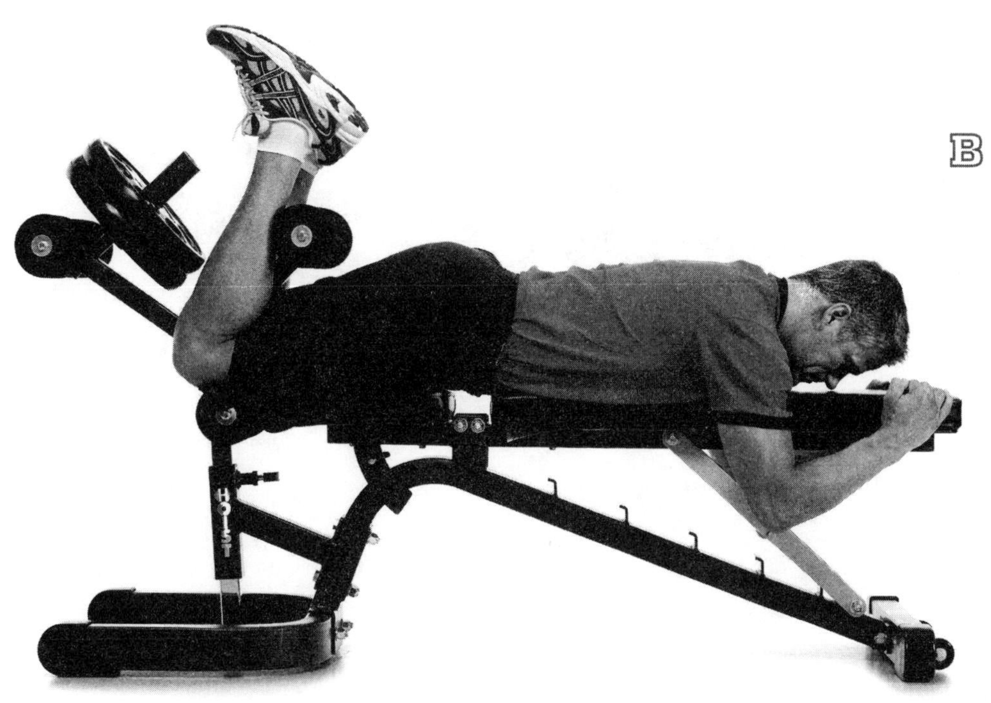

B

BARBELL BENCH PRESS

Grab the bar with your hands just wider than shoulder width. Lift the bar off the uprights and hold it over your chest.

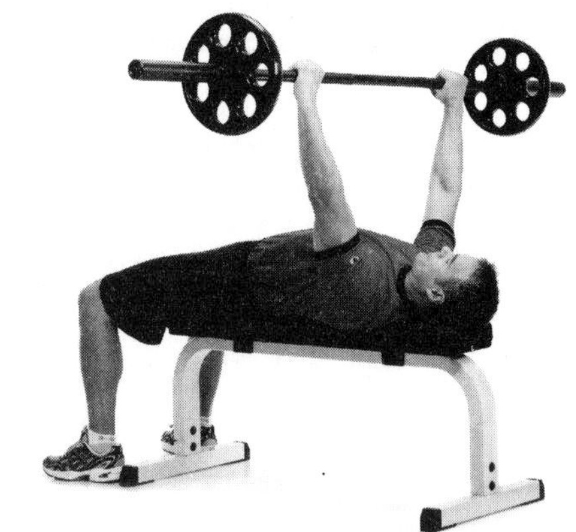

Next, lower the bar toward your chest, stopping when your upper arms are parallel to the floor. Pause there for a second and then push it back to the starting position. *Note:* You can make this exercise easier on your shoulders by using a closer grip and keeping your elbows in closer to your body.

B

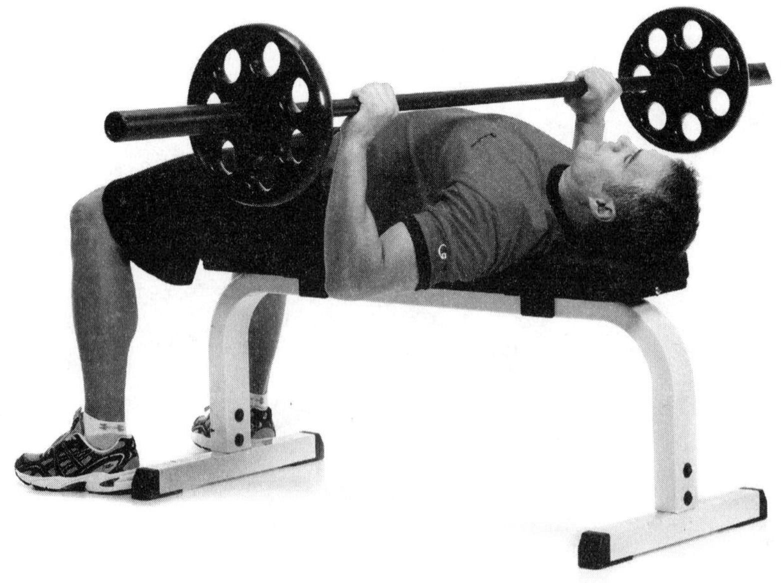

PRONE DUMBBELL ROW WITH ELBOWS OUT

Set an incline bench to a 45-degree angle and hold a pair of dumbbells with your chest against the pad. Let your arms hang straight down from your shoulders and turn your palms so that they face behind you.

Next, lift your upper arms as high as you can by bending your elbows and squeezing your shoulder blades together. Your upper arms should be almost perpendicular to your body at the top of the move, with your forearms pointing toward the floor. Pause and then slowly lower the weights to the starting position.

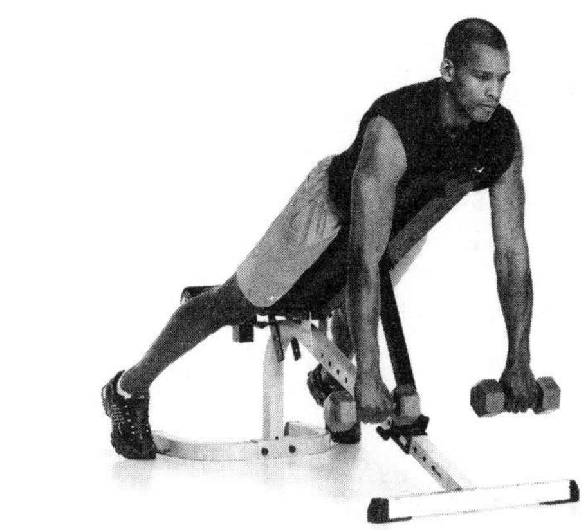

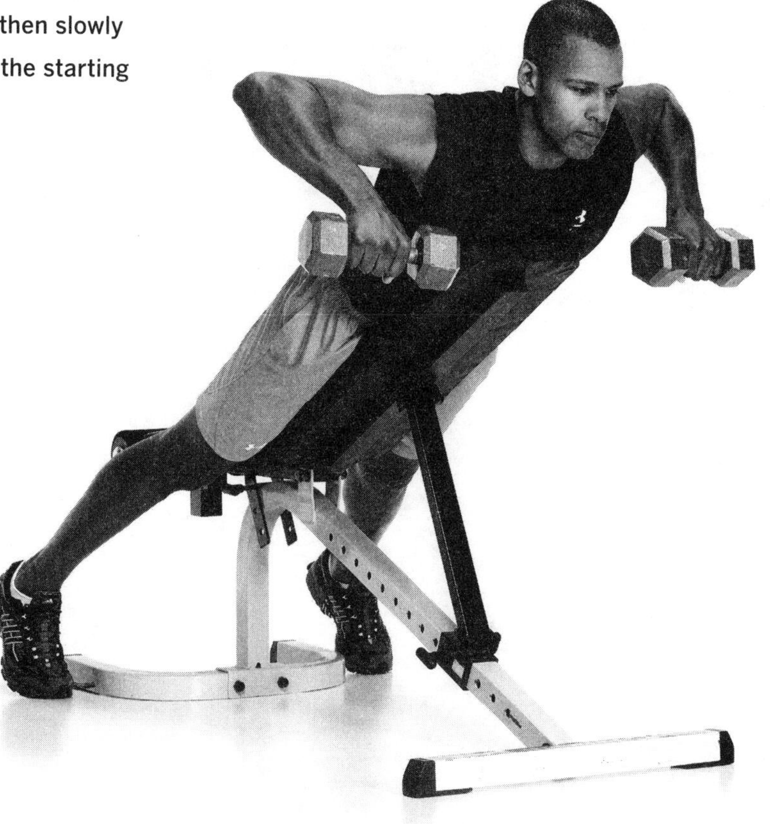

B

DUMBBELL CALF RAISE

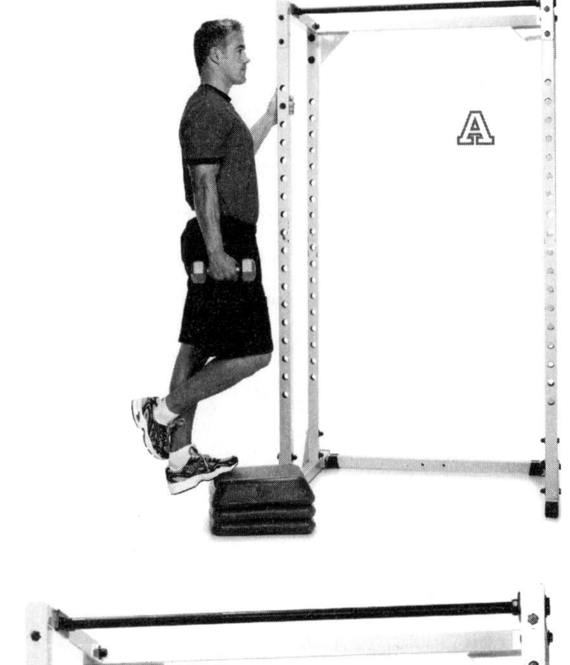

Grab a dumbbell in your right hand and stand on a step or a block. Put your left hand on something for balance—a wall or weight stack, for instance. Cross your right foot behind your left ankle and balance yourself on the ball of your left foot, with your heel hanging off the step. Lower your left heel as far as you can.

Pause, and then lift it as high as you can. Finish the set with your left leg and then repeat with your right (while holding the dumbbell in your left hand).

Note: If you train in a gym, this exercise can also be done using a calf raise machine.

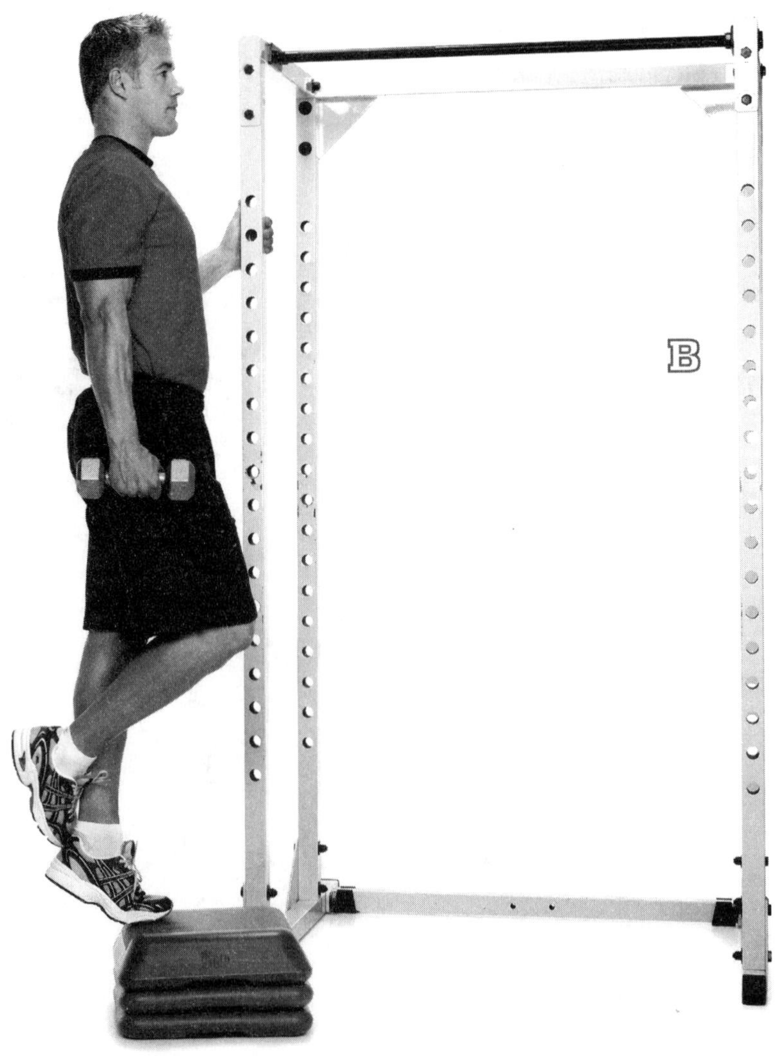

CABLE EXTERNAL ROTATION

Attach a stirrup handle to an adjustable cable station. Kneel sideways to the weight stack (or set the pulley at hip height and stand sideways to the machine) and grab the handle with the hand farthest away from it.

Maintaining a 90-degree bend in your working arm, rotate your forearm outward, as if it were a door rotating on a hinge. Be sure to keep your elbow as close to your hip as possible (using a rolled-up towel between your elbow and hip can help with this) and avoid extending your wrist by bending your knuckles back. Pause and then slowly return your arm to the starting position. Finish your set and then do the same number of reps with your other arm.

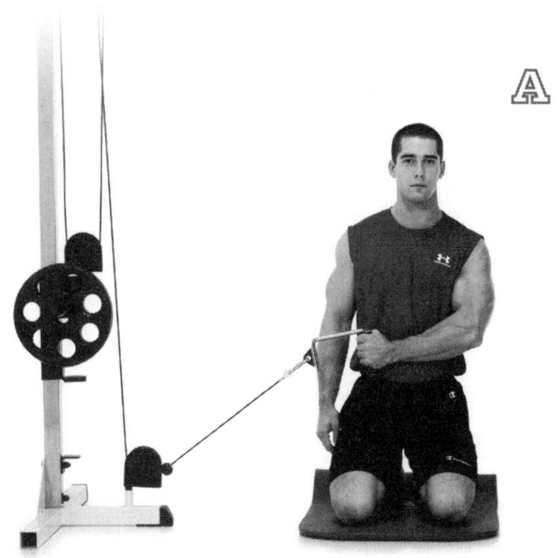

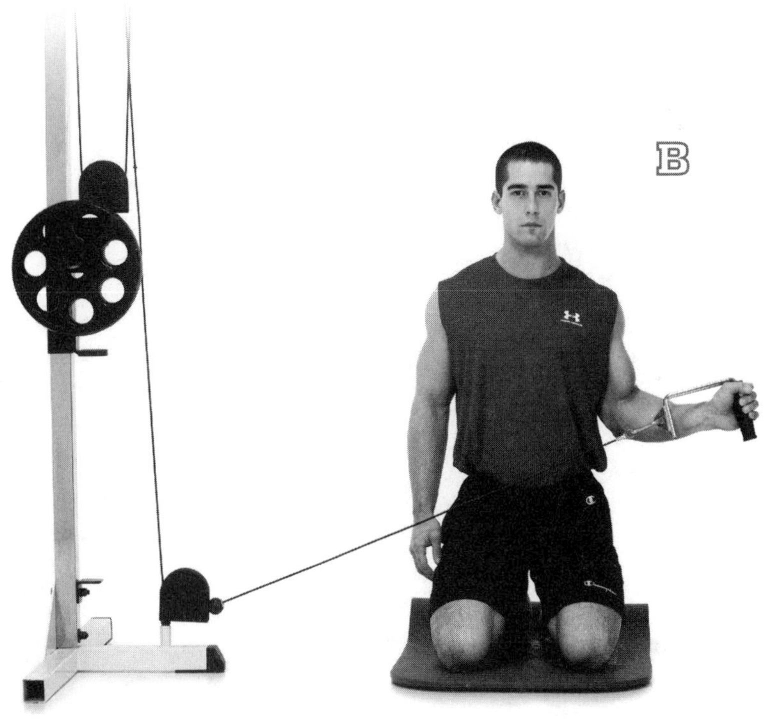

WEIGHTED RUSSIAN TWIST

Sit on the floor with your knees bent about 90 degrees and feet flat on the floor. Next, holding a light dumbbell, medicine ball, or weight plate between your hands, extend your arms and lean back until your wrists line up over your knees.

Hold this same trunk angle as you twist as far as possible to one side and then the other.

A

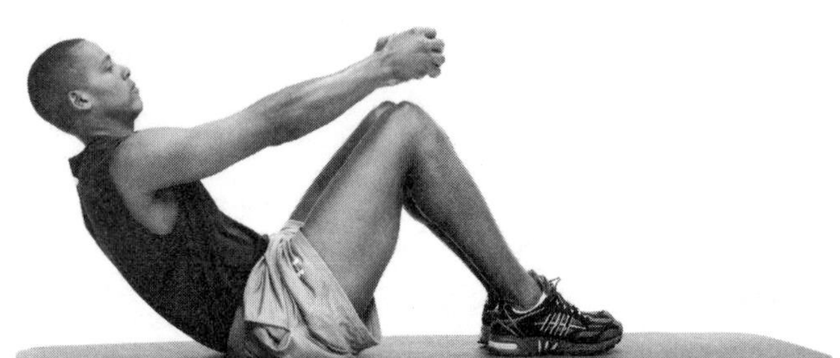

B

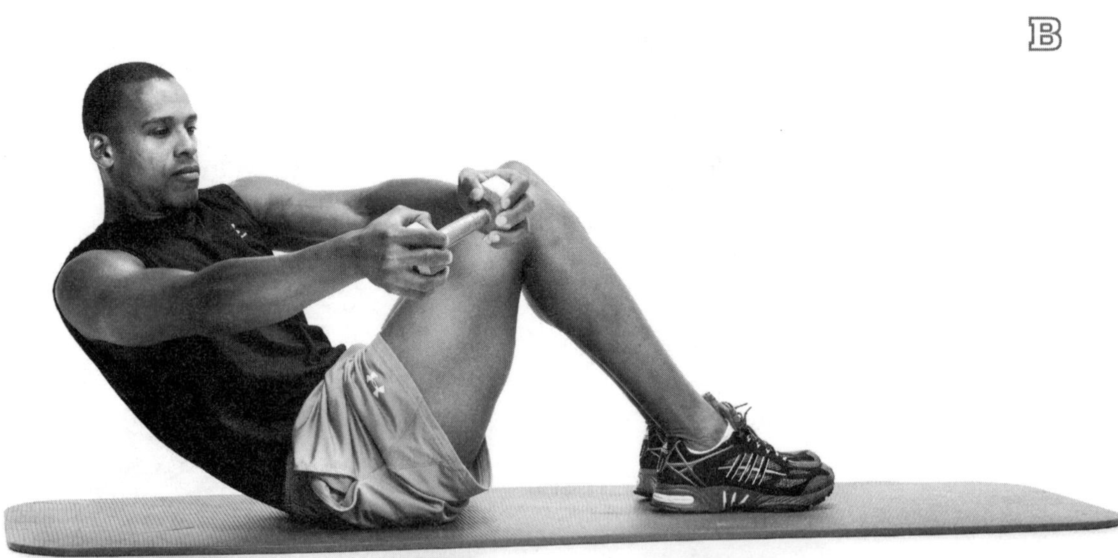

BARBELL DEADLIFT

Set a barbell on the floor and stand facing it. Squat down and grab it overhand, your hands just outside your legs.

With your back flat and head up, stand up with the barbell, pulling your shoulder blades back. Then slowly lower the bar to the starting position.

Note: Those of you who have lower-back issues may want to either start from the top position (by taking the bar off the supports in a squat rack) or not go as low. Or do the exercise with dumbbells held at your sides, which allows you to maintain a more upright posture and reduced lower-back strain.

A

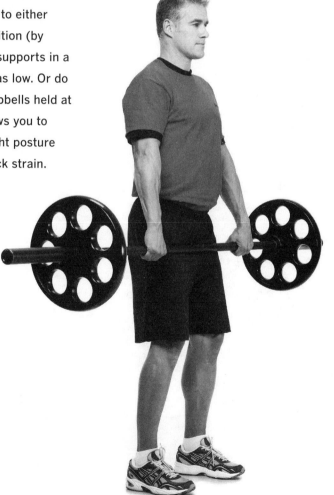

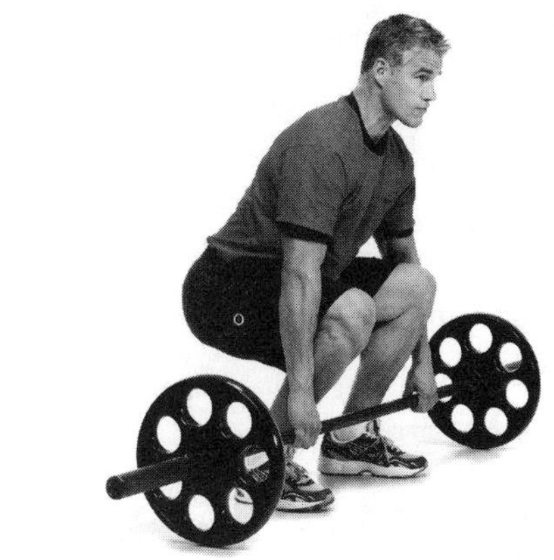

B

DUMBBELL DEADLIFT

Stand holding a pair of dumbbells at arm's length with your palms facing your thighs and a stance that's slightly wider than shoulder width. (The position of the weight here allows you to remain more upright and reduces lower-back strain as compared to the barbell deadlift.)

Keeping a slight arch in your back and your shoulders pinched together, begin to sit down and back until your thighs are parallel to the floor. Pause there for a second and then press back up to the starting position.

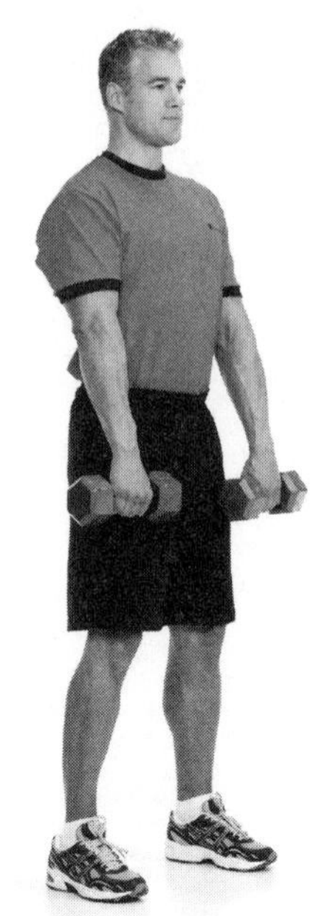

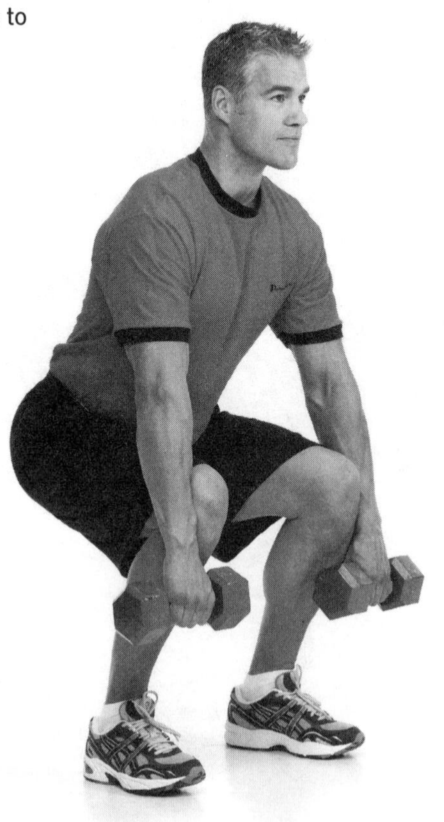

B

ROMANIAN DEADLIFT

Grab an unloaded barbell (feel free to add weight to it as you get stronger) with an overhand grip that's just beyond shoulder-width. Stand holding the bar at arm's length and resting on the fronts of your thighs. Your feet should be shoulder-width apart and your knees slightly bent. Focus your eyes straight ahead.

Slowly bend at the hips as you lower the bar to just below your knees. Don't change the angle of your knees. Keep your head and chest up and your lower back flat or slightly arched. Lift your torso back to the starting position, keeping the bar as close to your body as possible.

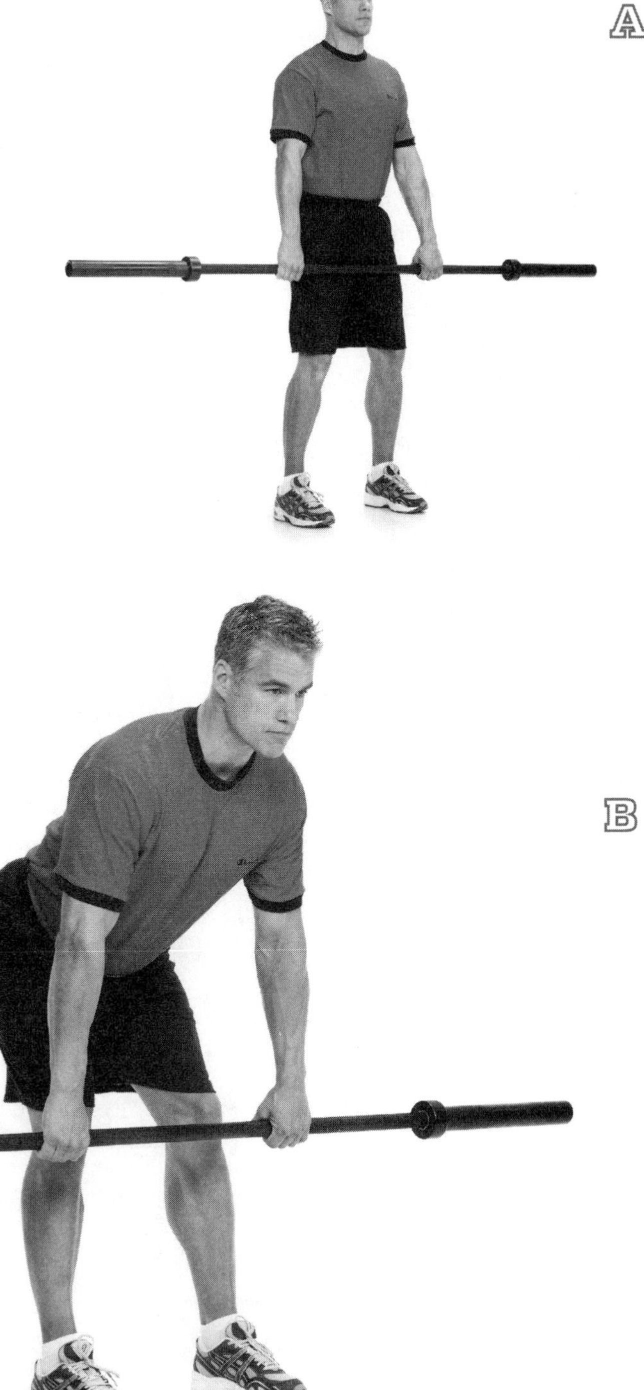

DUMBBELL LUNGE

Standing with your feet hip-width apart, grab a pair of dumbbells and hold them at your sides.

Step forward with one leg and lower your body until your front knee is bent 90 degrees and your rear knee nearly touches the floor. Your front lower leg should be perpendicular to the floor and your torso should remain upright. Push yourself back up to the starting position as quickly as you can and repeat with your other leg.

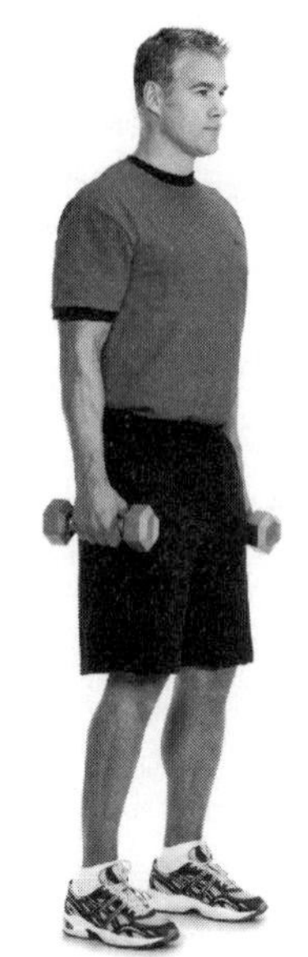

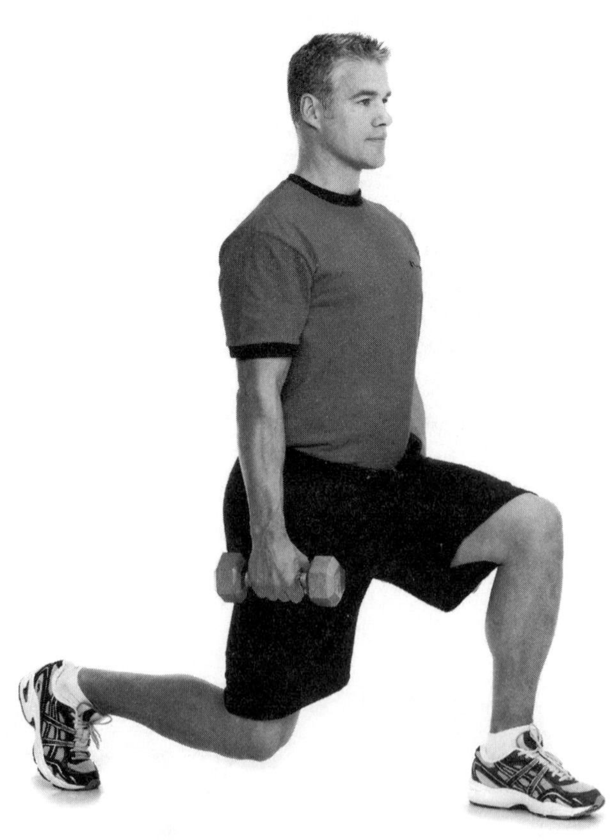

B

CHINUP

Grab the chinup bar with a shoulder-width, underhand grip, as you bend your knees and cross your ankles behind you to hang from it.

Keeping your chest out, pull yourself up until your chin clears the bar. Pause there for a second and then slowly return to the starting position.

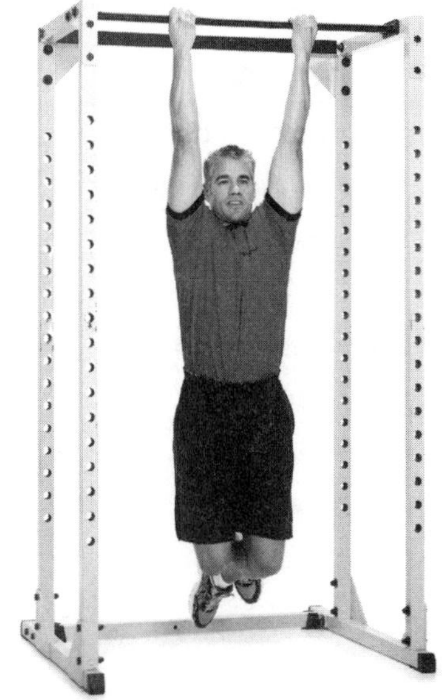

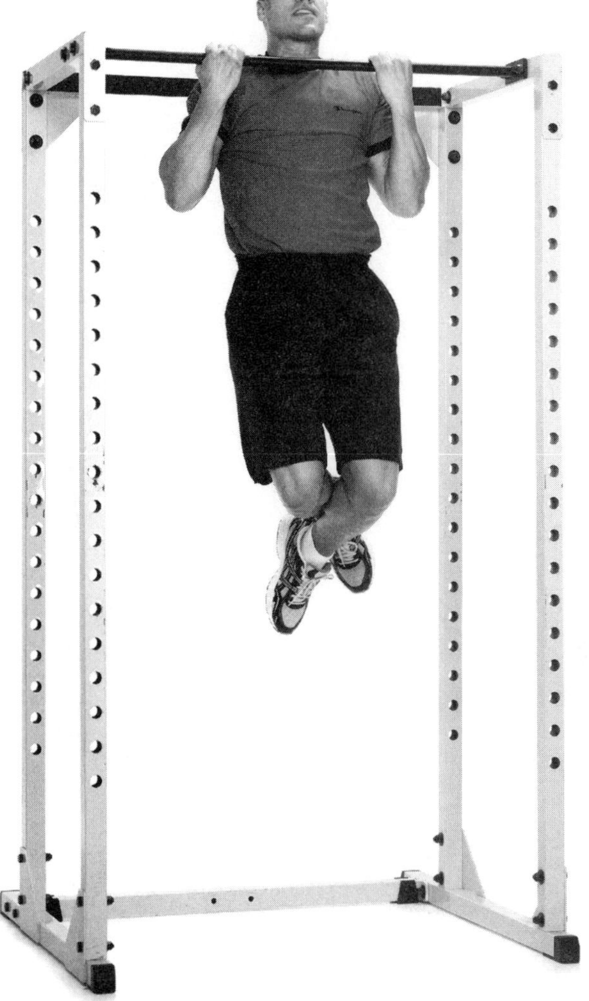

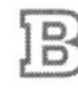

LAT PULLDOWN

Grab the bar of a lat pulldown machine (or a straight bar on the high pulley of a cable station) with a shoulder-width, overhand grip.

Moving only your arms, pull the bar down to your chest by squeezing your shoulder blades together. Hold for a second and then bring the bar back to the starting position.

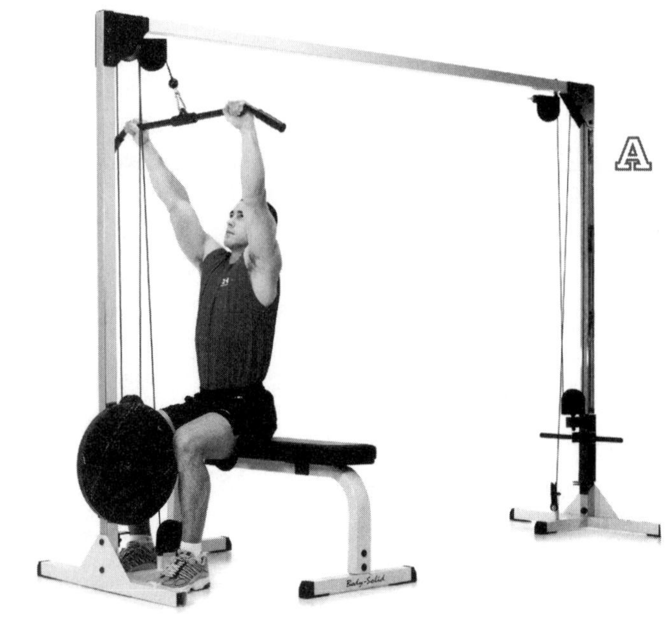
A

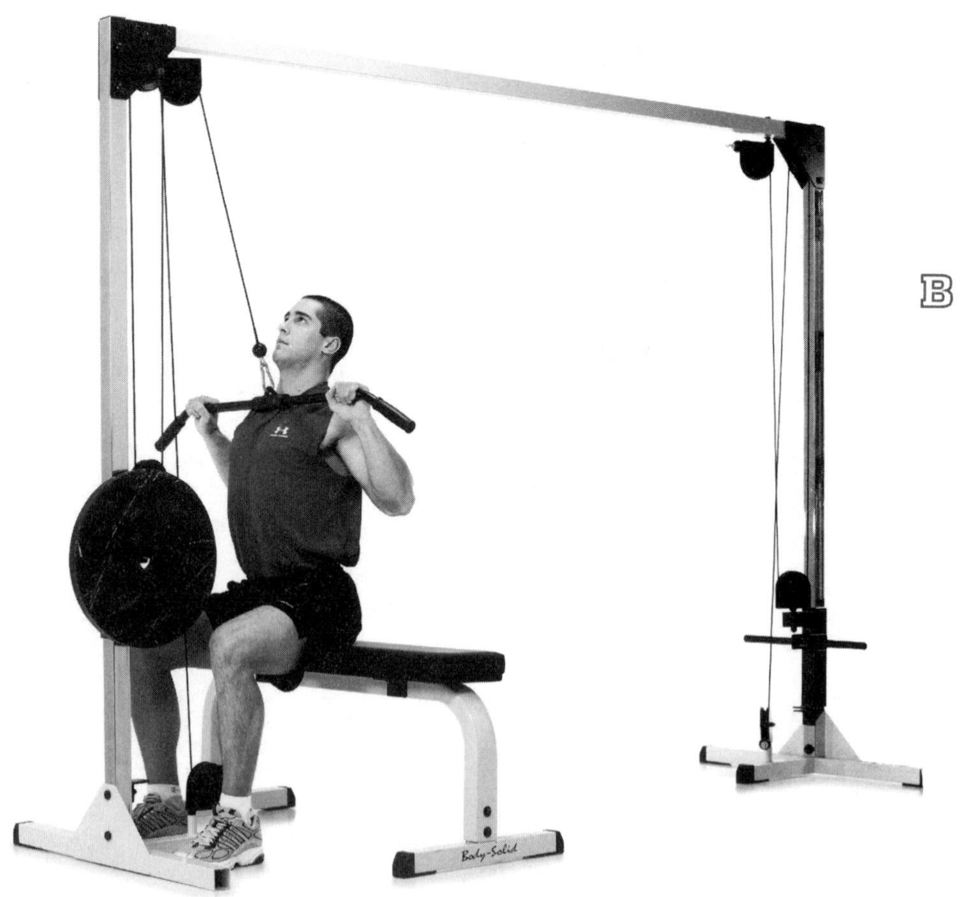
B

STANDING BARBELL SHOULDER PRESS

Grab a barbell with a shoulder-width, overhand grip. Stand holding the barbell at shoulder level, your feet shoulder-width apart and knees slightly bent.

Begin by pushing the weight straight overhead, leaning your head back slightly but keeping your torso upright. Pause and then slowly lower the bar to the starting position.

Note: This exercise can also be done with dumbbells, using a neutral grip to ease shoulder strain.

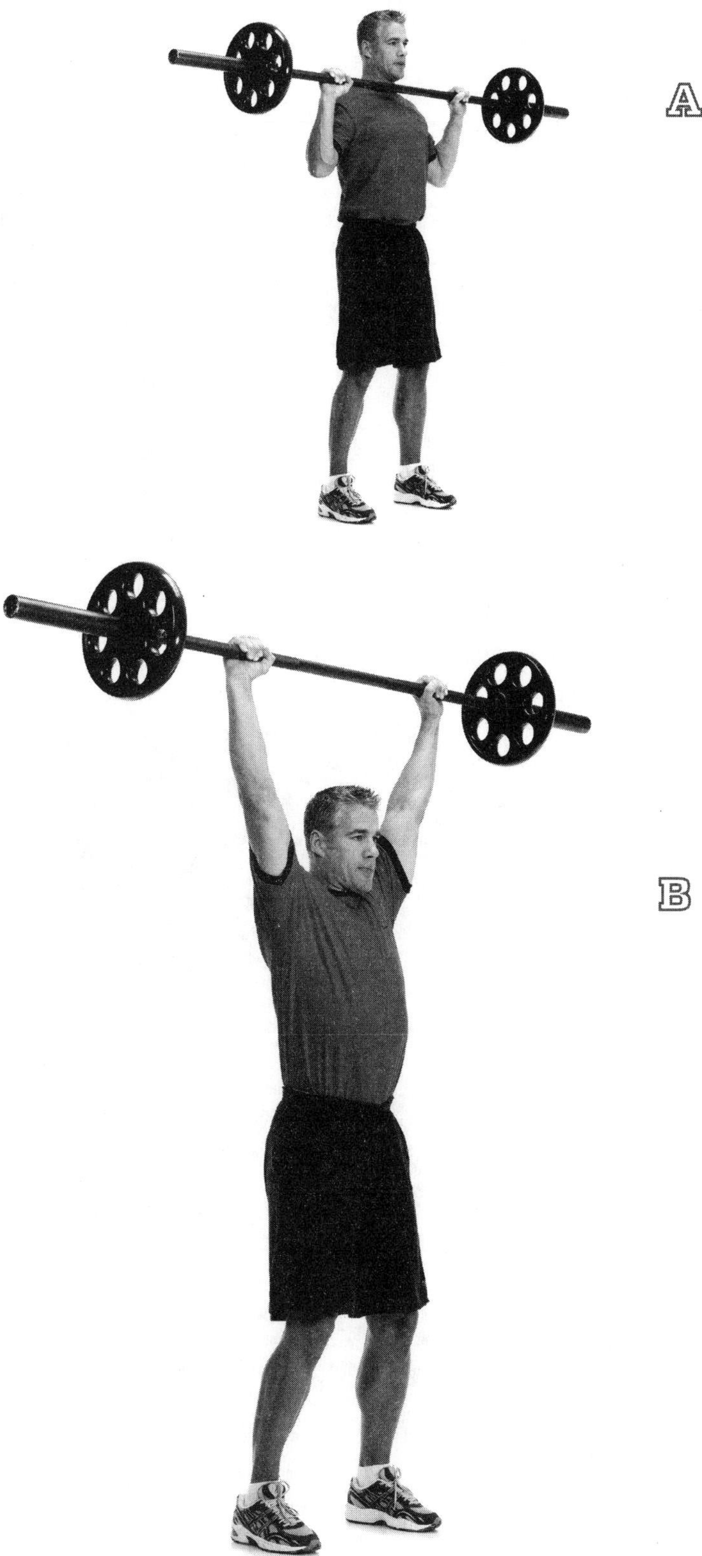

ONE-ARM ROW WITH ELBOW OUT

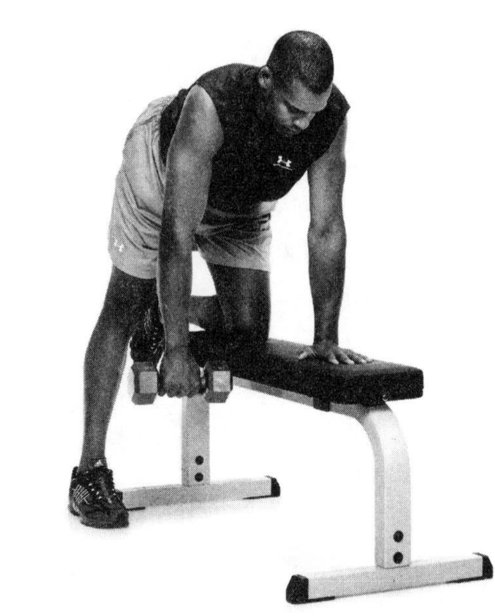

A

Grab a dumbbell in your right hand and place your left hand and knee on a bench. Keep your back flat and your upper body parallel to the floor. Let your working arm hang straight down at your side, with your palm facing behind you.

Pull the dumbbell up until your elbow passes your torso, making sure to keep your elbow away from your torso. Pause and then slowly return to the starting position. Finish your set and then do the same number of reps with your other arm.

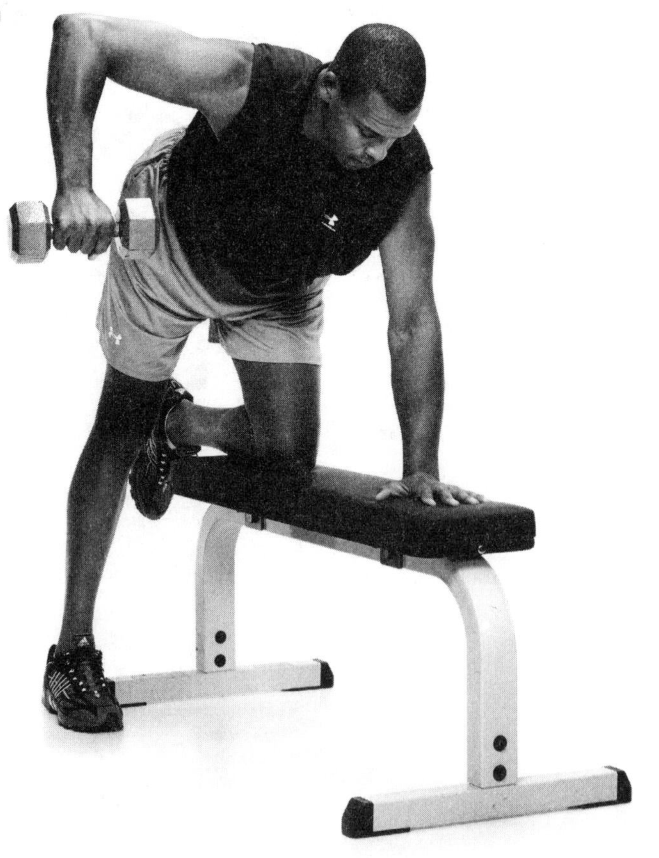

B

BACK EXTENSION

Position yourself in the back-extension station and hook your feet under the leg anchors. Cross your arms over your chest and lower your upper body, allowing your lower back to round, until it is just short of being perpendicular to the floor.

Raise your upper body until it is slightly above parallel. At this point you should have a slight arch in your back and your shoulder blades should be pulled together in back.

Note: This exercise can also be done using a Swiss ball if you don't have access to this kind of bench (See page 166.)

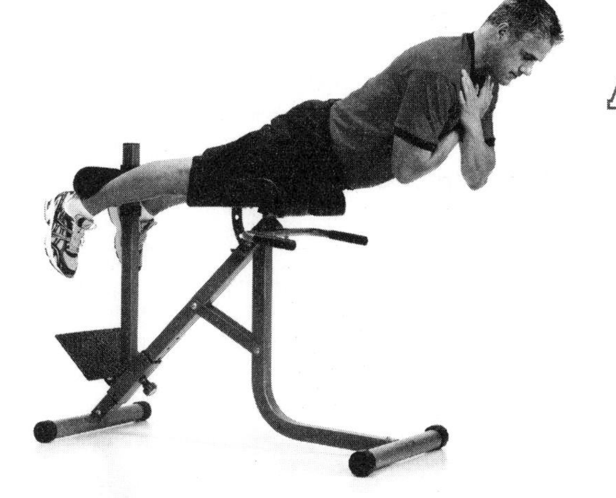

A

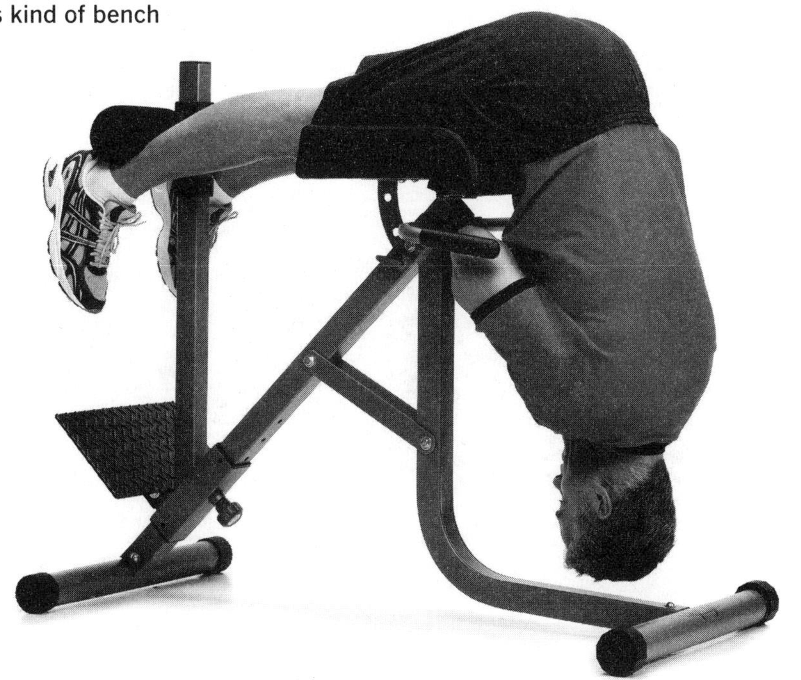

B

LATERAL BRIDGE

Lie on your side with your forearm lined up right beneath your shoulder, perpendicular to your torso.

Keeping your body totally straight, contract your abdominals and obliques as you raise your lower torso, hips, and legs off the floor. In the top position your body should form a diagonal line from your feet to your head. Return to the starting position and repeat. Finish your set and then do the same number of reps on your other side.

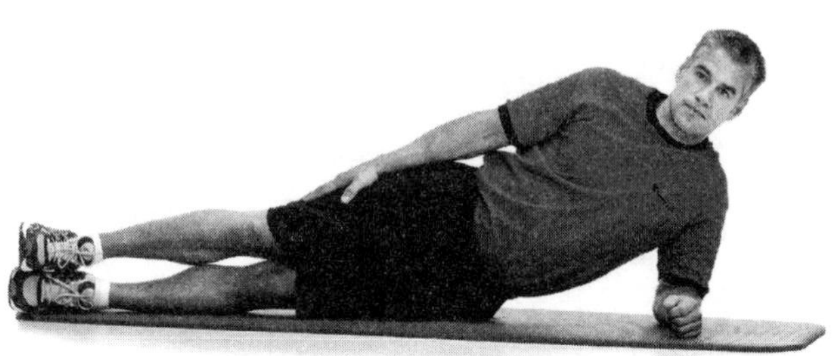

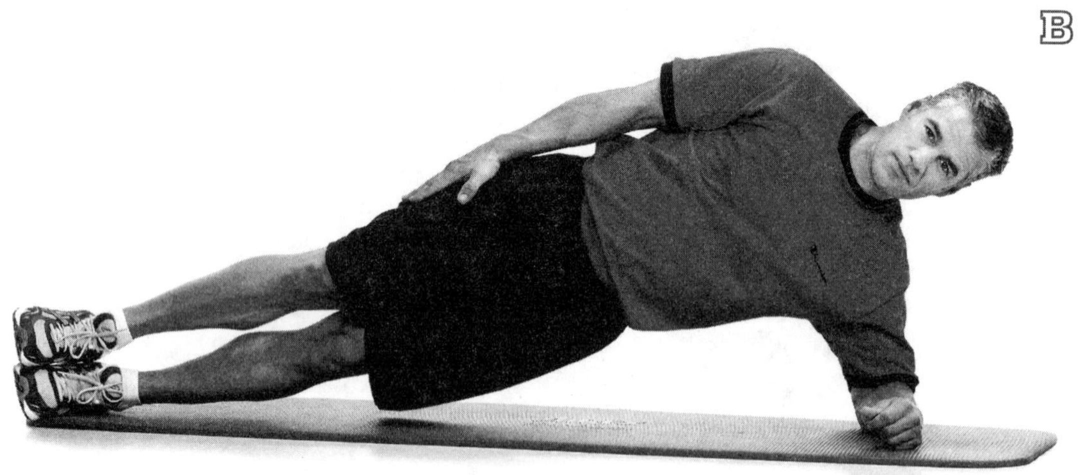

SWISS BALL CRUNCH

Lie back on a Swiss ball with your feet flat on the floor and legs bent at a 90-degree angle. As you lie back, allow your back to conform to the surface of the ball by arching your back.

From there, keep your lower body perfectly still as you use your abdominals to lift your shoulder blades off the ball. Pause for a second at the top and lower yourself back down to the starting position.

A

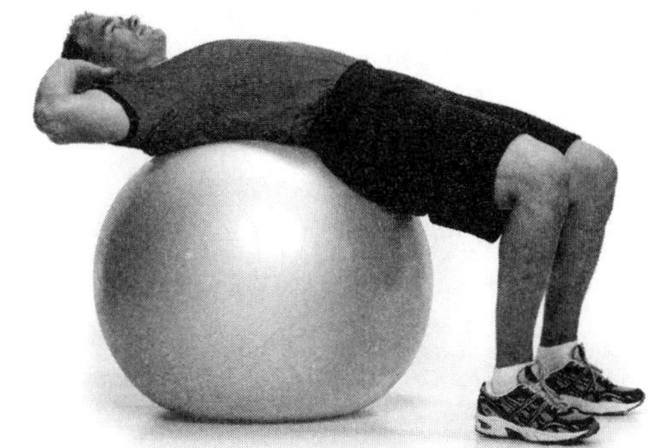

B

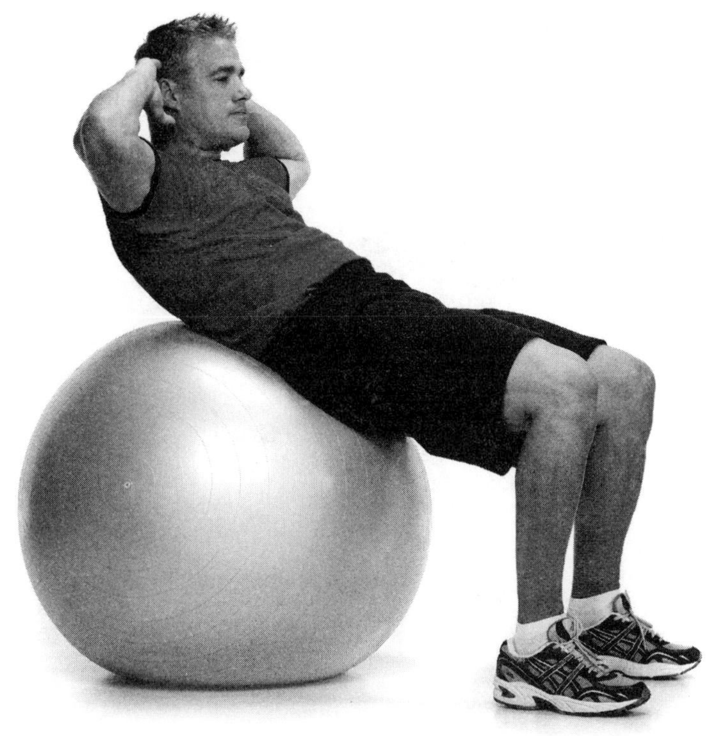

INCLINE DUMBBELL BENCH PRESS

Grab a pair of dumbbells and lie on your back on a bench set to a low incline (15 to 30 degrees). Lift the dumbbells so they're over your chin and hold them with your palms turned forward (thumbs facing each other). Slowly lower the weights to your upper chest, pause, then push them back up over your chin.

A

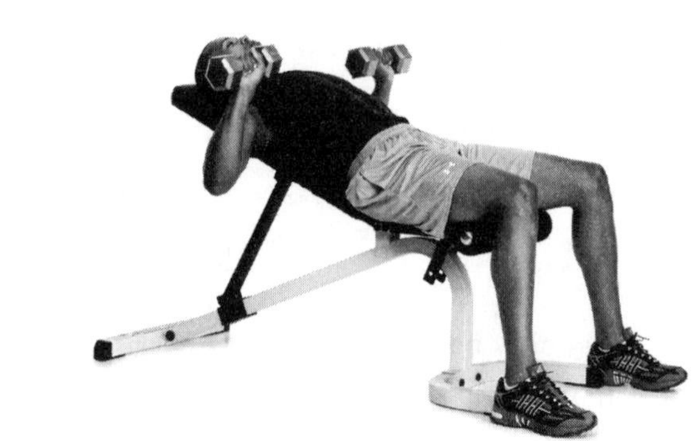

Note: This exercise can also be performed with a neutral grip (palms facing each other) and your elbows closer to your body to minimize shoulder strain.

B

REVERSE FLY

Lie prone over a 45-degree exercise bench holding a pair of dumbbells at arm's length.

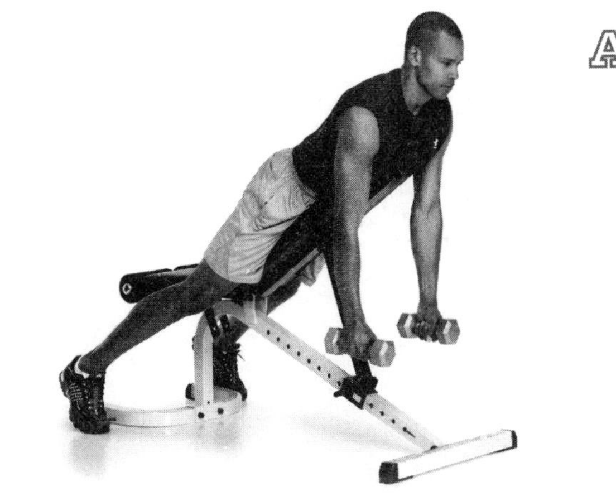

A

Keeping a slight bend in your elbows, pinch your shoulder blades together and work your arms up in a wide, arcing motion. At the top of the movement your elbows should remain slightly bent and you should see the weights out of the corners of your eyes.

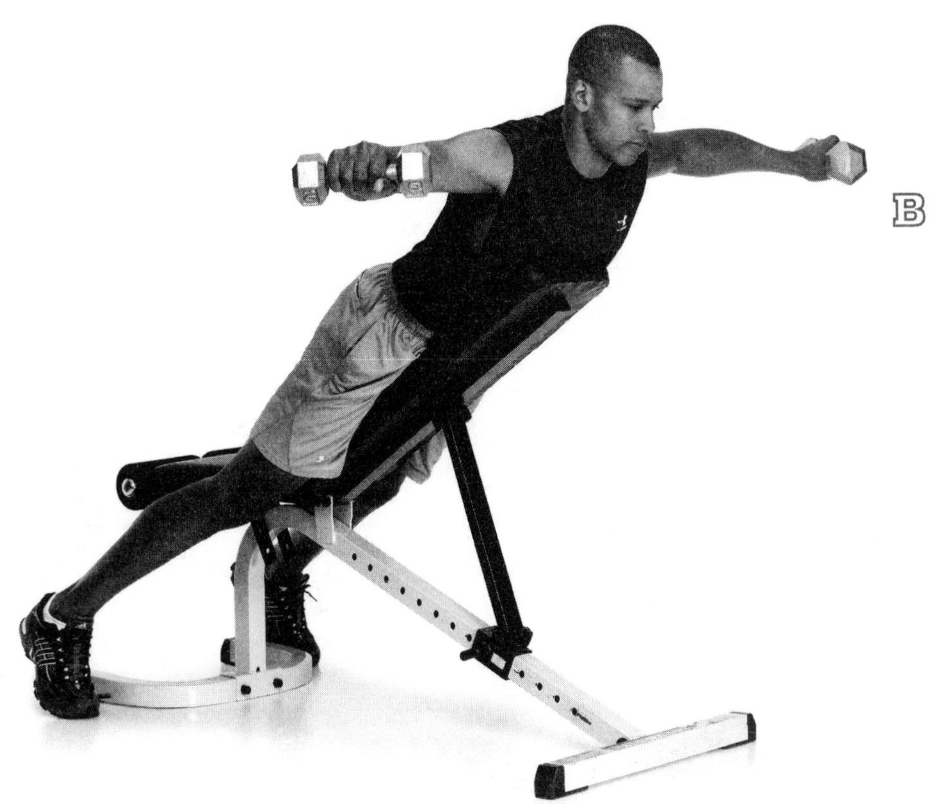

B

CHAIR DIP

Set up a couple of chairs or sturdy benches several feet apart. Begin by placing both hands on the seat of one chair or bench and your outstretched legs on the other one.

Keeping your torso as straight as possible, bend at the elbows and lower yourself until your upper arms are parallel to the floor. Pause for a second and push yourself back up to the starting position.

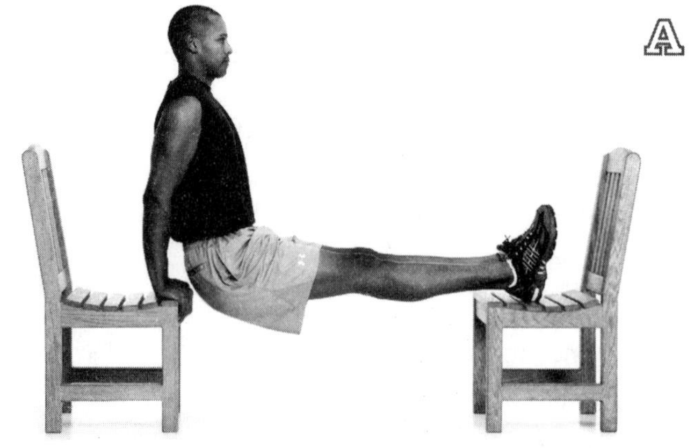

A

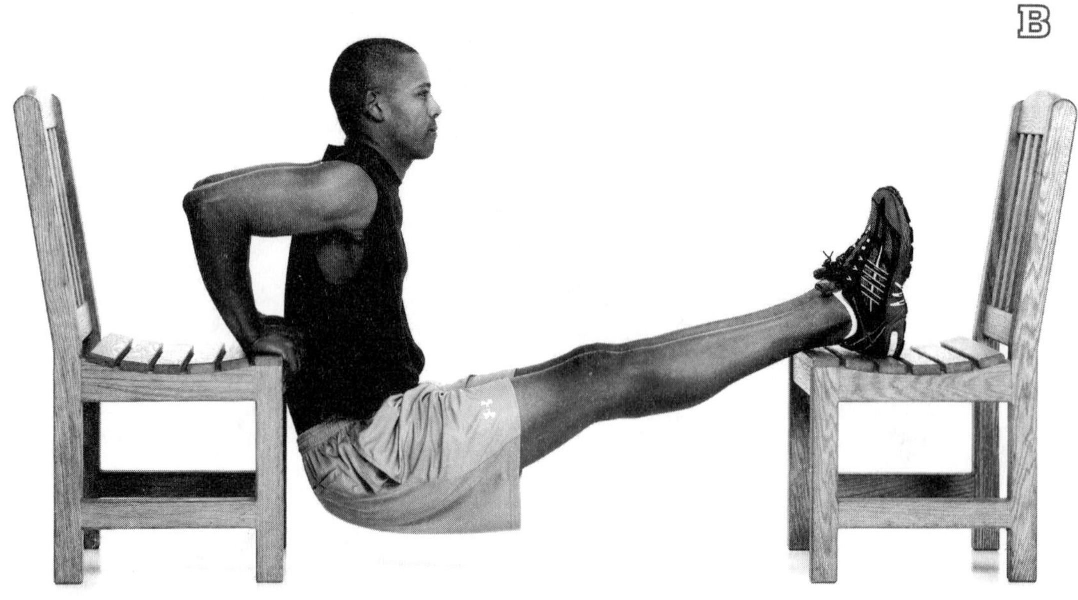

B

MODIFIED V-UP

Lie on the floor with your head up and your knees slightly bent so that only your heels, rear end, and shoulder blades are in contact with the floor.

Begin by contracting your abs as you bring your chest toward your thighs and your thighs toward your chest. In the contracted position, you'll be balancing on your rear end with your arms extended and your chest and thighs as close together as possible.

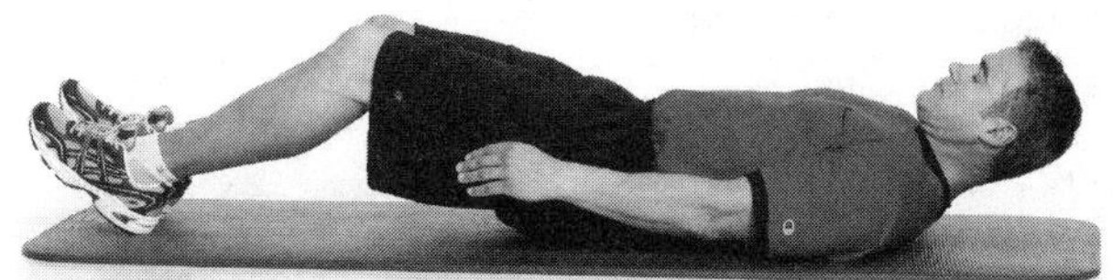

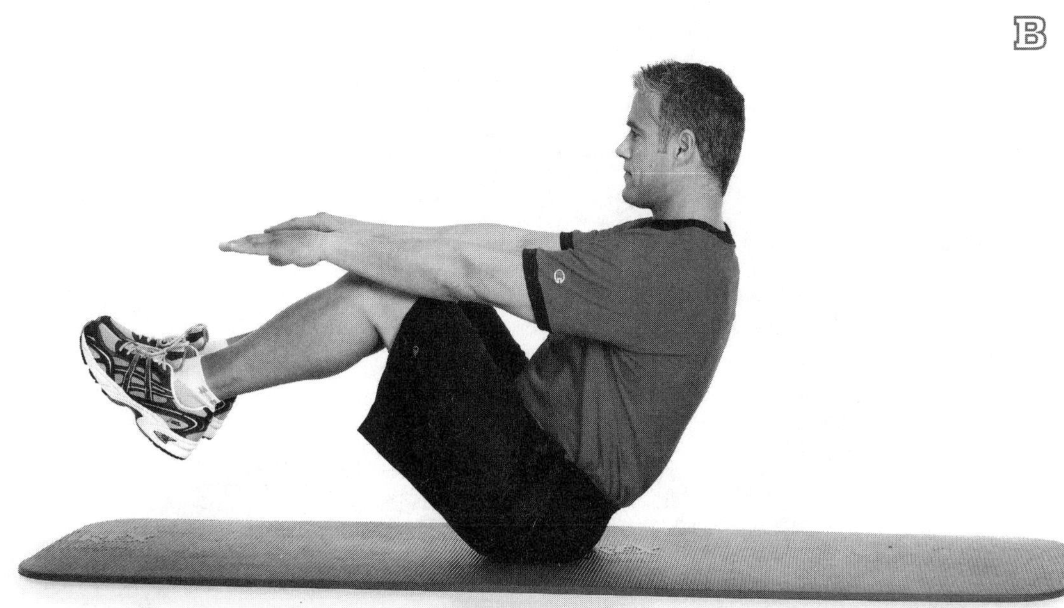

INCLINE REVERSE CRUNCH

Lie on a slant board with your hips lower than your head. Grab the bar behind your head for support. Bend your hips and knees 90 degrees.

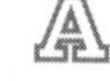

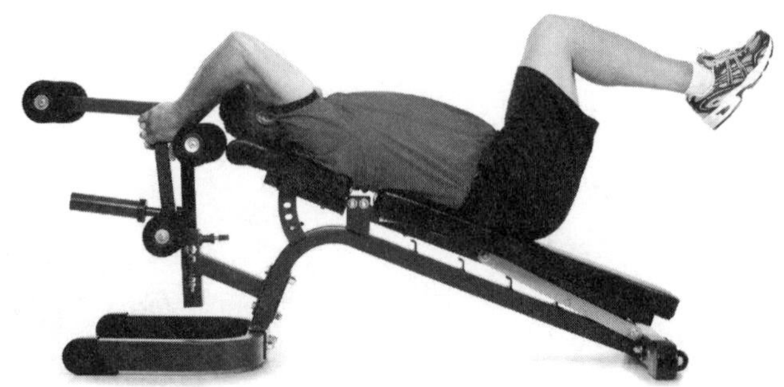

Pull your hips upward and crunch them inward, as if you were emptying a bucket of water that was resting on your pelvis. Keep your hips and knees at 90-degree angles throughout the exercise. Pause and then slowly lower your hips to the starting position.

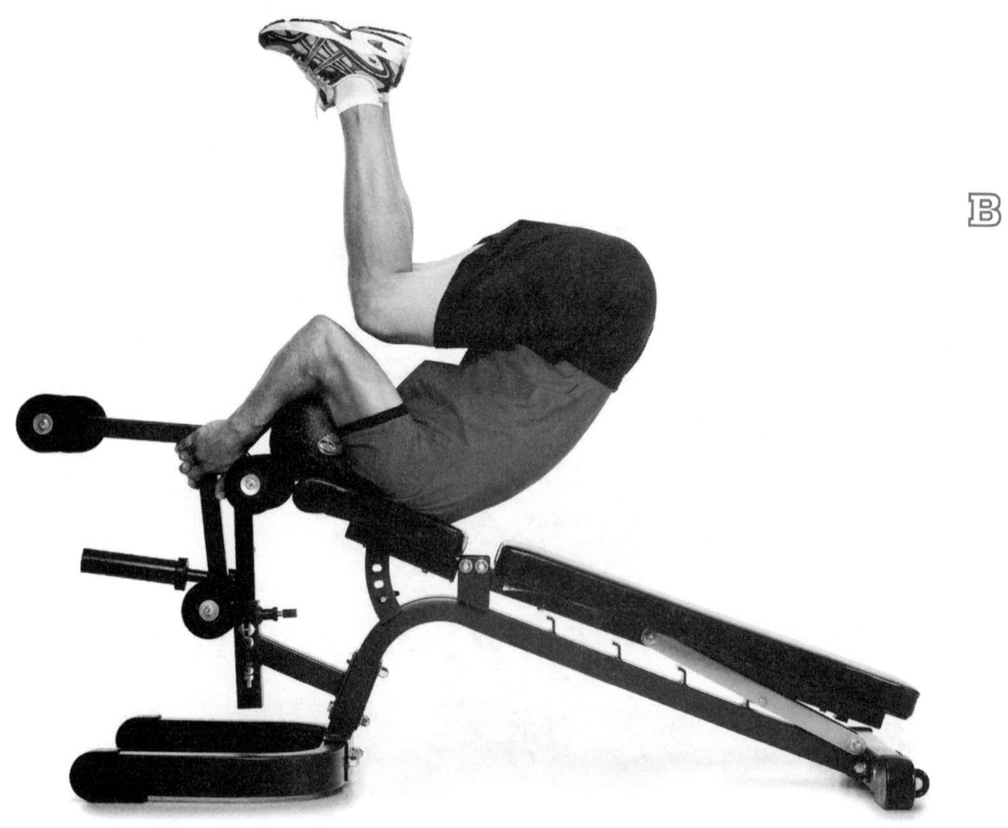

B

WEIGHTED SITUP

Lie on your back on the floor holding a weight plate across your chest, with your knees bent and feet flat on the floor.

Slowly lift your torso until your arms almost touch your thighs. Pause and then slowly lower yourself back down to the floor.

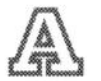

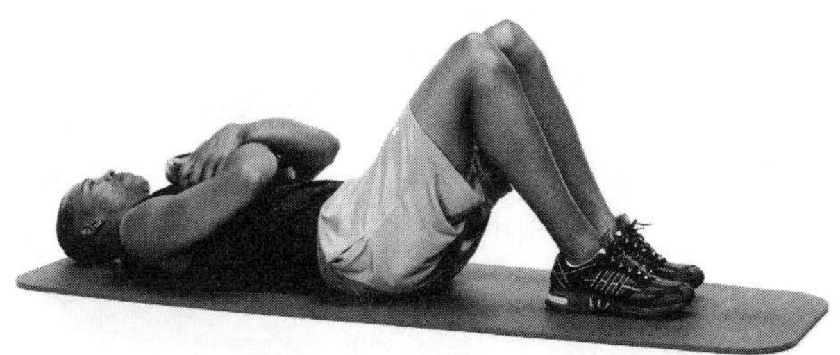

B

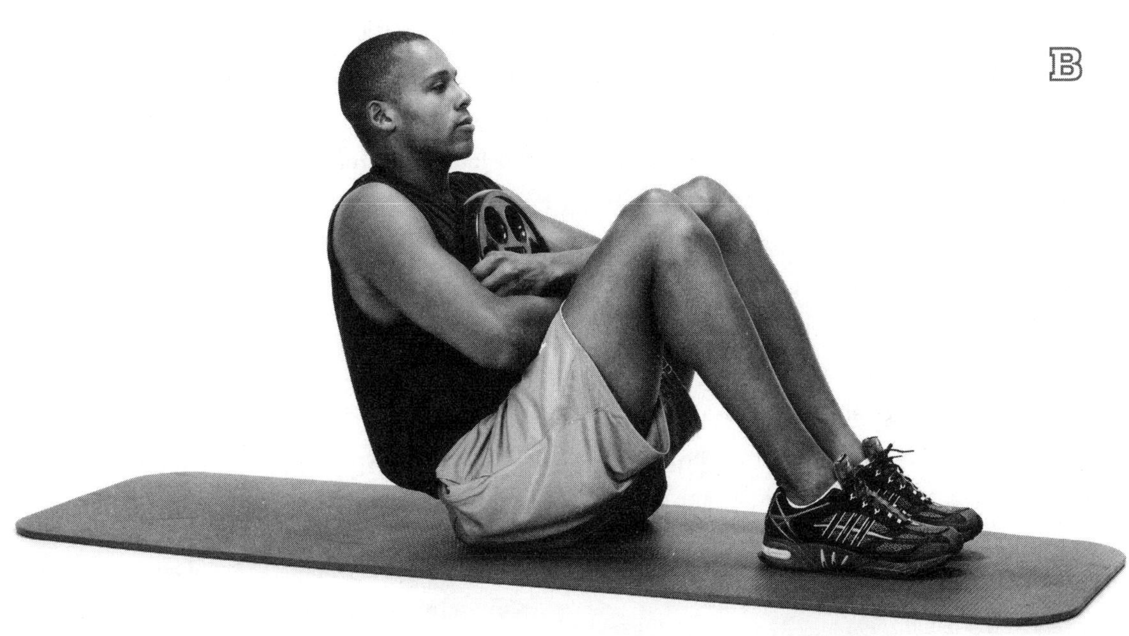

THE CARDIO CONUNDRUM

HOW MUCH IS TOO MUCH WHEN YOU'RE TRYING TO BUILD MASS?

Right about now you're probably wondering where you're supposed to work your heart in the midst of all this muscle building. After all, there's got to be some cardio in this routine, right? Of course there is; you just can't get carried away with it if you're serious about putting on some size. Remember, the primary goal during this phase is to build muscle. This requires not only lifting heavier weights—which, by the way, places a greater demand on your body's recuperative powers—but also eating a caloric surplus above your total daily energy requirement. Throwing a ton of cardio into the mix is a tad contradictory, to say the least.

Here's where being a rank amateur will actually work to your advantage. Those of us who've been training for several years find it almost impossible to burn fat and build muscle at the same time. From a nutritional standpoint, building muscle and burning fat are at opposite ends of the spectrum. The former requires you to consume more calories than your body needs on a daily basis, and the latter demands that you take in fewer. It simply isn't possible to simultaneously achieve both goals to any significant degree. Sure, you might make modest improvements in each area, but those of us who are looking to make wholesale changes in our physiques know that these two goals are best separated into different phases of training. In your case, though, because training of any type will still be perceived by your body as a relatively new stimulus, you may notice an increase in muscle mass accompanied by a slight reduction in body fat.

What I'm getting at here is that the amount of cardio you should do during this phase really depends on how much muscle you want to build. If you're content to keep muscle growth to a minimum, feel free to do the cardio workouts as often as 3 or 4 times per week, if you have the time. If, however, you're interested in adding several pounds of muscle, then you're going to have to keep the cardio to a minimum—say one to two brief, intense workouts per week. This will be just enough to maintain cardiovascular fitness and minimize any fat gain from the caloric surplus you'll be consuming. Don't kid yourself, though: You're not going to simultaneously pack on muscle mass as you strip away body fat. It just doesn't work that way.

Assuming that you are interested in getting a little bigger, you're going to have to pick your spots when it comes to getting in your cardio workouts. One strategy is to keep cardio sessions short and sweet and as far removed from your strength training as possible—like, say, doing them on off days from lifting. Another strategy is to do your cardio immediately following your weight workout. It won't zap your energy for the weights, and it has the added benefit of burning more fat for fuel since your body will want to preserve its carbohydrate stores following a tough session with the iron. Both of these strategies will reduce the likelihood of slowing down the muscle-building process.

The following two cardio workouts are brief yet intense and designed to maximize your recovery time between lifts. I recommend doing one or the other at least once and a maximum of three times per week. Simply follow the prescribed work and rest intervals while using the cardio modality of your choice.

Workout A: The Pyramid (12 minutes)

Work intervals: Follow a pyramid scheme of 15 seconds, 30 seconds, 45 seconds, 60 seconds, 45 seconds, 30 seconds, 15 seconds

Recovery intervals: 30 seconds, 60 seconds, 90 seconds, 120 seconds, 90 seconds, 60 seconds, 30 seconds

Intensity: 8 to 9 for the work intervals and 6 to 7 for the recovery intervals

So after a 3- to 5-minute warmup, up the intensity for a tough work interval of 15 seconds. Follow it with a recovery interval of double that length, or 30 seconds. Then push hard again, this time for 30 seconds, recover for 60, and so on, until you finish all the intervals. The premise is simple: escalating work intervals followed by recovery periods of double the length.

Workout B: The Yo-Yo (18 to 24 minutes)

Work intervals: 15 seconds and 45 seconds (6 to 8 rounds)

Recovery intervals: 30 seconds and 90 seconds (6 to 8 rounds)

Intensity: 8.5 to 9 for the work intervals and 6.5 to 7 for the recovery intervals

Alternate between extremely intense but brief work intervals (15 seconds) and somewhat less intense, longer work intervals. Follow each work interval with a recovery interval twice as long.

THE LAST REP

DON'T BE AFRAID TO STAND OUT

This phase is a prescription for building muscle that's far different than what the gang down at the local pump palace is doing. It's more balanced, a lot more time efficient, and much more comprehensive in its focus. Best of all, it's designed with you in mind. There's no need to punish yourself with maniacal training routines or go broke on high-priced supplements just to gain a little muscle. More than anything else, this chapter should have confirmed for you that it is possible for real guys to get real results by simply having the guts to go against the tide of popular thinking. Well, that plus a burning desire to improve, of course.

The workouts in this chapter definitely aren't easy. As you've probably noticed, that's a theme throughout this book. I'm urging you to stick with it because your results will be well worth it; you'll start to look visibly bigger after just 4 to 6 weeks on this phase of the program.

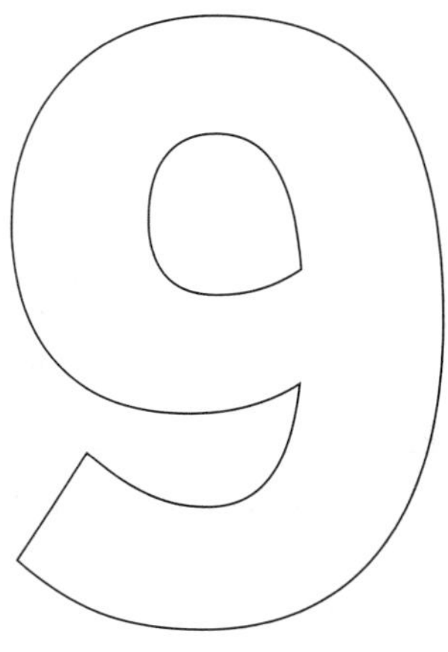

ONLY THE STRONG SURVIVE

PHASE 5: TRAINING TO GET STRONGER IS MORE IMPORTANT THAN YOU THINK

Training for strength is not normally associated with novice lifters. Hoisting heavy weights when you're light on experience is a pretty easy way to get hurt. It's also precisely why the phases in this book have been arranged in the order they appear in. Jump into this phase without doing any of the prep work leading up to it, and you're asking for trouble. Not bothering to identify and correct weak links or failing to add the muscle mass your body needs to facilitate increases in strength will leave you wide open to injury. Trust me on this one: I've seen it happen to even the most experienced of lifters.

Why even bother training for strength in the first place? You're just a beginner; what do you need to be that strong for? It's not like you're going to go around the office telling everyone how much you can bench. Okay, maybe that was a bad example given the fragility of the male ego and its constant need for reassurance. My point is, the ability to move heavy objects may not be all that important to you. You might be content with bigger arms, a smaller waist, and the ability to walk from the couch to the refrigerator without getting winded.

Well, I'm here to tell you that as lofty as those goals may be, you're doing yourself a real disservice if you don't include increasing total body strength among them. Because aside from the whole not-getting-winded thing, none of those aesthetic goals can have as much of an impact on your daily life as getting stronger can.

STRONG ASSOCIATIONS

BEING STRONG IS ABOUT MORE THAN JUST LOOKING THE PART

When most people hear the word *strength*, they conjure up images of well-muscled individuals lifting unfathomable amounts of weight. We've all seen those strongman competitions on ESPN where guys with necks the size of tree trunks run with refrigerators on their backs or press gigantic logs over their heads. While that's certainly impressive in a freakish sort of way, there are far more diverse and realistic ways to express strength. Like, say, lifting the spare tire out of your trunk without throwing out your back. Or stepping down from a porch or high step without fear of your leg giving way. These are just a couple of examples of how having the ability to generate a little more force could come in handy.

Think about it for a minute. I'm sure if you tried you could come up with several instances throughout the day where you're called upon to display strength in some manner. If you're a manual laborer, it could involve loading and unloading heavy equipment or supplies into and out of your truck. This would require strength endurance, or the ability to utilize strength repeatedly over a given time frame. Then there's the ability to turn on the ball and drive one up the gap at the company softball game, which requires explosive strength. Finally, there's maximal, also known as absolute, strength, which you might need to loosen a stubborn lug nut when changing a tire or to lift a fallen tree off of a stranded hiker. What? It could happen.

Unfortunately, you don't necessarily improve your ability to carry out these types of tasks by engaging in the moderate-load, high-repetition training programs that most beginners gravitate toward. Sure, moderate weight with high reps can improve strength to some degree; the mere fact that you're working against some form of external resistance is going to make you stronger. The problem is that it won't necessarily be the type of strength that allows you to do the activities listed above. The repetitious nature of this type of training *might* have a favorable impact on strength endurance, but it'll have little if any effect on explosive or absolute strength. That's because training adaptations are extremely specific to the form of training used to bring them about. And when you lift only moderate loads at controlled speeds, you don't improve to any significant degree your ability to develop force quickly or substantially.

GETTING ON YOUR NERVES

WORKING ON A WORKOUT FOR YOUR NERVOUS SYSTEM

The reason that traditional types of "strength training" are so ineffective for improving either explosive or absolute strength is because they don't cause sufficient stimulation of your type IIb fast-twitch muscle fibers, the ones you need for quick, intense bursts of strength, like sprinting down the block or hoisting a heavy suitcase into your trunk. In most traditional lifting programs, your nervous system senses that you don't need either maximal or explosive force to overcome a given resistance. So it recruits those motor units (each comprised of a nerve cell and all of the muscle fibers it stimulates) it needs to get the work done: type IIa fast-twitch fibers, which are better suited to working against moderate loads for higher reps.

If you want to exert maximal or near-maximal force and/or contract your muscles rapidly, you need to provide your nervous system with the stimulus it needs to recruit type IIb fibers. Not that your nervous system won't be stimulated by training with lighter loads; the main reason most beginners experience strength gains early on in a training program is because their nervous systems become better at stimulating their muscles to contract. Where in the beginning your nervous system may be able to stimulate only a few of the motor units responsible for activating a given muscle, the more you train, the more motor units are called into play. It's just that the only way to tap into the motor units that activate those powerful type IIb muscle fibers is through both heavy and explosive lifting.

So why should you care about any of this? Because the ability to recruit type IIb fibers can come in awfully handy, whether you're helping your buddy move a sofa bed or sprinting after a toddler who's gone astray. And no matter how diligent you are about your workouts, continually focusing on just type IIa muscle fibers with bodybuilding-inspired workouts will never prepare you to meet these IIb demands. (For more on the differences between type IIa and IIb muscle fibers, see "Typecasting," below.) The best you can hope for is a body that looks good and may stand up to some light wear and tear. As soon as you're called upon to face one of life's little unexpected physical demands, chances are you won't be ready. Unless, of course, you embrace the idea of becoming stronger right now.

Training for strength is a lot more than some narcissistic pursuit designed to inflate your ego. It's a key element of any well-rounded fitness program that, in my opinion, ranks right up there with cardiovascular fitness and flexibility in terms of relevance to daily living and long-term health. It's amazing how relatively few people

TYPECASTING

Which muscle fibers are best suited for certain tasks?

Although there are various subdivisions of human muscle fibers, fibers are most commonly classified into three different groups: the fast-twitch types IIa and IIb and the less powerful type I's that are used more for endurance work. The chart below will help you distinguish which fibers are called upon most during specific activities, as well as what the ultimate work capacity of each fiber is. Keep in mind that all of these fibers work on a continuum, meaning that no particular task relies exclusively on one type of fiber. Your body first recruits type I's, and then if the task is difficult enough, quickly calls in type IIa's and finally type IIb's if needed. While no one type of fiber works completely on its own, the intensity you're working at determines which type predominates.

Fiber Type	Contraction Speed	Work Capacity	Sample Activities
IIb	Fast	0 to 8 seconds	Short-distance sprints, vertical jumps, and heavy/explosive weight training
IIa	Moderate-fast	8 to 90 seconds	Moderate-repetition weight training and middle-distance running
I	Slow	90 seconds +	Walking, jogging, and long-distance training, i.e., marathons and triathlons

seem to realize that. Everyone knows about the importance of cardiovascular exercise, and most folks include some amount of stretching in their routines. But the number of people who lift weights with the goal of becoming stronger is extremely limited. If you ask me, that has to do with the aura of danger that surrounds the idea of training for pure strength.

THE FEAR FACTOR

TRAINING FOR STRENGTH IS ONLY AS DANGEROUS AS YOU MAKE IT

Now don't get me wrong, I'm not saying that lifting heavy loads or moving lighter loads quickly and explosively isn't at least potentially dangerous. Obviously it's much easier to injure yourself lifting this way than by doing slow, controlled repetitions while sitting on a machine. The fact is, though, the only things that make training for strength dangerous are performing your exercises with sloppy technique or using too much weight. In and of themselves, few if any exercises are "dangerous"—not even those that have a high degree of difficulty, like the Olympic clean and press. This extremely complex, total-body movement is a fantastic way to improve explosive strength. It also, believe it or not, has far more application to daily living than a machine chest press (see page 177) or leg press (see page 196) does.

If you've ever bent over to scoop up your toddler and raise her overhead or in one motion picked up a heavy object off the floor and hoisted it onto a high shelf, you've already done a version of the clean and press. Granted, you weren't wearing a little unitard and there was no panel of judges to signal whether the lift was successful. But you still did it, and in all likelihood you will do it again at some point.

Yet it's rare to see anyone other than high-level athletes performing a formal clean and press exercise. Which is too bad really, because speed-based movements like this, hang cleans, and push presses, as well as near-maximal lifts on exercises like deadlifts and squats, have loads of application for the average person.

Now, I am by no means advocating that beginners rush right into doing any of the aforementioned exercises. I'm merely pointing out that after first improving flexibility, core strength, and the strength of some of the smaller, more intricate muscles that help stabilize joints—as you have done in the previous phases—training to develop explosive and absolute strength isn't the no-no many beginners perceive it to be. Not that you should train this way all the time, mind you. Routinely engaging in this type of training can be very stressful to your nervous system, joints, and connective tissues. But as part of properly organized periodized training, it can be extremely beneficial to people of all ages.

That said, for some people certain movements may prove problematic. Those with lower-back problems (i.e., disc herniations) or chronic knee or shoulder problems may find that the risks of lifting heavy or explosively far outweigh the benefits. I'd be pretty reluctant to attempt a set of heavy deadlifts with a herniated disc or to thrust weights explosively over my head if I suffered from chronic shoulder pain. If you fall into this category, aside from recommending that you seek proper medical attention to alleviate the problem, I've also included some alternative exercises you can do to replace any of those a bit beyond your reach right now.

As for the rest of you, if you're still a little skittish about training to increase strength, you needn't be. So long as you have done the necessary prep work and follow the directions for correctly performing the exercises, you should be fine.

THINK BIG

MORE STRENGTH = MORE MUSCLE

Besides improved nervous system function, another benefit of getting stronger is that it enables you to put on muscle mass at a much quicker rate. As I've already mentioned, both heavy loads and quick, explosive muscle actions stimulate your type IIb muscle fibers. Well, as luck would have it, these also happen to be the fibers that have the greatest potential for growth. Unfortunately, they go largely unchallenged when you continually work with loads light enough to allow for reps in the 8-to-15 range. Oh sure, your type IIa fibers get plenty of work, but the real powerhouses pretty much lay low. Therefore, if your goal is to get bigger, it only makes sense to dedicate at least some time to targeting those fast-twitch fibers.

Secondly, increasing your strength means that you'll be able to lift more weight for the same number of reps. Let's say that you can bench-press 185 pounds for 10 reps. Then, after a 4- to 6-week strength phase like the one contained in this chapter, you can suddenly bench 200 pounds for those same 10 reps. More weight being moved for the same number of reps over the same time frame will equal more muscle mass.

In case you're more interested in being stronger than in looking the part, don't sweat it. If you're not interested in picking up added size, simply stay at or slightly below your calculated daily caloric needs. That way you'll get the strength boost without the extra bulk.

TAKES A LICKING . . .

A STRONGER BODY IS MORE RESISTANT TO INJURY

Last but not least, allow me to hit you with perhaps the most important reason why you need to get stronger. The stronger you are—provided, of course, that strength is accompanied by sufficient flexibility—the more resistant you'll be to injury. Just about any weight room injury you can name (aside from dropping a weight on your foot) can be linked to a lack of strength somewhere on the body. Just because the prime movers of a given exercise can handle the load doesn't mean all the support structures necessarily can. Some of the more common examples of this include shoulder injuries, which are almost always due to insufficient rotator cuff strength. Also prevalent are knee injuries brought on by strength imbalances of various lower-body muscles—like, for instance, a knee that buckles inward when squatting because of insufficient strength in the glutes on that side. Gee, where have you heard that one before?

This reduced injury potential extends beyond the gym walls. How many times have you seen a guy bend over to pick something up and throw out his back? Now, I know what you're going to say, and I agree: Backs are tricky that way. Sometimes it's just a matter of moving the wrong way; no matter how strong you are, you're doomed. But it also stands to reason that a stronger core would, at the very least, reduce your chances of sustaining such an injury. And what about your legs? Do you have any idea how much you ask them to do in an average day? From lunging and stepping to quick starts and rapid decelerations, your legs need to be able to withstand an awful lot. Strengthening the muscles that surround and support the various joints of your lower body is your best defense against things like ACL tears, shin splints, and even hip fractures.

HOW MUCH, HOW HARD, AND HOW OFTEN?

QUANTIFYING YOUR STRENGTH-TRAINING PROGRAM

Now that I've calmed your fears and convinced you that training for strength can actually be beneficial, it's time to address some of the other concerns you may have. Namely, how heavy, how intensely, and how often should a virtual neophyte like you (remember, you still have only a couple of phases of training under your belt) engage in this type of training? That's a fair question. After all, it's one thing to realize that this is a worthwhile way to train; it's another entirely to do it with any sort of confidence. So before I get you started on the actual programs, let's first go over all of the parameters you'll need to follow for a safe and productive experience.

Loading: For all of the heavy-lifting exercises, like squats, deadlifts, bench presses, and rows, select a load that allows for 3 to 5 reps per set with proper form. Be sure not to go to the point of muscular failure. Training to increase strength is stressful enough on your central nervous system; the last thing you want is to push to the point where you're about to pass out. Besides, training to the point of failure is an inefficient way to improve strength because it extends your recovery time between workouts considerably. You're much better off stopping when you think you might have been able to get one more rep with good form.

So how will you know if you've selected the appropriate weight? One of the best ways to gauge your progress is by monitoring the speed at which the weight travels. If the bar starts to slow considerably as you get deeper into the set, you won't get as good a strength-building stimulus from the exercise. Whatever speed that bar starts at, make sure it stays right around that speed for best results. You don't have to use a stopwatch or anything, just eyeball it. Better yet, count in your head as you raise and lower the bar. Try to keep both the lowering (negative) and raising (positive) phase of each lift to about 2 seconds max. As soon as that weight starts to slow down, simply stop the set. This will help ensure that your strength levels continue to climb and you're not overtaxing your nervous system.

For the explosive exercises, the weight needs to be considerably lighter to allow for speed of movement. This is slightly different from the example provided above. Heavy loads can actually move somewhat slowly due to the amount of weight you'll be using (although in reality you'll be pushing them as hard and fast as you can to recruit those fast-twitch fibers like nobody's business); it's just that as soon as the speed of the weight decreases from what it was at the start of the exercise, it's time to stop the set. With the explosive lifts, the weight will literally be moving quite fast. If you can't move it quickly, you'll know you've gone too heavy. You just want to maintain the same speed throughout the set. Stay in the 3- to 5-rep range with these exercises as well, only using a much lighter weight—one that you could normally lift 8 to 10 times.

Volume: Because you'll be lifting the weights for relatively few reps, to create enough of an overload for improvement you'll need to do more sets than in previous phases. So where you've been doing 2 or 3 sets per exercise, in this phase you'll be doing 4 to 6. Additionally, because your nervous system takes longer to recover than your muscles do, when doing heavy and explosive exercises you'll extend your rest intervals to as long as 3 minutes between sets. I know that sounds like a long time, but you need to ensure that you adequately recover between efforts. The stored chemical energy you'll be calling on to carry out these exercises requires ample time to regenerate inside your body. Start your next set too soon and you probably won't complete the desired rep range. One final note: There are bodyweight strengthening exercises in this phase that require only 60 to 90 seconds of rest after each set, because they don't subject you to anywhere near as much loading as the heavy and explosive moves.

Frequency: As far as how often you should train, go with 3 days per week, for a couple of reasons. First, since you're a beginner you really won't be using all that much weight. That means your recuperative powers won't be taxed to the same extent as a more experienced lifter's would, so you can train with greater frequency. Secondly, to help build "real world," aka functional, strength, I've included either 1 or 2 days per week (depending on your level of training experience) of less familiar, calisthenic-type exercises that are designed to improve total-body strength and mobility at the same time. Some will use additional weight, while others will be difficult enough to perform using just your own body weight for resistance.

Make no mistake, these are challenging exercises that will have a major impact on the way your body functions outside of the gym. Approach them with an open mind and plenty of humility, because they're a lot different from many of the exercises you've done in past phases. Just because they may seem a bit foreign to you—and to your fellow gym members—that doesn't mean they aren't effective.

THE STRENGTH WORKOUTS

STRENGTH TRAINING BY THE NUMBERS

In keeping with our theme of matching appropriate workouts to specific types of beginners, there are two different routines featured in this phase: one for those who are over 35 and/or completely inexperienced and one for those under 35 with some former exposure to training. The most significant differences between the two are that the former stresses total-body strength and mobility to a greater degree, while the latter requires a bit more heavy lifting. In both instances, I've included alternative exercises in the event that some of you have preexisting orthopedic limitations that may prevent you from attempting some of the primary exercises listed.

Workout #1

Target population: Newbies of all ages, as well as ex-jocks and seasonal lifters over age 35

Frequency: 3 lifting days per week on a rotating schedule, i.e. workout A on Monday, workout B on Wednesday, and workout A again on Friday

Number of sets per exercise: 3 or 4 for mobility exercises (workout A); 4 to 6 for traditional lifts (workout B)

Number of reps per set: 4 to 6 per set for mobility exercises; 3 to 5 (with each limb, where applicable) for traditional lifts (except for prone external rotation, for which you should do 10 to 12)

Rest intervals between sets: 60 to 90 seconds for mobility exercises; 2½ to 3 minutes for traditional lifts

Workout A (Monday and Friday): Strength and Mobility

Turkish get-up

Reverse pushup (supinated grip)

Elevated one-leg squat (off step, or bench)

Overhead squat

Lower-body rotation

Workout B (Wednesday): Pure Strength

Barbell deadlift or dumbbell deadlift

Barbell push press or incline dumbbell bench press

Split squat

One-arm row

Prone external rotation

This isn't a typical workout, where your body is divided into different segments. There are no specific exercises for smaller muscle groups like the arms and calves; these muscles will be doing their fair share of work during some of the other lifts. You may also notice that between the reverse pushups and the one-arm rows, there's some form of upper-back strengthening each time you train. That's because most guys tend to neglect this area in favor of doing too much chest work. The heavy rowing emphasis combined with the external rotations is intended to balance the muscles that surround the shoulder.

Although both the Turkish get-up and the elevated one-leg squat involve a speed component during the upward phase of the movement, I've included only one true "explosive" exercise here: the barbell push press. The overhead squat and lower-body rotation are holdovers from the self-assessment phase (so is the one-leg squat, although this time you'll be performing it a little bit differently). The only difference is that this time you'll be doing the overhead squat and lower-body rotation as actual exercises, not as assessment tools. They'll also serve as a nice gauge of whether you did all your homework during your corrective phase.

Workout #2

Target population: Ex-jocks and seasonal lifters under age 35

Frequency: 3 days per week, i.e. workout A on Monday, workout B on Wednesday, and workout C on Friday

Number of sets per exercise: 4 to 6 for traditional lifts (workouts A and C); 3 or 4 for mobility exercises (workout B)

Number of reps per set: 3 to 5 (with each limb, where applicable) for traditional lifts, except for reverse flies and prone external rotations, for which you should do 10 to 12; 4 to 6 for mobility exercises

Rest intervals between sets: 2½ to 3 minutes for traditional lifts; 60 to 90 seconds for mobility exercises

Workout A

Squat or leg press

Barbell push press or incline dumbbell bench press

Prone dumbbell row with elbows out

Split squat

Reverse fly

Workout B

Turkish get-up

Reverse pushup (pronated grip)

Overhead squat

T-pushup

Lower-body rotation

Workout C

Chinup or lat pulldown

Clean pull or dumbbell deadlift and shrug

Barbell bench press

Swiss ball leg curl or lying leg curl

Prone external rotation

As with workout #1, I've supplied you with a couple of alternative exercises in the event that you can't execute certain movements due to preexisting injuries. I've also given you a couple of explosive strength exercises: the push press and the clean pull. While the dumbbell deadlift and shrug should also be performed explosively, the main difference between it and the clean pull is that holding dumbbells at your sides, instead of a barbell in front of you, will allow those with lower-back issues to maintain a more upright posture. This will help keep unnecessary strain off your lower back. Using a neutral grip when doing both the push press and the incline press is another useful strategy for taking strain off joints, as your shoulders will find this to be more comfortable.

Something else that warrants mention is the higher-repetition range used for both the prone external rotation and reverse fly. Since both exercises strengthen the muscles that act on the posterior (rear) aspect of the shoulder, they help improve structural balance. Both also play an important role in promoting proper posture, which makes them more responsive to higher-rep ranges since postural muscles are highly fatigue resistant and respond best to reps in the 10-and-up range.

Finally, a word of warning about the Swiss ball leg curl that appears in workout C. Although this is one of the most effective hamstring exercises you can do, the eccentric phase of the exercise, where you bring the ball back out away from your body, is very challenging. Be sure your hamstring flexibility is up to par before attempting this. Being able to straighten your leg directly above your hip when lying on your back is a good gauge.

TURKISH GET-UP

Lie on your back holding a light dumbbell in your right hand directly over your shoulder.

Begin by sitting up to the left and propping yourself up on your left forearm. As you do this, bend your knees and bring your feet in toward your rear end as you look to plant your right foot into the floor.

Keeping the dumbbell perpendicular to the floor throughout all of this, shift most of your weight to your right foot.

Stand, reaching the dumbbell towards the ceiling. Slowly reverse the steps and get back down on the floor, completing the desired number of reps with your right side before moving on to your left.

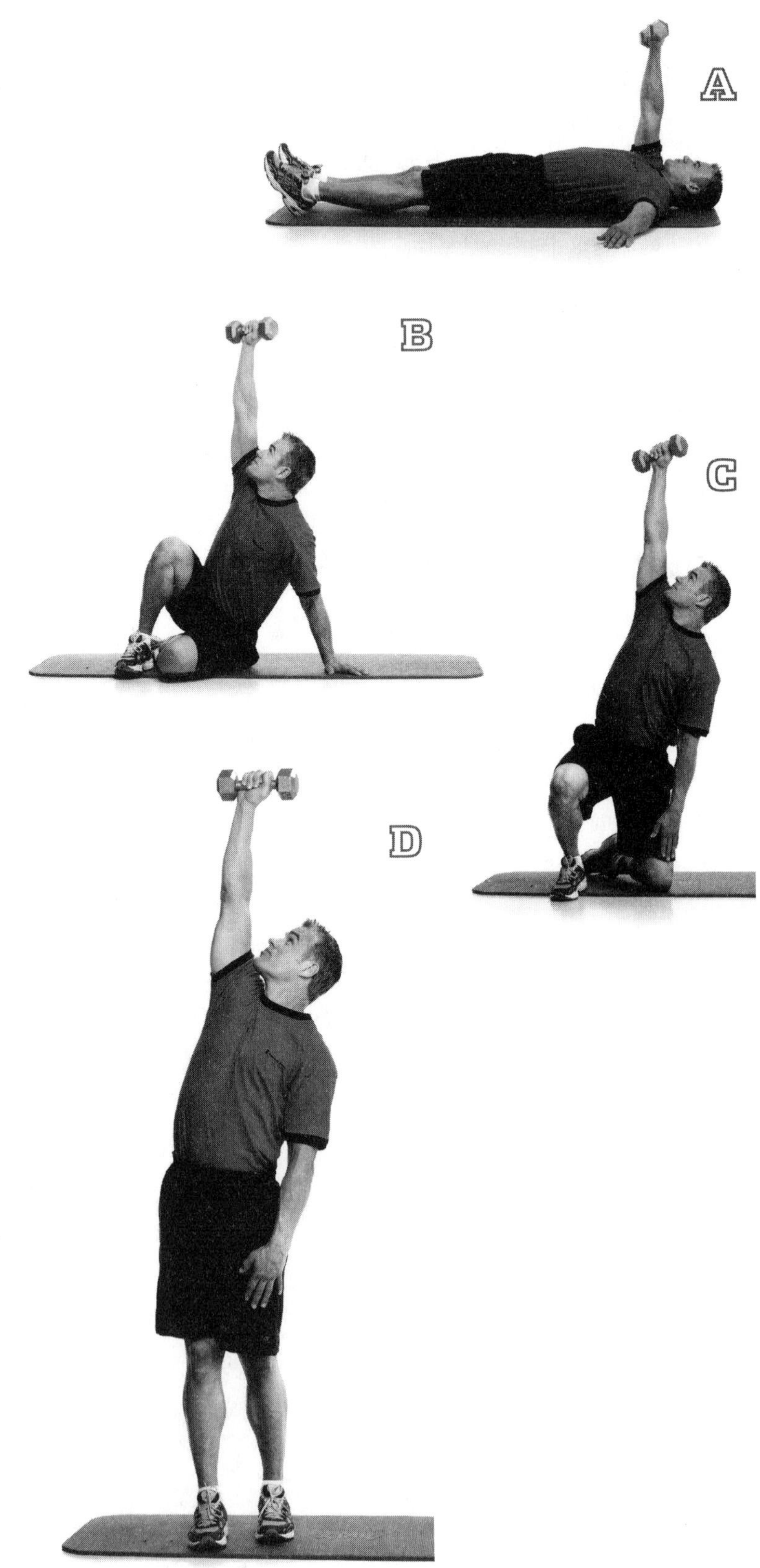

REVERSE PUSHUP (SUPINATED GRIP)

Lie underneath a barbell set in the supports in the squat rack (how high the bar is depends on how strong you are; the higher up you place it, the easier the exercise is to do). Grasp the bar with a palms-up, or supinated grip, and support your weight on the backs of your heels as shown.

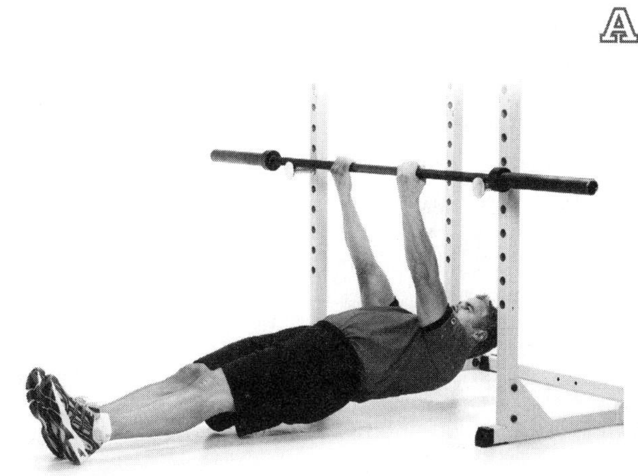

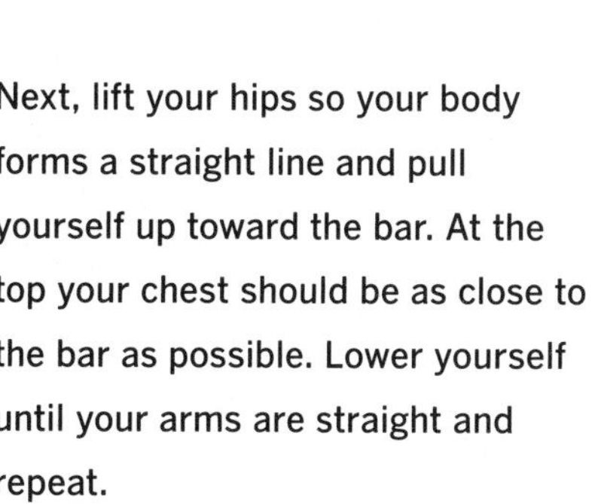

Next, lift your hips so your body forms a straight line and pull yourself up toward the bar. At the top your chest should be as close to the bar as possible. Lower yourself until your arms are straight and repeat.

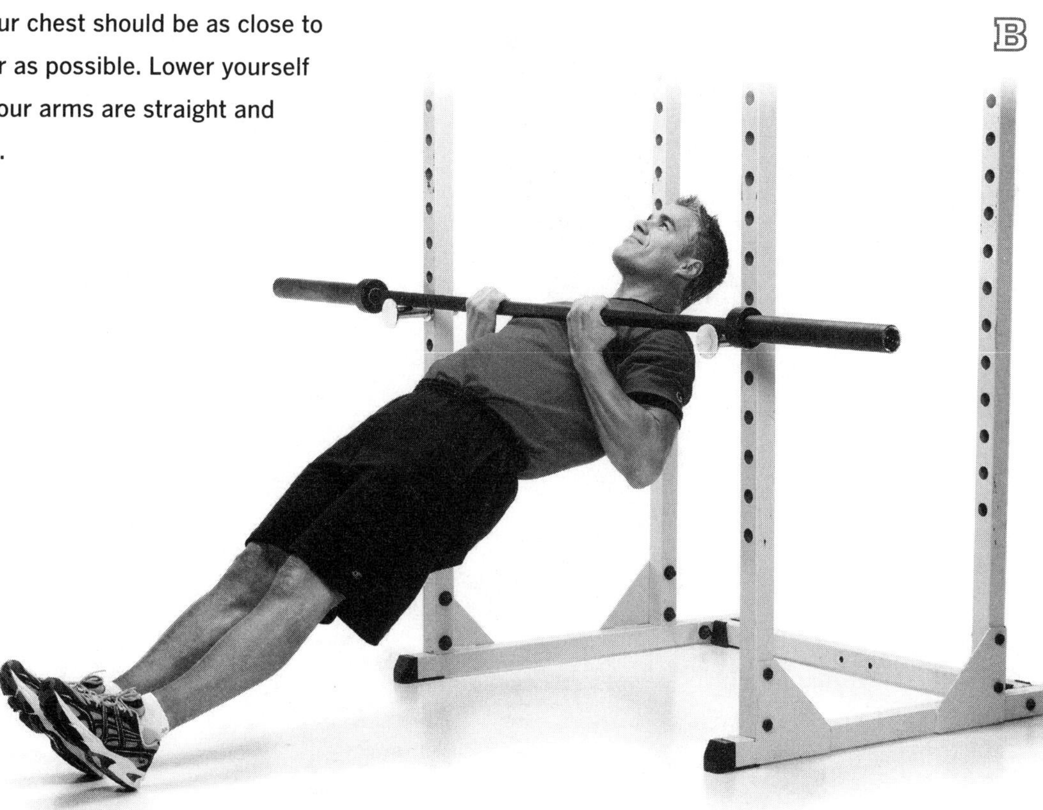

ELEVATED ONE-LEG SQUAT

Stand on a bench or sturdy step, allowing one leg to hang off the side.

Next, hold that leg out slightly in front of you as you allow your arms to come forward and bend your supporting knee and hip to lower yourself down as far as possible. Once there, pause and press back up, making sure to hold the other leg out in front of you the entire time. Finish your set and then do the same number of reps with your other leg.

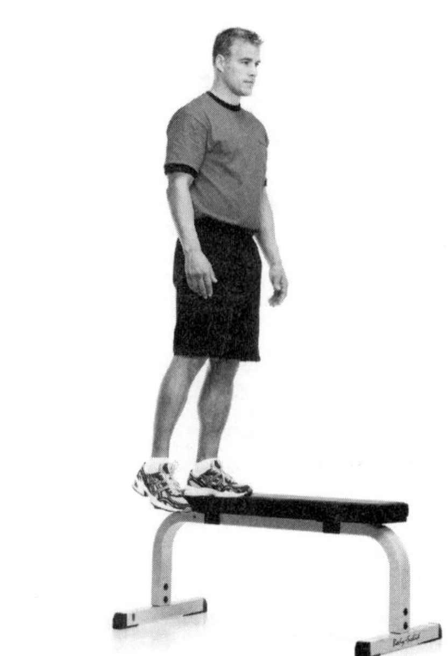

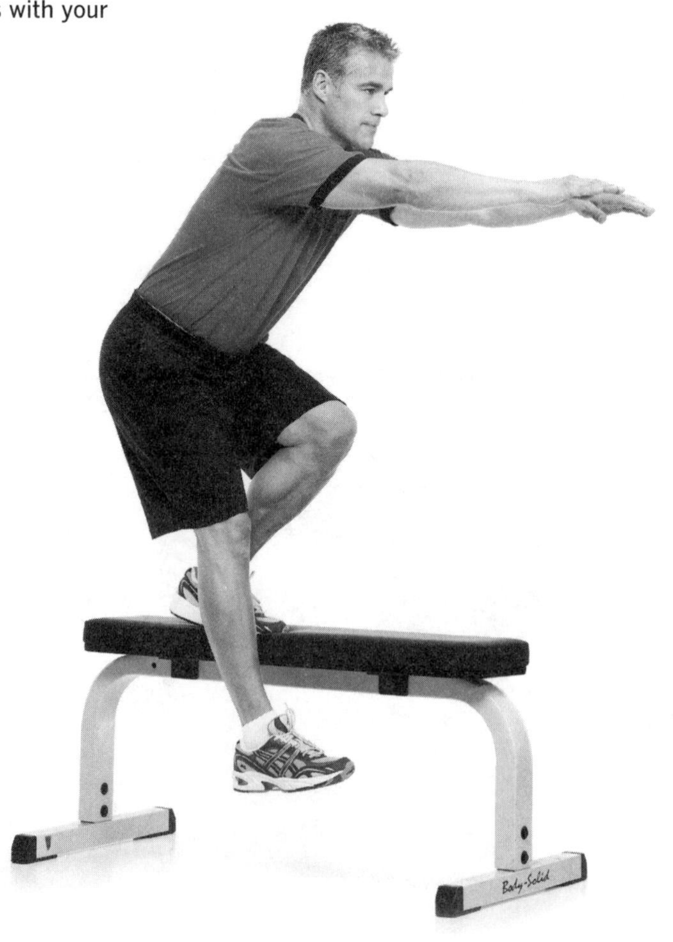

B

OVERHEAD SQUAT

Hold a light barbell with a wide overhand grip and press it up so that your arms are fully extended above you. The bar should be directly over your shoulders. Set your feet shoulder-width apart, knees slightly bent, back straight, eyes focused straight ahead.

Next, slowly lower your body as if you were sitting back into a chair, keeping your back in its natural alignment. When your upper thighs are parallel to the floor, pause, then return to the starting position.

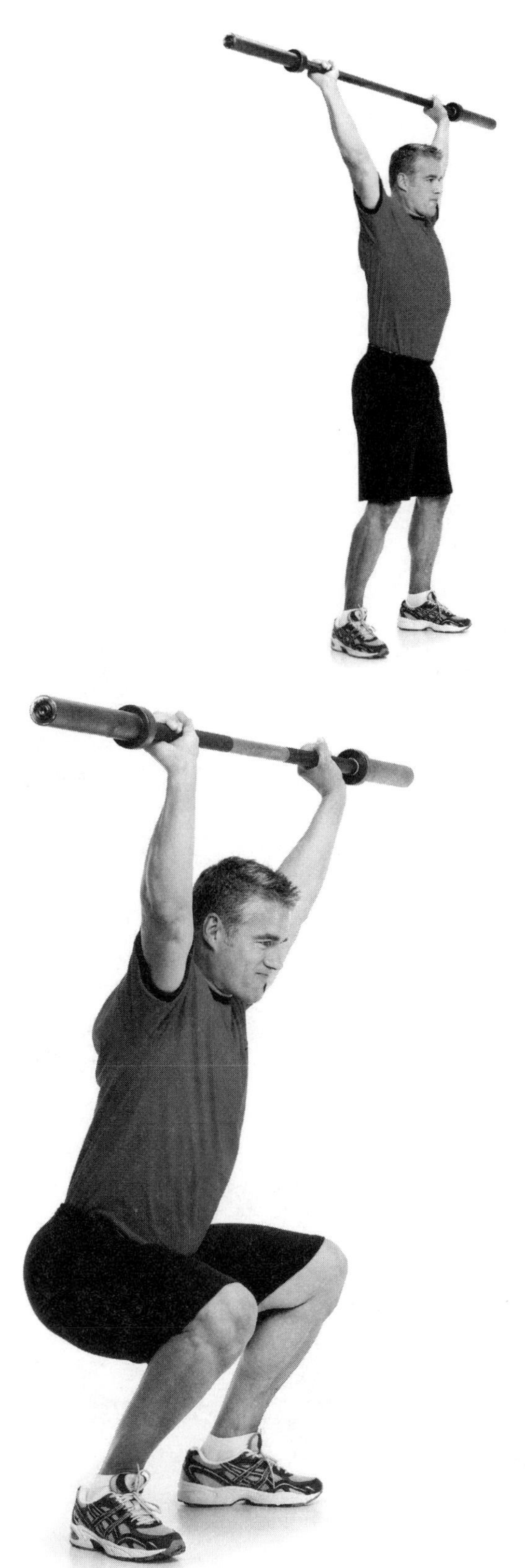

A

B

LOWER-BODY ROTATION

Lie on your back on the floor with your arms outstretched to the sides and your legs stacked over your hips.

Keeping both shoulders in contact with the floor throughout the movement, allow your legs to drift over to one side as far as possible. Pause in the lowest position and use your core muscles to bring your legs back to the starting position and then repeat to the other side.

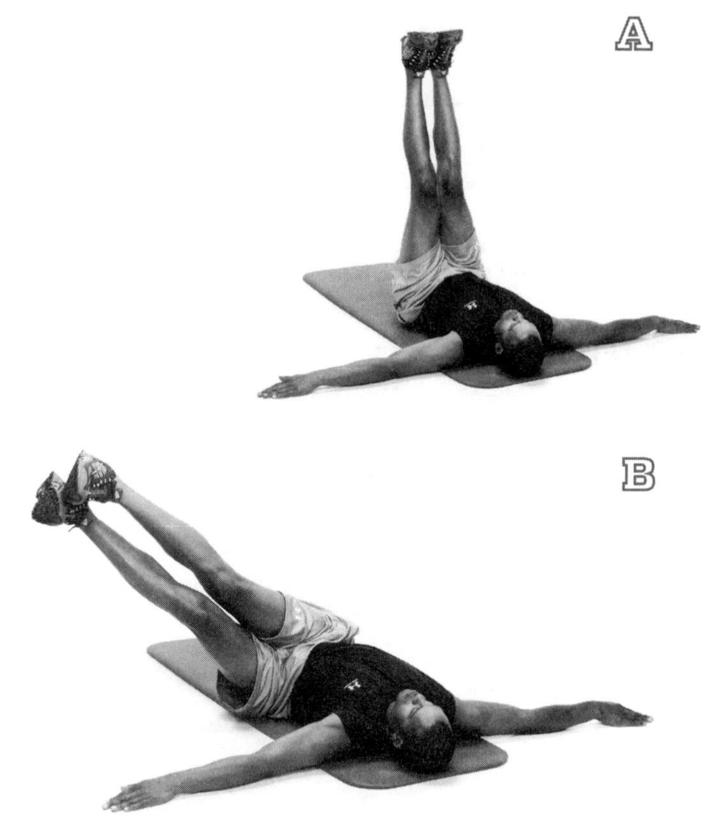

A

B

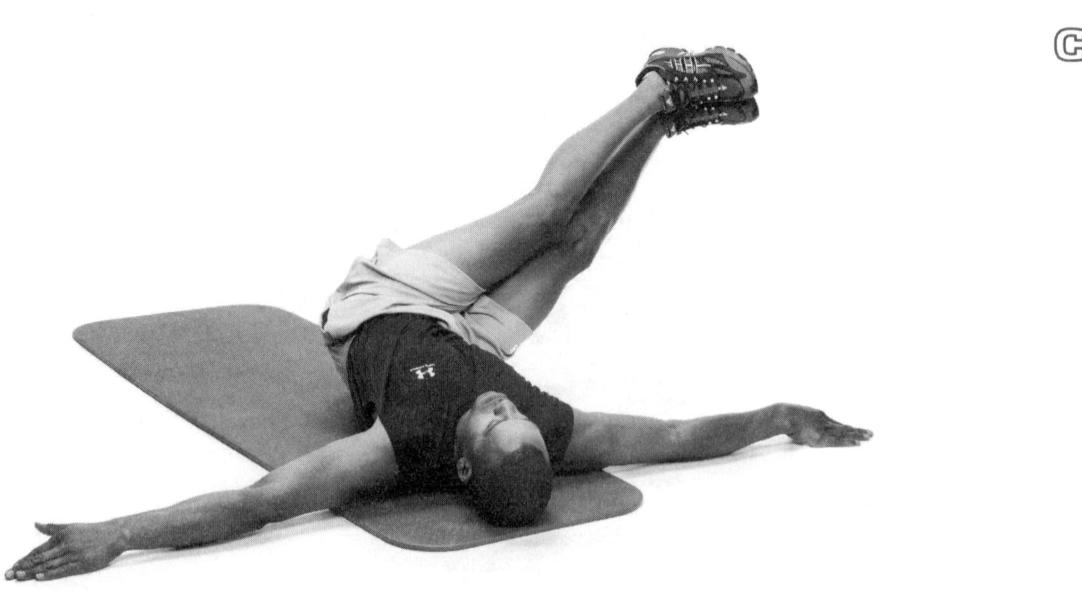

C

BARBELL DEADLIFT

Set a barbell on the floor and stand facing it. Squat down and grab it overhand, your hands just outside your legs.

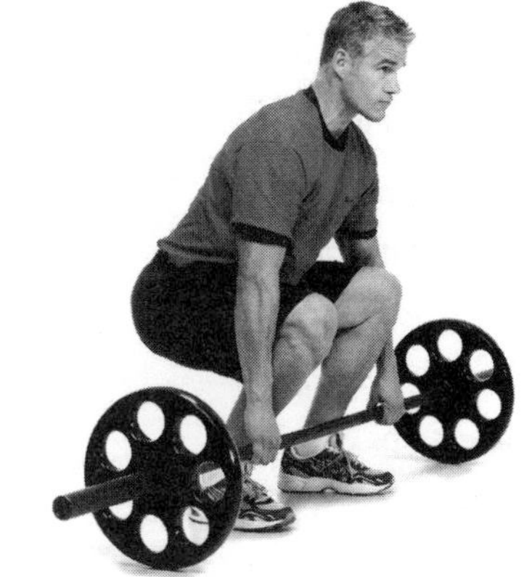

With your back flat and head up, stand up with the barbell, pulling your shoulder blades back. Then slowly lower the bar to the starting position.

Note: Those of you who have lower-back issues may want to either start from the top position (by taking the bar off the supports in a squat rack) or not go as low. Or do the exercise with dumbbells held at your sides, which allows you to maintain a more upright posture and reduced lower-back strain.

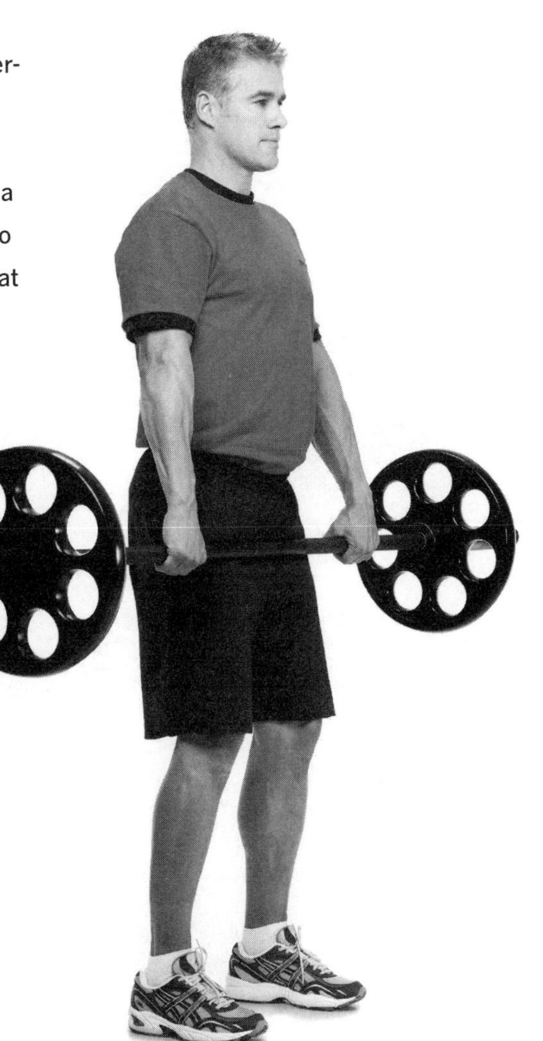

B

INCLINE DUMBBELL BENCH PRESS

A

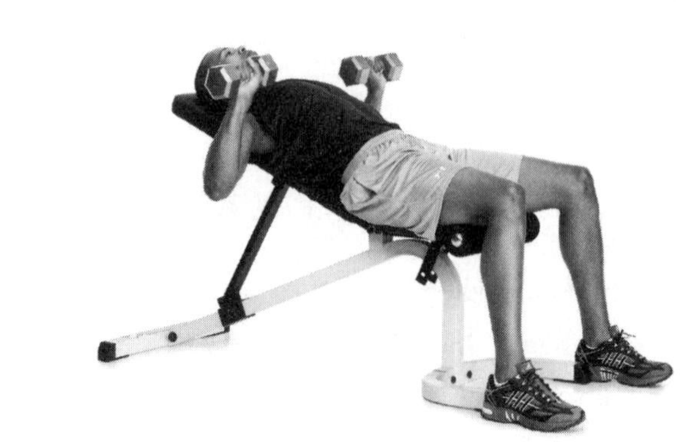

Grab a pair of dumbbells and lie on your back on a bench set to a low incline (15 to 30 degrees). Lift the dumbbells so they're over your chin and hold them with your palms turned forward (thumbs facing each other). Slowly lower the weights to your upper chest, pause, then push them back up over your chin.

Note: This exercise can also be performed with a neutral grip (palms facing each other) and your elbows closer to your body to minimize shoulder strain.

B

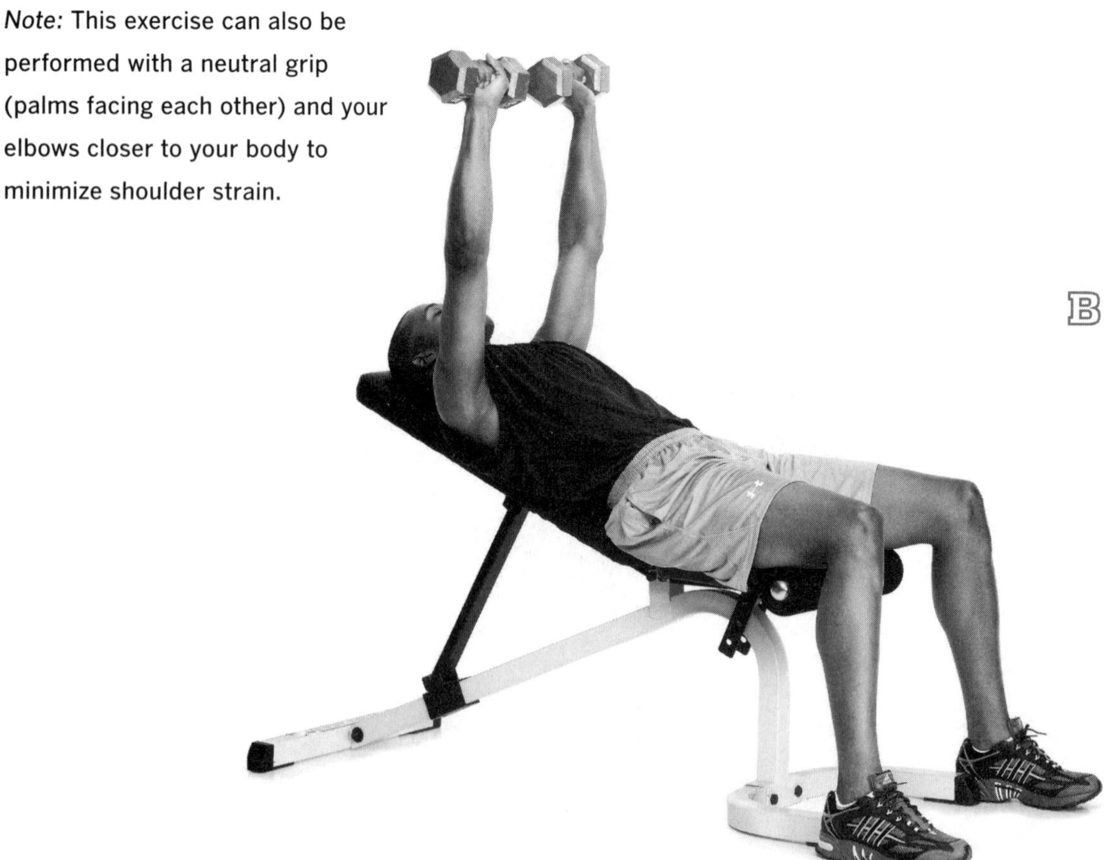

BARBELL PUSH PRESS

Grab a barbell with a shoulder-width, overhand grip. Stand holding the barbell at shoulder level, your feet shoulder-width apart and knees slightly bent.

Dip your knees slightly and push up with your legs as you press the barbell over your head. Lean your head back slightly as you push the barbell above you, but keep your torso upright. Lower the barbell to the starting position.

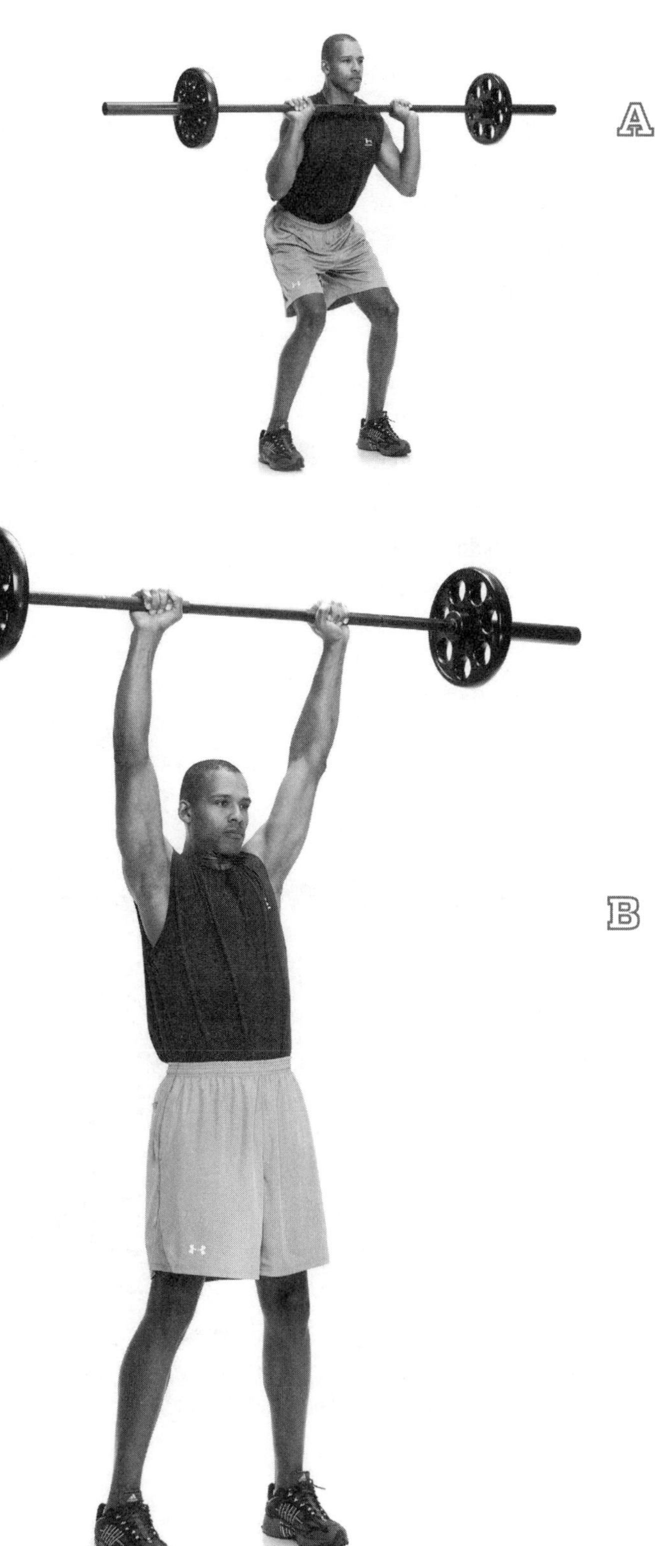

SPLIT SQUAT

Stand with a barbell across your upper back and one leg approximately 2 to $2^1/_2$ feet in front of the other, with only the ball of your back foot in contact with the floor.

Keeping your torso as straight as possible, bend both knees and descend toward the floor so that in the bottom position your lead leg forms a 90-degree angle. Pause and press back up to the starting position.

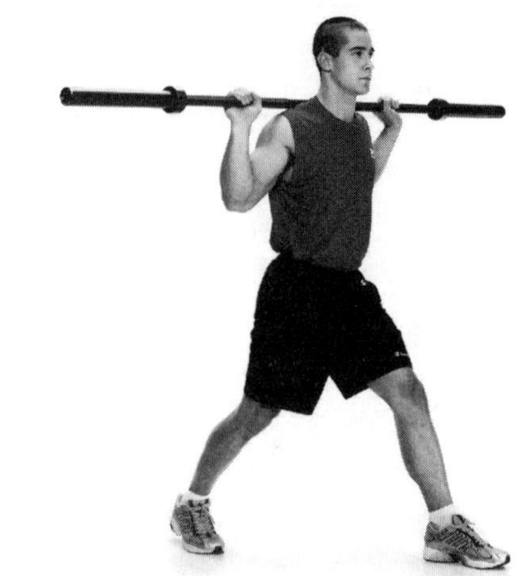

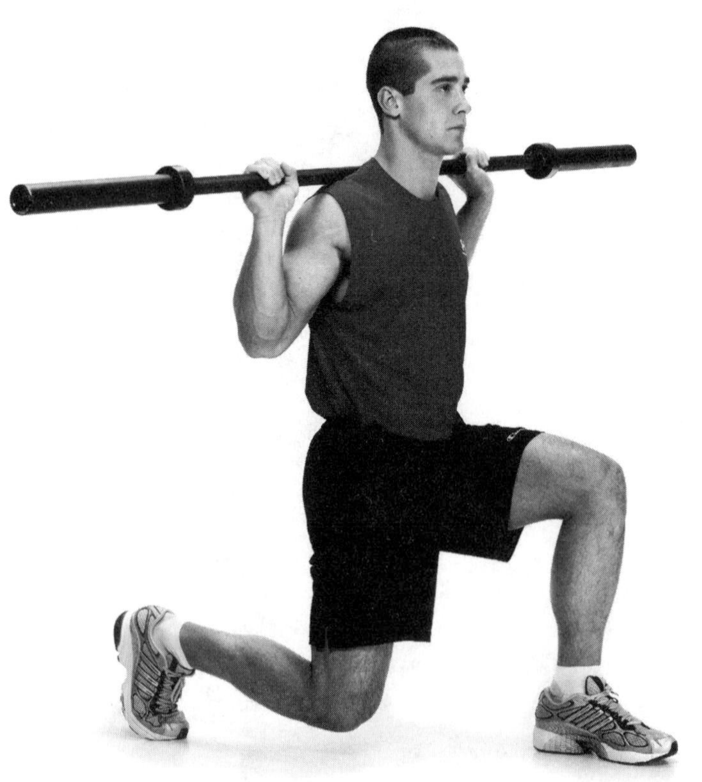

B

ONE-ARM ROW

Grab a dumbbell in one hand and place your opposite hand and knee on a flat bench. Keep your back flat and your upper body parallel to the floor. Let your working arm hang straight down at your side. Turn your palm so that it's facing your other arm.

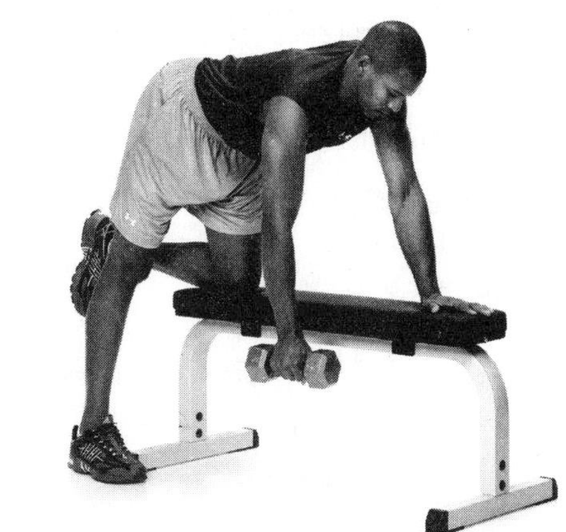

Pull the dumbbell up to the side of your chest and back toward your hip by bending your arm and squeezing your shoulder blade toward the middle of your back. Pause and then slowly return to the starting position. Finish your set and then do the same number of reps with your other arm.

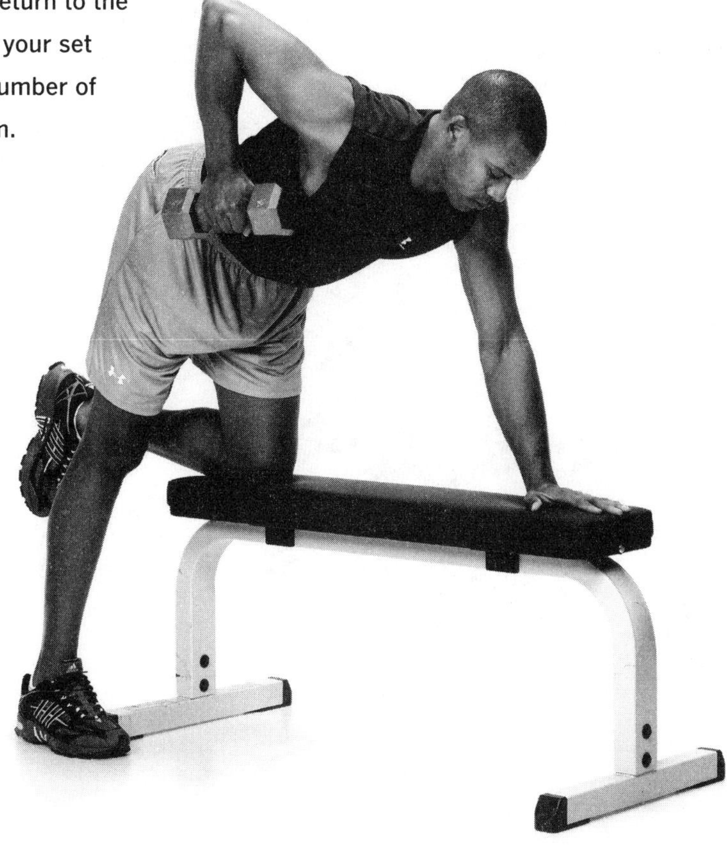

B

PRONE EXTERNAL ROTATION

Set an incline bench to a 45-degree angle and lie facedown on it holding a pair of light dumbbells. Begin by raising your upper arms so they're perpendicular to your torso and parallel to the floor. Next, bend your elbows 90 degrees, so your forearms hang straight down toward the floor and your palms face back.

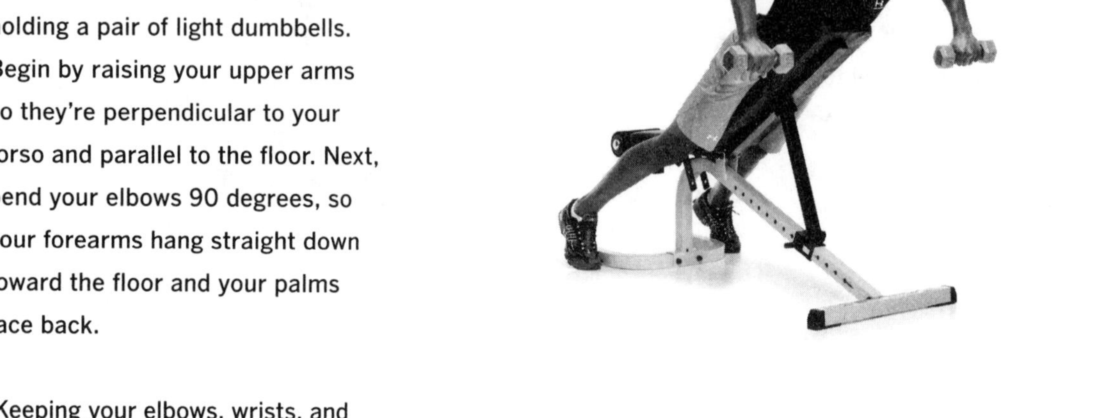
A

Keeping your elbows, wrists, and upper arms in fixed positions, rotate the weights up and toward you as far as you can—you want your shoulders to act like hinges, your arms like swinging gates. Pause and then slowly lower the weights to the starting position.

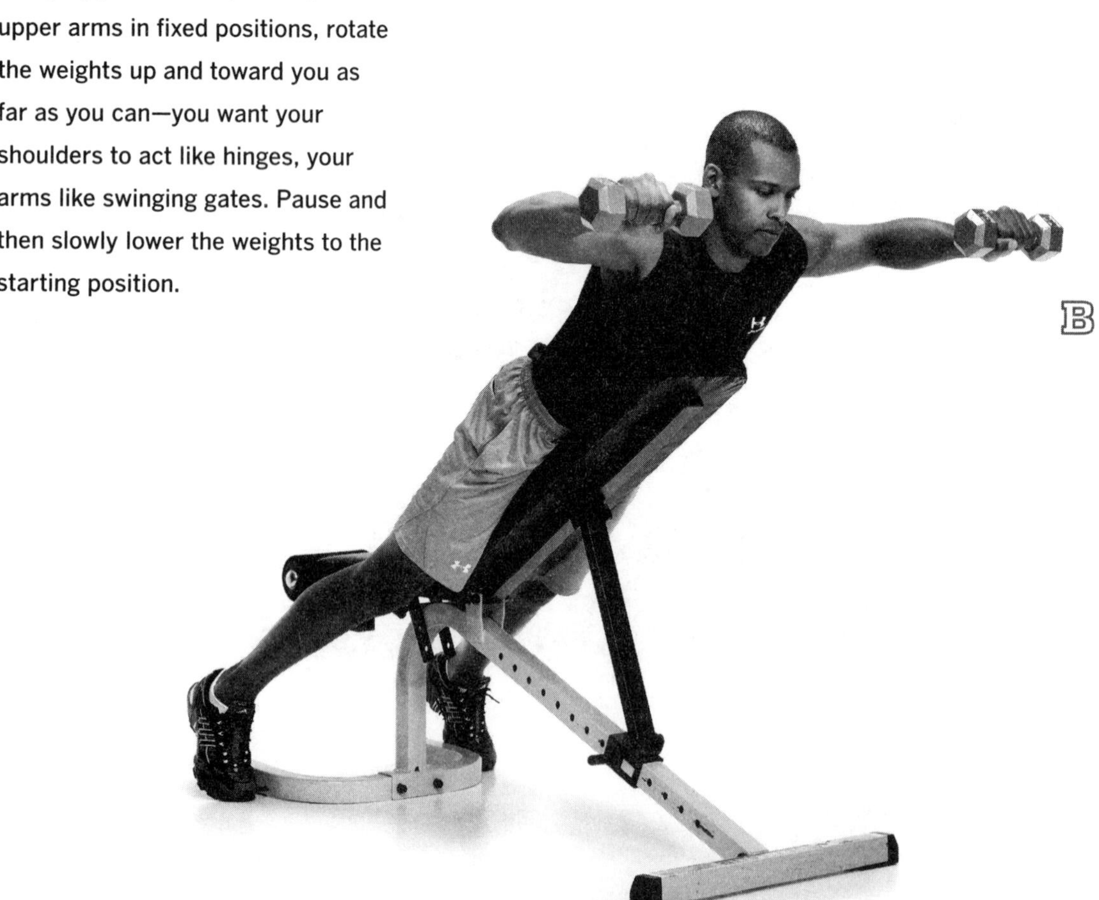
B

BARBELL SQUAT

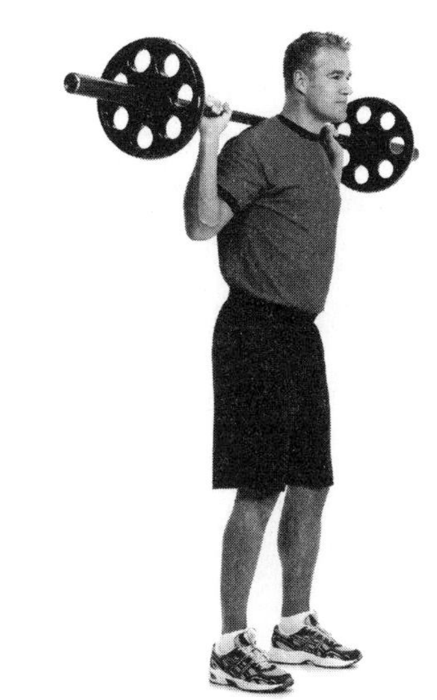

Hold a barbell with an overhand grip so that it rests comfortably on your upper back (not on your neck). Set your feet shoulder-width apart, knees slightly bent, back straight, eyes focused straight ahead.

Next, slowly lower your body as if you were sitting back into a chair, keeping your back in its natural alignment and lower legs nearly perpendicular to the floor. When your thighs are parallel to the floor, pause, and then return to the starting position.

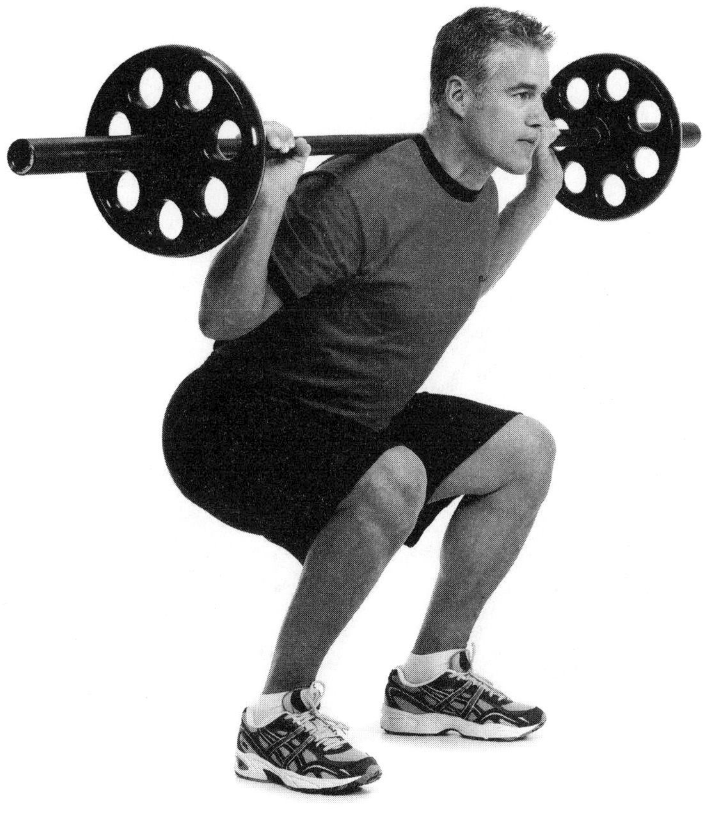

B

LEG PRESS

Position yourself in a 45-degree plate-loaded leg press sled with your feet about shoulder-width apart and your lower back pressed into the pad.

Begin by unlocking the sled and slowly lowering the weight down toward your chest. Once your thighs are parallel to the force plate, pause for a second and push back up to the starting position.

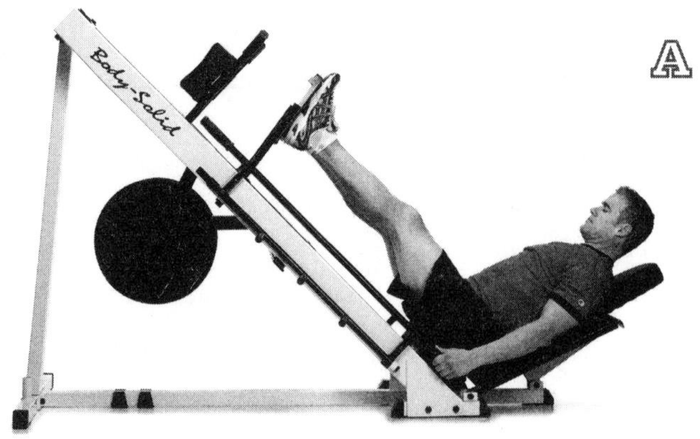

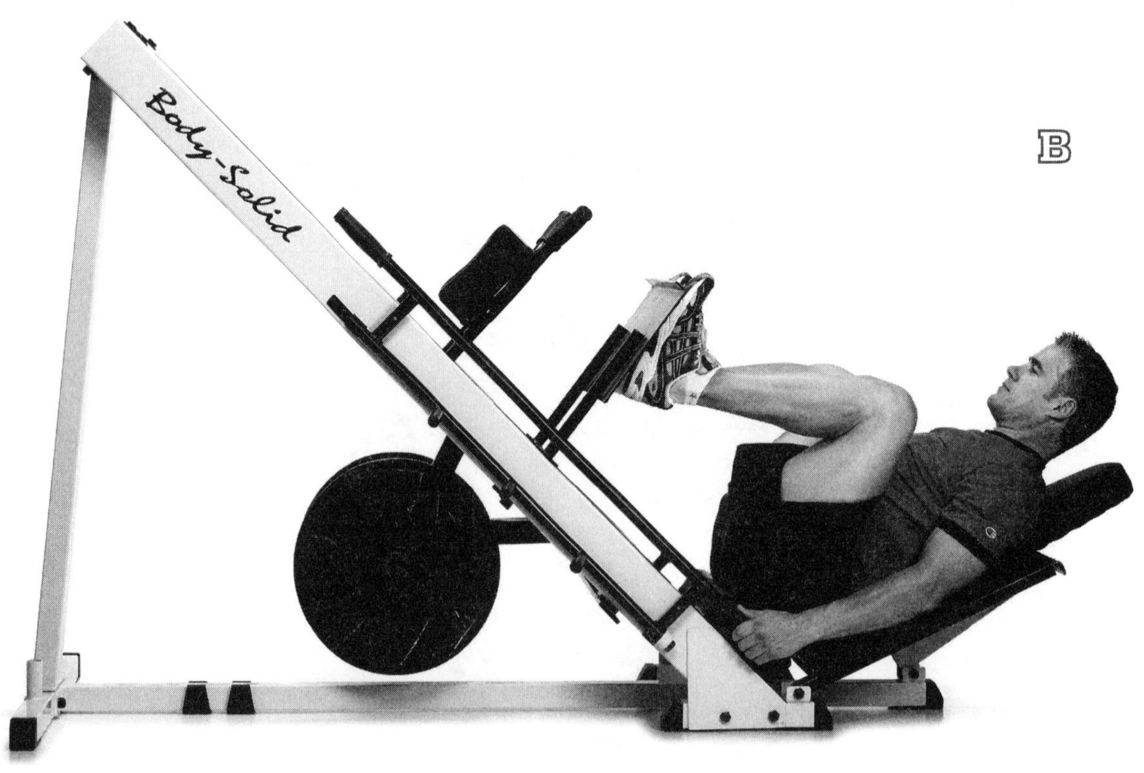

PRONE DUMBBELL ROW WITH ELBOWS OUT

Lie facedown on an incline bench set to a 45-degree angle holding a pair of dumbbells down at arm's length and turn your palms so that your thumbs are facing each other.

Lift your upper arms as high as you can by bending your elbows and squeezing your shoulder blades together. Your forearms should be pointing toward the floor throughout the movement. Pause, then slowly lower the weights to the starting position.

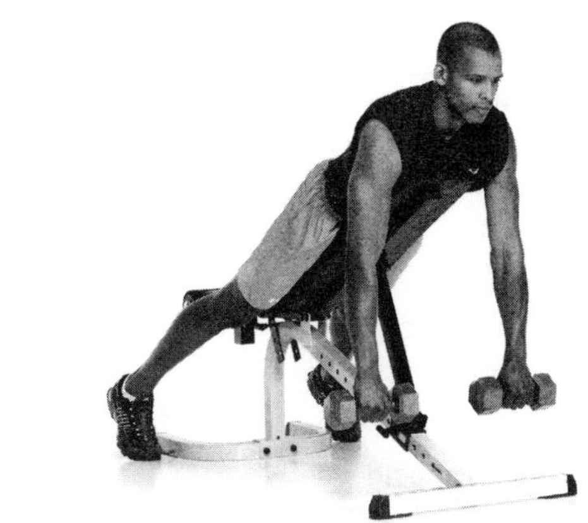

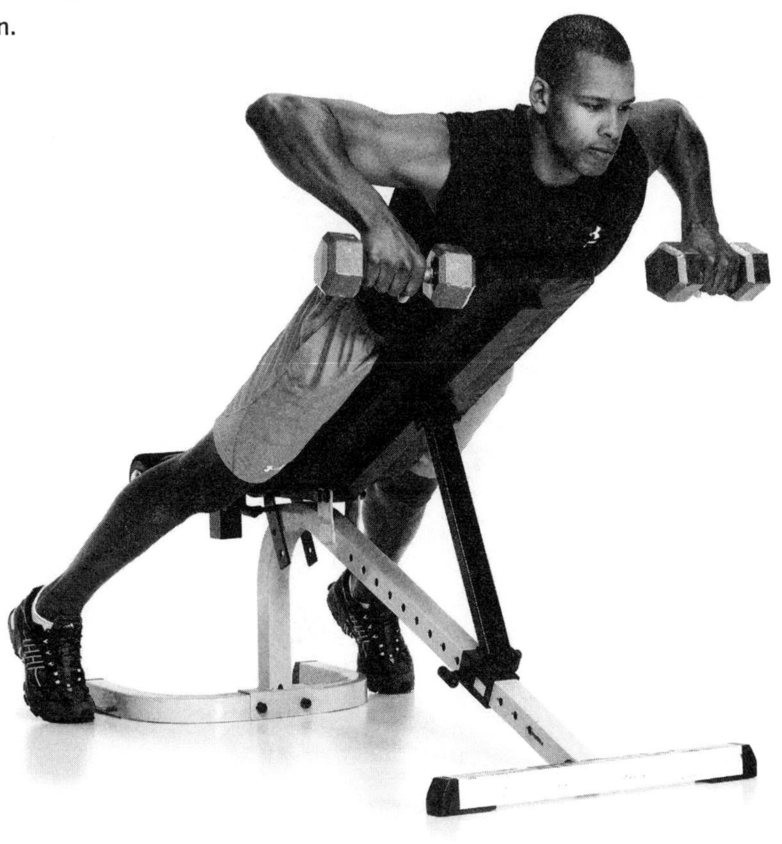

B

REVERSE FLY

Lie prone over a 45-degree incline bench holding a pair of dumbbells down at arm's length.

Keeping a slight bend in your elbows, pinch your shoulder blades together and work your arms up in a wide, arcing motion. At the top of the movement your elbows should remain slightly bent and you should see the weights out of the corners of your eyes.

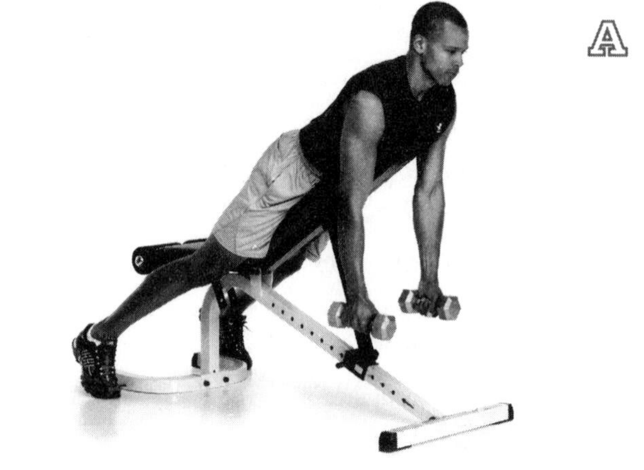

A

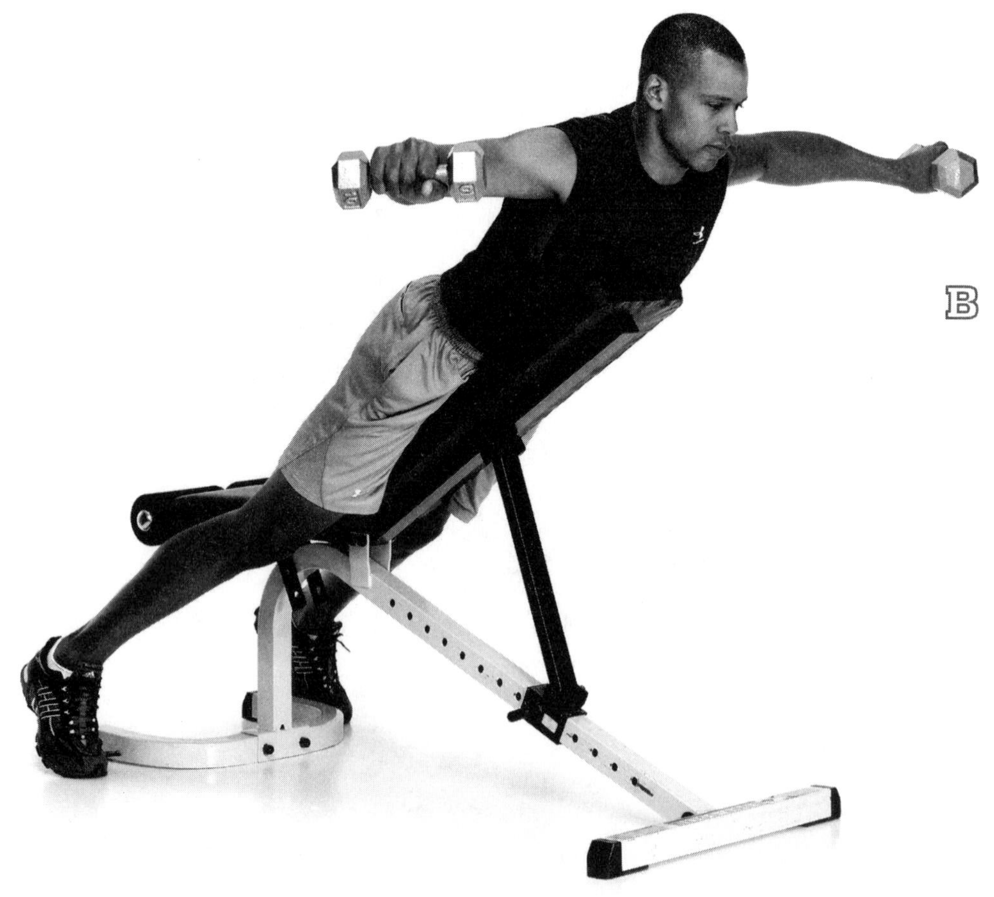

B

T-PUSHUP

A

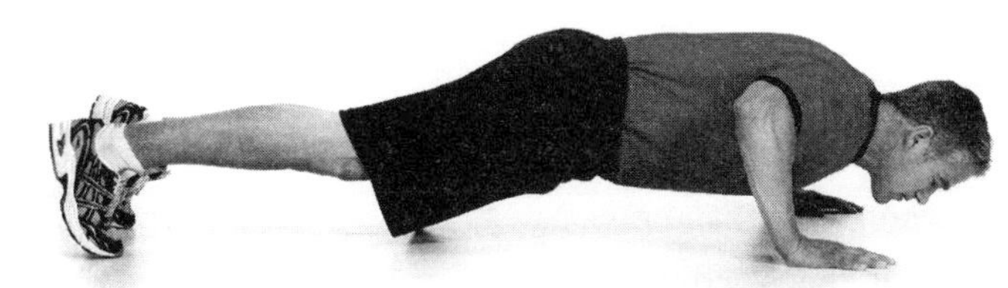

Begin as you would a regular pushup, only with your feet spaced slightly wider apart, say just outside shoulder width.

B

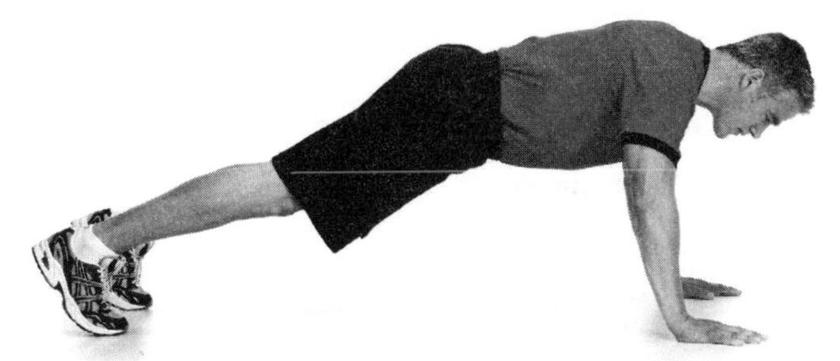

Push up and, as you near the top of the pushup, immediately rotate one arm toward the ceiling as you simultaneously turn your hips and legs to the same side. At the top you should end up with your arms in a straight line, pointing from ceiling to floor, and your weight resting on the sides of your feet. Return to the starting position and execute another T-pushup before repeating to the other side.

C

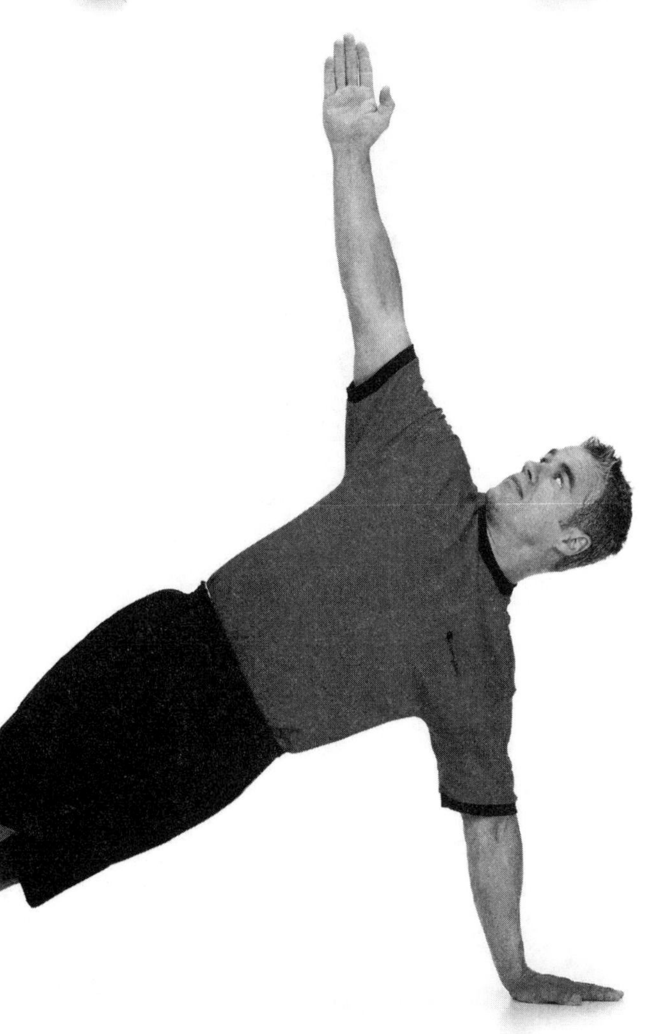

CHINUP

Grab the chinup bar with a shoulder-width, underhand grip, as you bend your knees and cross your ankles behind you to hang from it.

Keeping your chest out, pull yourself up until your chin clears the bar. Pause there for a second and then slowly return to the starting position.

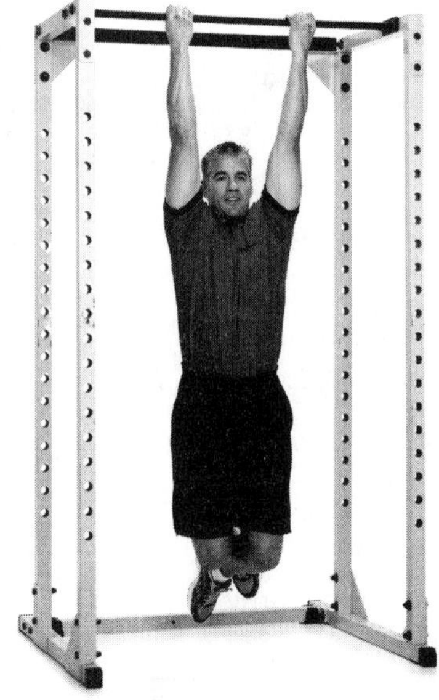

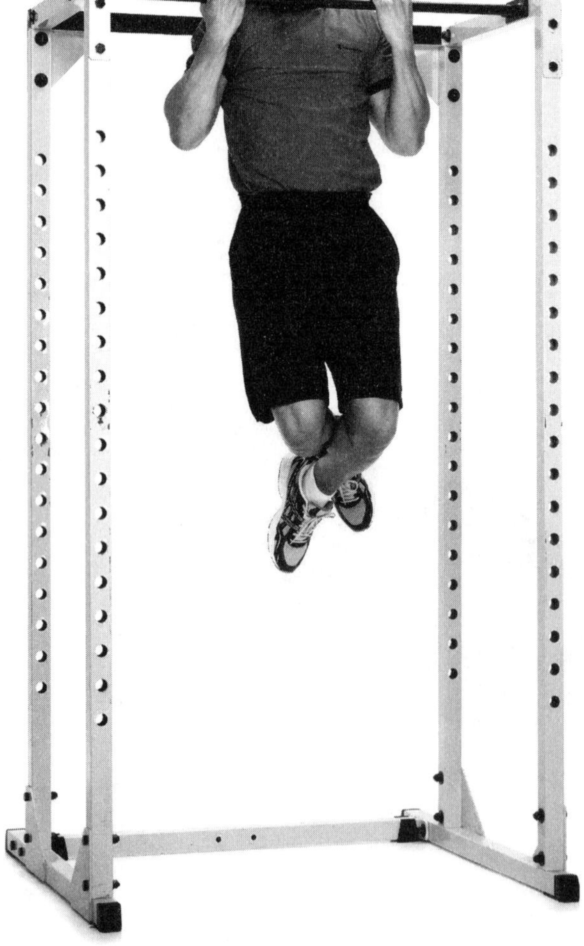

B

CLEAN PULL

Position yourself as you would if doing a barbell deadlift: standing over a loaded barbell that's on the floor. Squat down, and grab the bar with a grip that's just outside your legs.

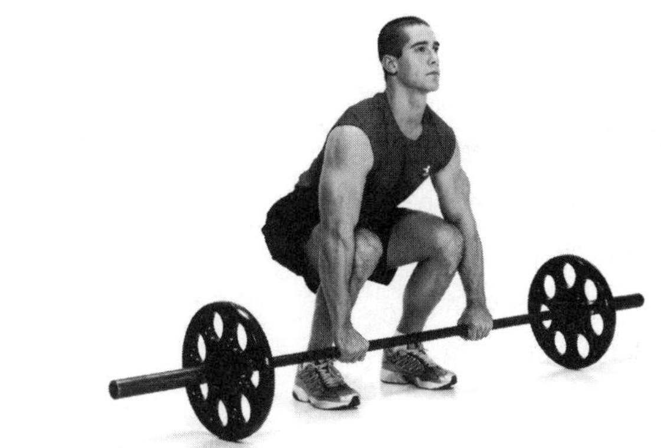

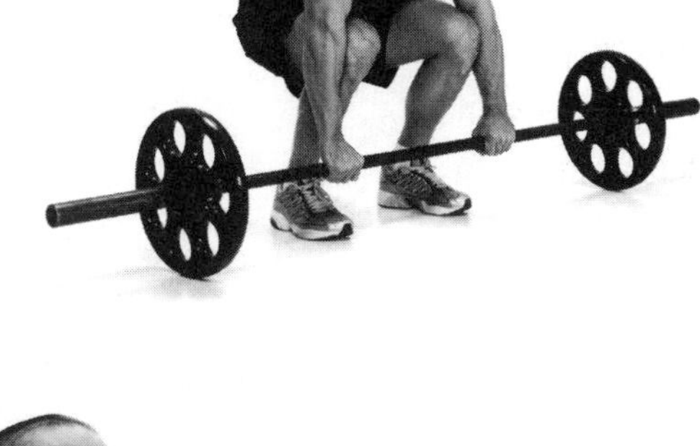

A

In one explosive movement, stand up and shrug your shoulders toward your ears. Try to hold the top position for a second before you lower the weight back to the starting position. Be sure to drive the weight with your legs and not pull it up with your upper body.

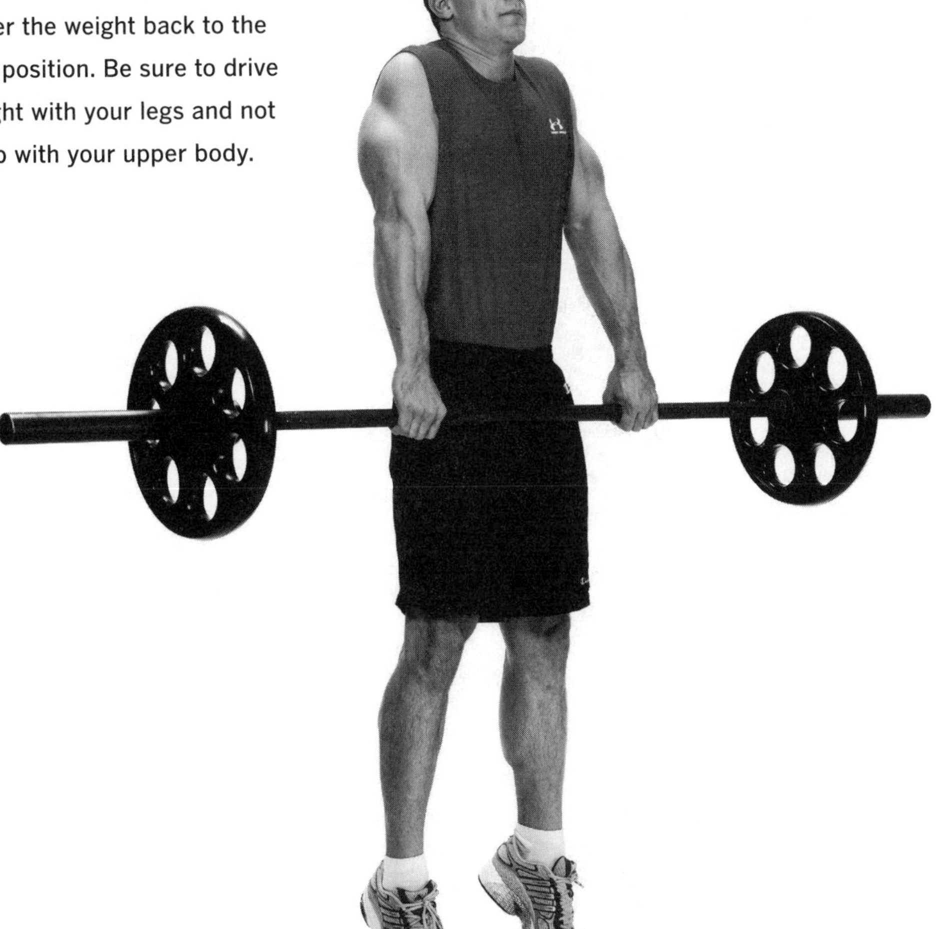

B

DUMBBELL DEADLIFT AND SHRUG

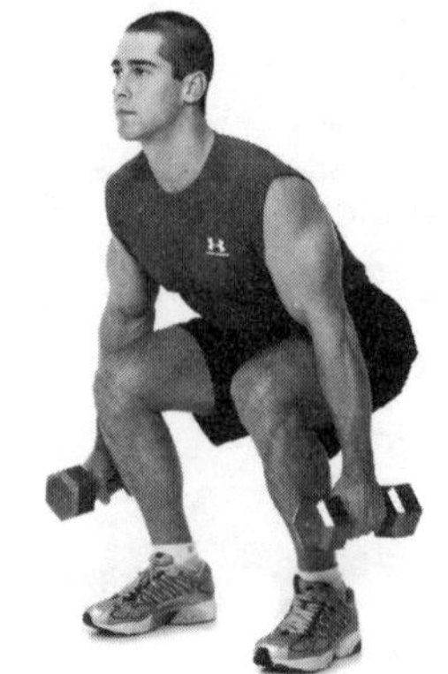

Stand holding a couple of heavy dumbbells at arm's length with a shoulder-width stance. Keeping the dumbbells at your sides, begin by sitting down and back as you lower your hips toward the floor.

When your thighs are parallel to the floor, immediately reverse the movement and stand back up as you shrug your shoulders toward your ears.

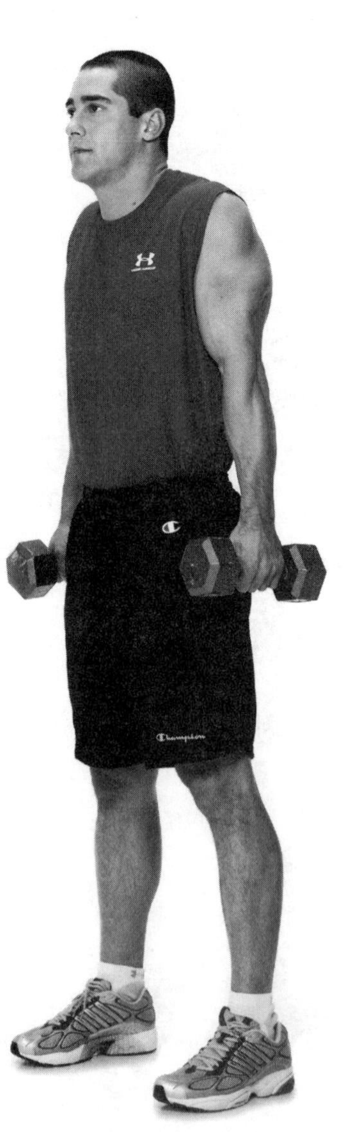

B

BARBELL BENCH PRESS

Grab the bar with your hands just wider than shoulder width. Lift the bar off the uprights and hold it over your chest.

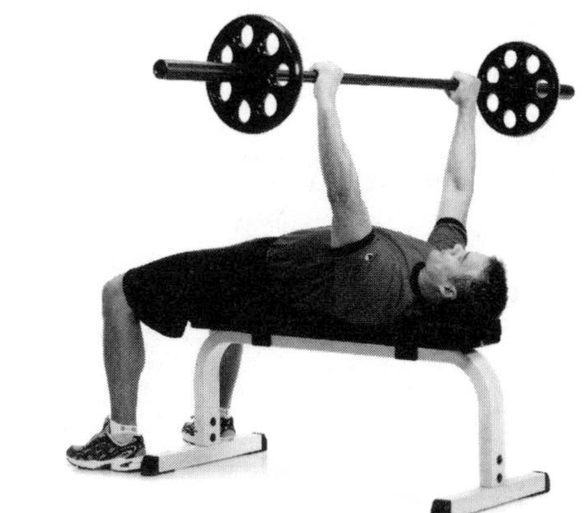

Next, lower the bar toward your chest, stopping when your upper arms are parallel to the floor. Pause there for a second and then push it back to the starting position. *Note:* You can make this exercise easier on your shoulders by using a closer grip and keeping your elbows in closer to your body.

B

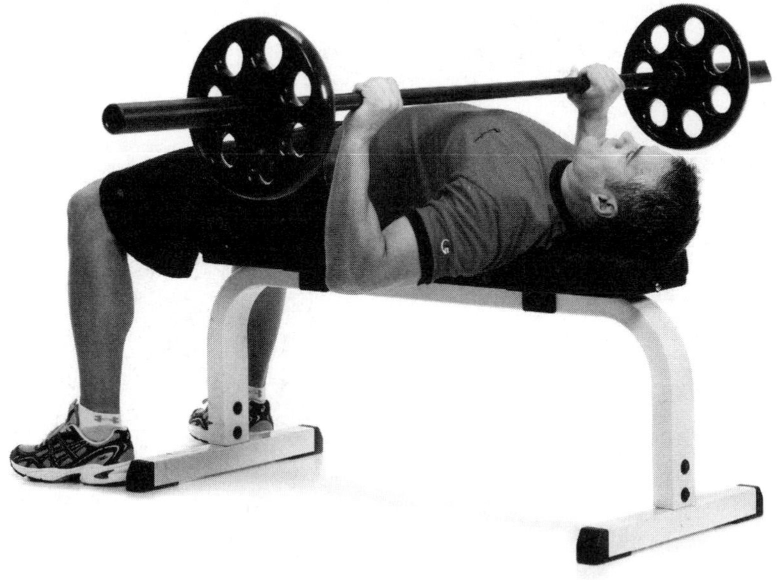

SWISS BALL LEG CURL

Lie on your back on the floor with your arms out to the sides and place your lower legs on a Swiss ball. Begin by pushing your hips up so that your body forms a straight line from your shoulders to your knees.

Next, pull your heels toward you and roll the ball as close as possible to your rear end. Pause, then reverse the motion—roll the ball back until your body is in a straight line, then lower your back to the floor and repeat.

A

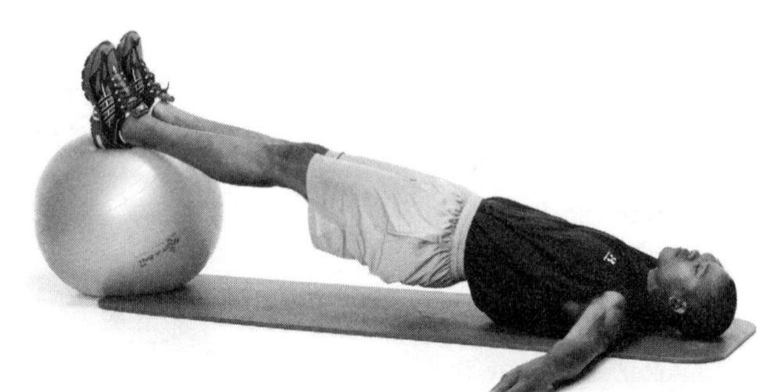

B

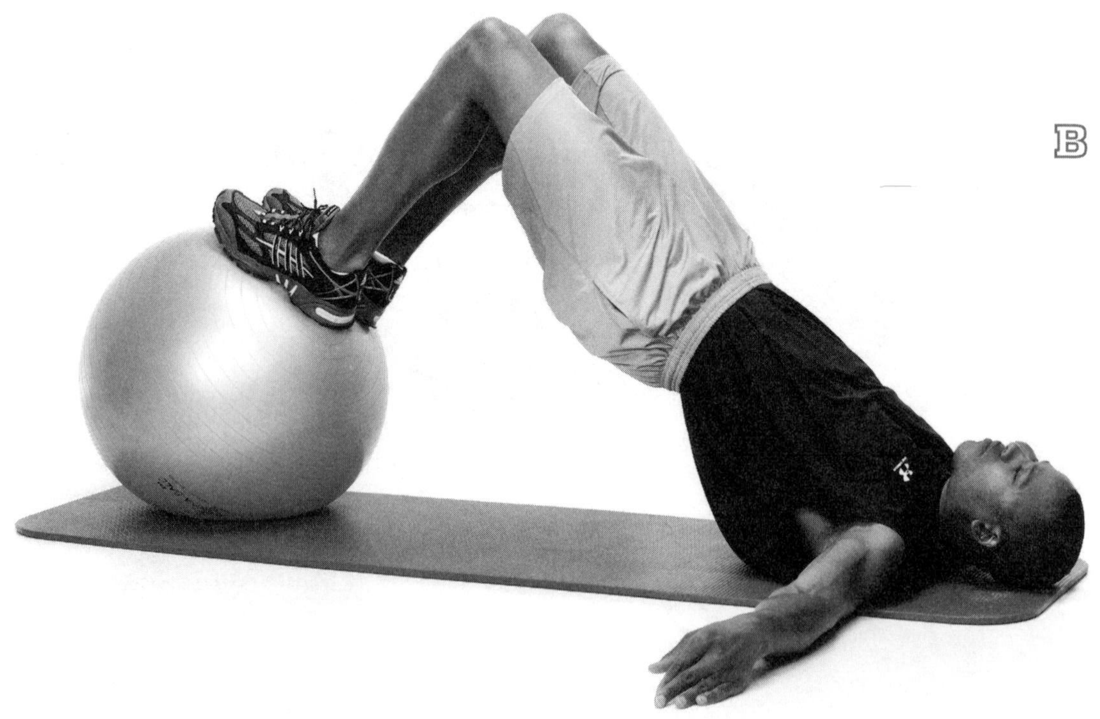

CORE CONCEPTS

STRENGTHENING YOUR BODY FROM THE INSIDE OUT

With the exception of the lower-body rotations, there is no direct core work in the previous workouts. I stress the word "direct" because your core will be working extremely hard during most of these lifts. You simply can't perform an overhead squat or a Turkish get-up without activating your core, and squats and push presses would be pretty much impossible if your core wasn't working at some level. I realize that some of you are still going to want to throw in some additional core work, either on off days or immediately following your workouts. That's fine. Just don't do it out of some misguided belief that it will miraculously burn fat from around your waist. It won't!

So please, can the crunches and broomstick twists. Just as you did more muscle-building-type core exercises in phase 4, I'd rather you do more strength-based core work to complement the rest of this phase. The list below will provide you with some suitable exercises. As I already mentioned, they are best done on off days or immediately after your workouts. Try 2 or 3 sets of 5 to 8 reps of each.

High-chair leg raise
Pike walk
Cable rotation
Weighted situp

HIGH-CHAIR LEG RAISE

Position yourself in a high-chair station with your arms on the elbow supports.

Keeping your back flat against the pad and body straight, begin by bending your knees slightly and lifting your thighs toward your chest. As you do, think of "folding" your body in half and allowing your hips to roll forward underneath you; do not just simply lift your knees up.

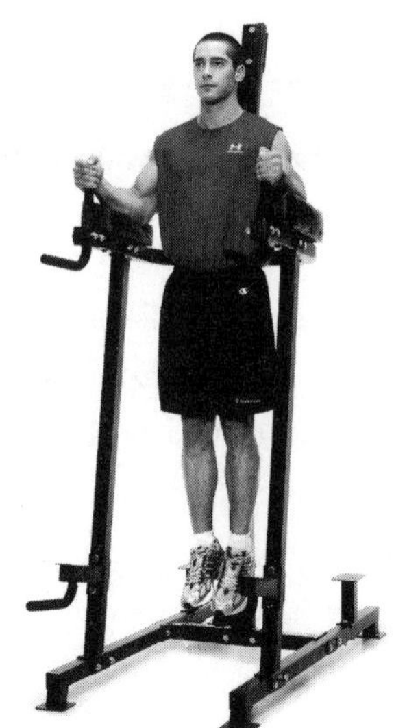

A

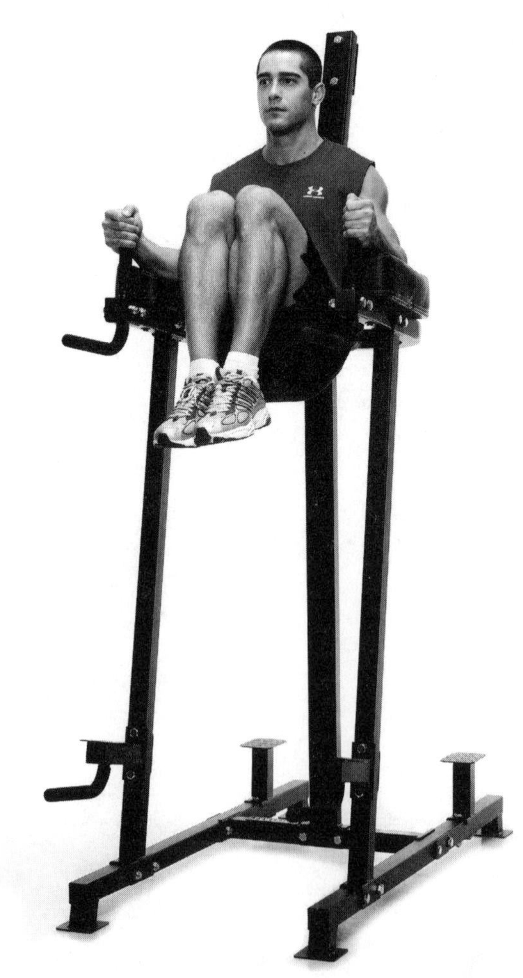

B

PIKE WALK

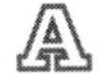

From a pushup position, walk your arms out in front of you until your hands are in front of your head. Be sure to maintain a neutral spine in this position—no arching your back.

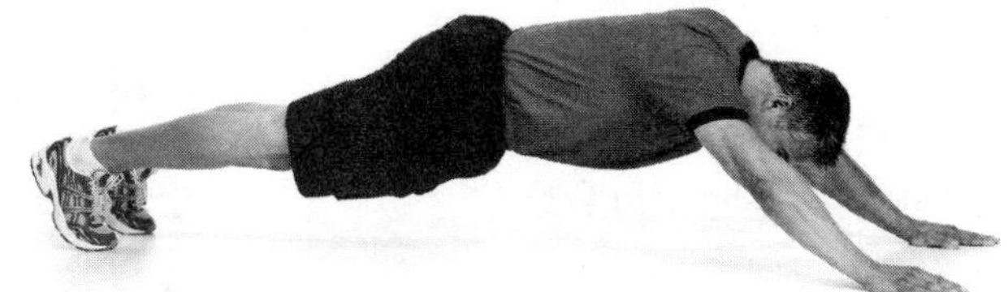

From there, keeping your legs completely straight, begin walking your feet up toward your hands as you lift your butt toward the ceiling. When you've gone as far as you can, slowly walk your arms forward and lower your hips until you reach the starting position.

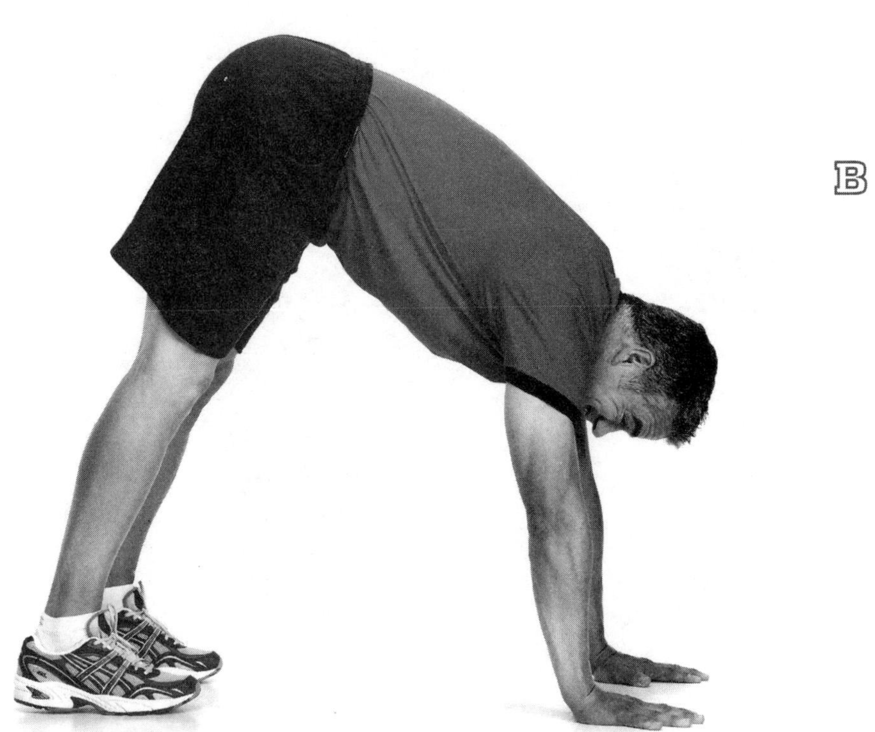

B

CABLE ROTATION

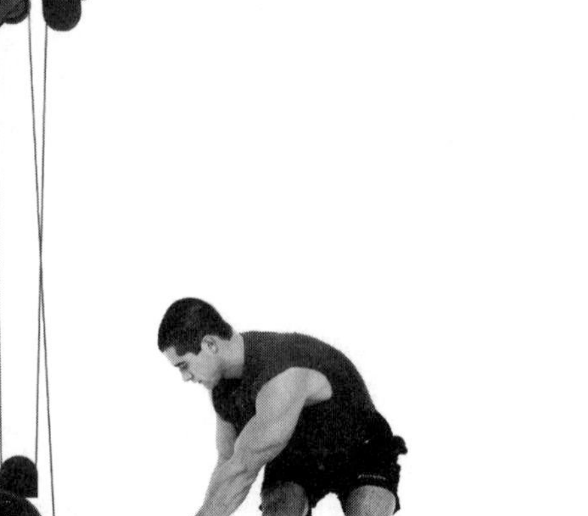

A

Stand sideways next to an adjustable cable station with a handle attached to a low pulley and grab the handle with your opposite hand (if the cable station is on your right, grab it with your left).

Wrap your other hand over the first and, with your knees slightly bent and arms straight, keep your lower body still as you rotate as far as you can to the opposite side. Pause for a second and lower the weight back to the starting position.

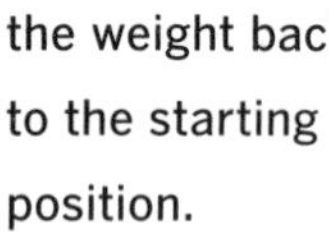

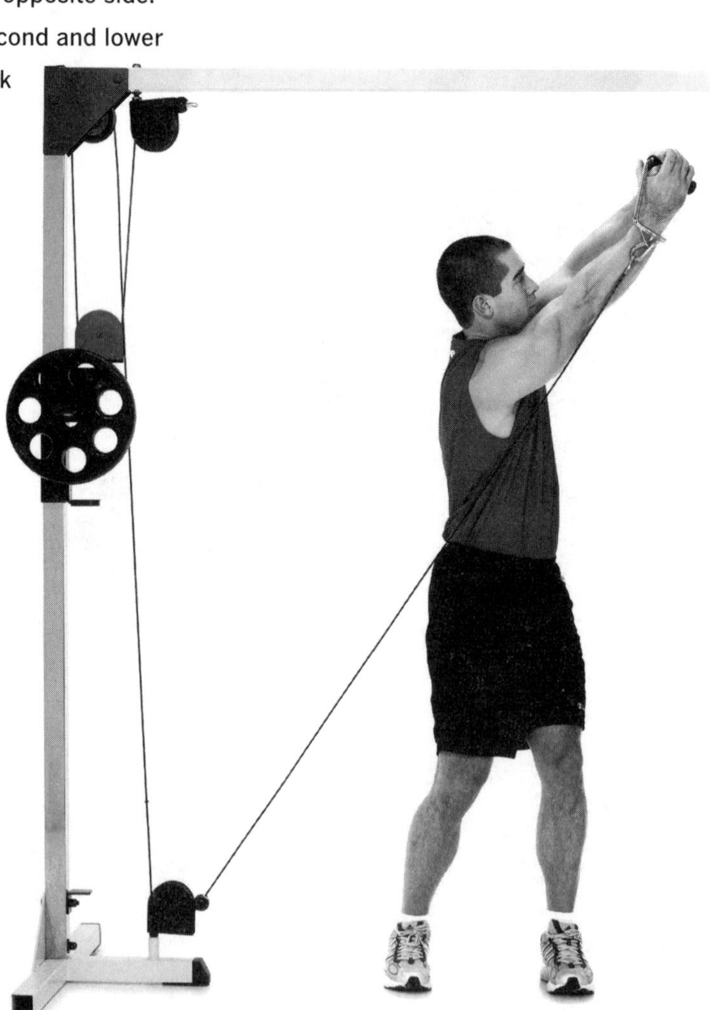

B

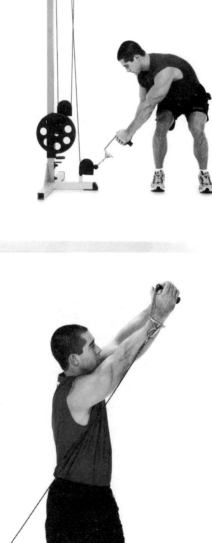

WEIGHTED SITUP

Lie on your back on the floor holding a weight plate across your chest, with your knees bent and feet flat on the floor.

Slowly lift your torso until your arms almost touch your thighs. Pause and then slowly lower yourself back down to the floor.

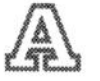

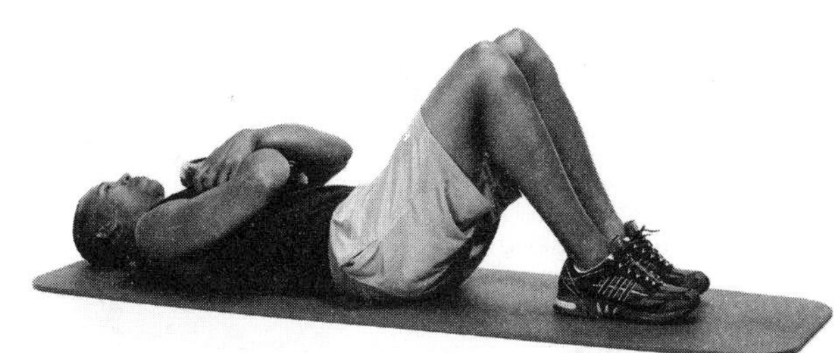

B

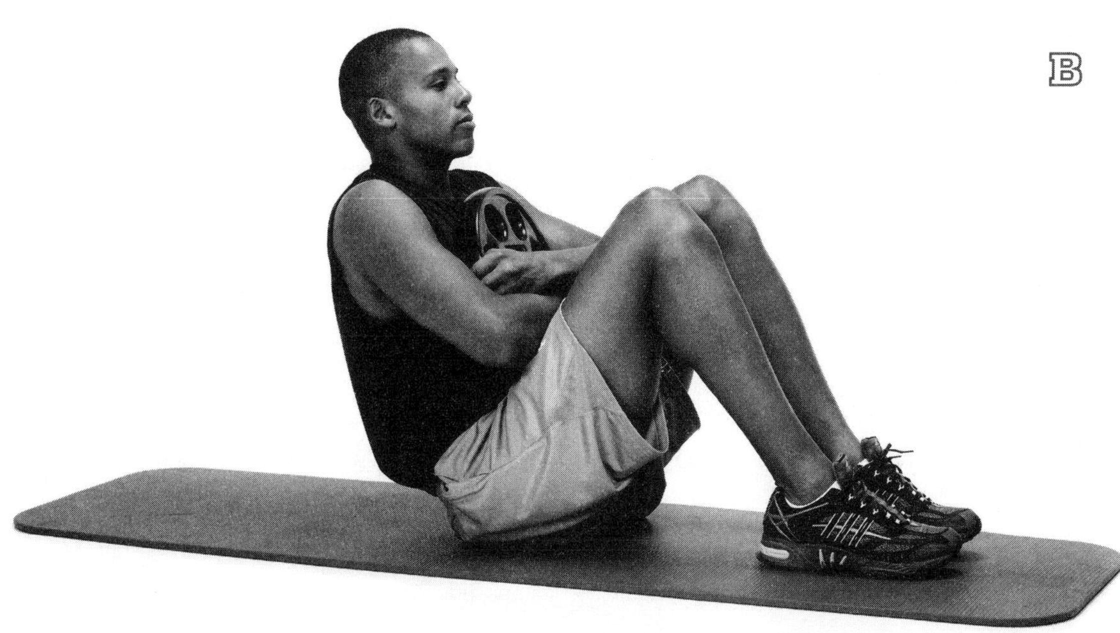

STRONG AT HEART

CARDIO TRAINING DURING YOUR STRENGTH PHASE

Just as during the muscle-building phase, where you opted for cardio workouts designed to complement that type of training, so too will you here. The difference is that since there's less overall volume in these workouts, you can select cardio workouts of slightly longer duration without the negative impact on strength development that they may have had on building muscle. That being the case, the following workout will work well on off days from lifting or immediately following your strength workouts. I recommend doing it anywhere from two to four times per week depending on how much time you have.

We're still going to go with intervals here, but this time let's extend their duration a bit to include some work for your aerobic energy system. In order to do this, the work intervals will be less intense but longer than those you've endured up to this point. The recovery intervals will also be the same length as the work intervals—and not all that much easier. I'm sure you'll find it to be a nice change of pace from the extremely winding work intervals you've done in every other phase.

Work interval: 3 minutes

Recovery interval: 3 minutes

Number of intervals: 4 to 5

RPE levels: 7 to 8 for work intervals; 5.5 to 6.5 for recovery intervals

This protocol is best suited to activities like cycling, running, and the elliptical trainer, due to their rhythmic, continuous nature. It probably wouldn't work well with things like jumping rope and various calisthenic drills. A work interval of that duration would likely be too difficult with higher-intensity/higher-impact drills such as those.

DOING A SLOW BURN

SELECTING THE RIGHT TYPES OF FOODS

In terms of nutritional recommendations for a strength-building phase, there's really not all that much to cover. You certainly don't need to consume a caloric surplus the way you did during the muscle-building phase. The neural aspects of strength development make it possible to increase strength without developing appreciable amounts of muscle. And in fact, some research has demonstrated that it's even possible to increase strength during a moderate energy deficit. Meaning that it may even be possible to lose fat while increasing strength.

About the only recommendation I would make is to pay strict attention to the types of carbs you consume, especially in the couple of hours leading up to your workout. Perhaps more so than any other type of training, strength work, be it explosive or heavy, requires tremendous mental focus. Consuming too many fast-acting carbs like pasta, fruit juices, and bagels can lead to large increases in blood sugar levels followed by subsequent drops, causing you to feel lethargic and making it difficult to concentrate. Needless to say, this is the last thing you need when you're attempting to lift heavy loads or recruit your muscle fibers to contract as quickly as possible. Therefore, be sure to refer back to the glycemic index on page 189 for good, slow-acting carb sources.

STRONG OPINIONS

GAINING A NEWFOUND RESPECT FOR TRAINING TO BECOME STRONGER

If you ask me, training for strength is the most misunderstood, underappreciated aspect of fitness. Fat burning and muscle building may get all the headlines, but you won't be able to do either for very long if you don't eventually become stronger. Strength gives you more confidence and self-esteem and immeasurably improves the quality of your daily life. For that reason alone it's a more effective way to promote program adherence and long-lasting results than the aesthetics-first approach that's become altogether too popular.

I know that training to produce wholesale increases in strength isn't something that most people associate with beginners, but when you think about it, neither is most of what we've covered up until this point. At the very least, training to become stronger will provide you with a truly unique challenge—one that will end the monotony often associated with the more traditional approach to working out. And when it comes to beginners, keeping workouts as mentally stimulating as possible is a definite plus.

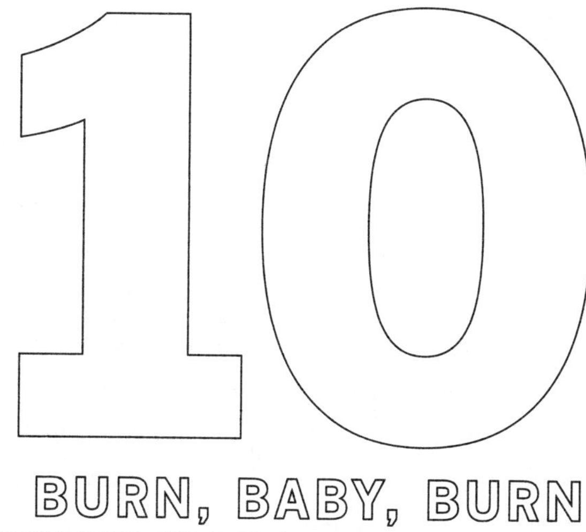

BURN, BABY, BURN

PHASE 6: THESE FAT-LOSS STRATEGIES REALLY WORK

So you want to burn some fat, huh? Well, you've come to the right place. This chapter is chock-full of all sorts of different ways to incinerate that pesky flab. It doesn't matter if you're looking to lose in excess of 20 pounds or just fine-tune your physique to get that coveted six-pack—all of the information you need to achieve your goal is literally right at your fingertips. All you have to provide is effort and dedication. Well, that and an open mind, of course. By now it should come as no surprise that you're going to go about achieving your goal in a somewhat unconventional fashion.

Take heart; this seemingly unorthodox approach is all about results . . . *fast* results. While building muscle may take a little more time, if done properly, burning fat can be a pretty quick proposition. How quick? Well, that really all depends on you and how much fat you're looking to lose. Follow the advice in this chapter to the letter and shaving 2 to 3 inches off your waist inside a month is certainly within reason. Not that it's all about vanity. Training in the manner outlined in this chapter will make you more resistant to fatigue, allow you to maintain or even increase your strength levels, and best of all, give you a whole new appreciation of the power of anaerobic exercise.

Yep, you read that correctly. Despite its long having been touted as the "best" way to burn body fat, aerobic exercise (long endurance workouts where your body uses oxygen as its means of providing the energy you need) isn't the only game in town when it comes to getting lean. Activities like sprinting, interval cardio work, and even strength training can burn fat at an astounding rate. They can also give your cardiovascular system a pretty tough, albeit different, kind of workout than it gets from traditional aerobic exercise like jogging and cycling.

Starvation diets and endless hours of aerobic training are no longer the preferred way to lose that gut. You'll now have a seemingly endless array of workout options at your disposal—options that can be easily modified to meet your needs regardless of your current physical condition. And you'll get the quickest and most dramatic results you've ever experienced. I've had clients who've dropped as much as 6 inches off their waists in as little as 8 weeks using this approach, without working anywhere near their alleged "fat-burning zone."

Before you can completely buy into what is likely an extreme departure from your current mind-set, we need to examine why the traditional approach to fat loss leaves so much to be desired. As you'll soon learn, much of the reason why so many people continue to employ outdated fat-loss strategies like high volumes of low-intensity aerobic training and radical caloric restriction has more to do with tradition than with physiology. We've been brainwashed into thinking that there's only one way to burn body fat and improve cardiovascular health. As you're about to read, that's far from the case.

DON'T BELIEVE THE HYPE

AEROBIC EXERCISE: FITNESS PANACEA OR CULTURAL HOAX?

Everybody knows that while weights are great for building size and strength, aerobic exercise (aka cardio) is what sheds that pesky body fat. What's more, aerobic exercise needs to be of a specific intensity and time frame in order for you to get into that vaunted fat-burning zone—otherwise, it's just wasted effort. Unless you work at 60 to 85 percent of your maximal heart rate for at least 20 minutes, you can basically forget about burning any body fat.

The preceding paragraph represents an archaic form of thinking that unfortunately still reigns supreme in health clubs, personal training studios, and basement gym setups far and wide. Used to be that if you mentioned fat loss, one word popped into everybody's mind: cardio. Who am I kidding, "used to be"? This still holds true, but believe me, I'm working on it. While I've got nothing against your doing aerobic exercise if you so choose, slow, steady-pace cardio is not the be-all and end-all most people make it out to be. When getting lean is the goal, there's a lot to be said for short-burst, anaerobic forms of exercise like sprinting and strength training, as well as interval work where your level of intensity varies throughout the workout. Besides the greater fat-burning potential, these anaerobic activities also present your cardiovascular system with a more potent training stimulus.

That last line may come as a shock, given the strong association between aerobic exercise and good cardiovascular health that's been established over the past few decades. Ever since Dr. Kenneth Cooper first introduced the idea of aerobic exercise to the American public back in the early 1970s, people have bought into the concept that moderate-intensity, oxygen-consuming activities like jogging, bike riding, and swimming are the best way to burn fat and keep the ol' ticker in good working order. While there's no arguing the obvious impact this type of training can have on weight control and long-term cardiovascular health, what is questionable is whether cardio is the best or most efficient way to achieve these goals.

Twenty years ago, when I first started out in this industry, it was absolutely unimaginable that another form of exercise could burn fat or improve cardiovascular function better than aerobics could. Emaciated marathoners and aerobicizers in leg warmers and matching headbands wouldn't even entertain the notion that sprinting or lifting weights could produce similar—if not better—results in some instances than their beloved aerobic exercise. Fast-forward to today. Attitudes have changed somewhat. Over the past several years, more and more people have begun to discover the powerful fat-burning properties and numerous cardiovascular benefits of more anaerobic forms of exercise.

WHAT'S IN A NAME?

IDENTIFYING THE VARIOUS FORMS OF ENERGY METABOLISM

Before we go any further, let me clarify a couple of terms at the very heart of this whole controversy. I'm talking specifically about the words *aerobic*, *cardio*, and *anaerobic*. I'll start with the first two because this is really where all of the confusion lies.

Contrary to popular belief, these two terms do not mean the same thing and shouldn't be used interchangeably. The term *aerobic* refers to a type of energy metabolism where oxygen is consumed and utilized in order to create the fuel necessary to perform a given task. The term *cardio* is short for "cardiovascular," which refers to your heart and circulatory systems Now, aerobic exercise does offer tremendous cardiovascular benefit, but so do other forms of training, albeit in a slightly different manner.

When you're exercising aerobically, it basically means that there's a balance between oxygen supply and oxygen demand. A nice, steady, paced jog and a leisurely bike ride are both good examples of aerobic exercise. Ramp things up to the point where you're sprinting or out of the bike saddle and stomping the pedals to get up a hill, and aerobic metabolism can no longer power this effort by itself. At this point you need to rely more heavily on anaerobic metabolism (meaning that energy is produced with very little oxygen), where the fuel to power your efforts is supplied through the breakdown of carbohydrates and stored chemical energy. This is a lot more taxing on your heart, muscles, and energy reserves.

Most people tend to favor aerobic metabolism because, besides being an easier way to train, it uses predominantly fat to power its energy demands (especially when you're working at lower levels of intensity). Anaerobic exercise uses primarily carbs. Naturally, this has prompted various training and nutrition experts to tout the effectiveness of low-intensity aerobic exercise as a means of burning excess body fat. I can't tell you how many times I've heard misguided trainers and nutritionists advise their clients to work at lower intensities so they can "burn fat, not sugar." Unfortunately, besides being erroneous, this mind-set has also blinded many people to the numerous cardiovascular and fat-fighting benefits that anaerobic exercise has to offer.

PEDAL VERSUS METAL

WHICH WORKS BETTER, AEROBICS OR STRENGTH TRAINING?

I know what you're thinking: How can anaerobic exercise like weight training be good for burning fat when in virtually any weight room you enter there are guys with huge guts? Fair point. The kind of weight training most guys do is not the type that brings about the benefits I've been talking about. Lifting a heavy weight for a few reps and then walking around and chatting with your buddies for several minutes isn't exactly going to melt the fat off you. Nor will it do much to improve resting blood pressure or blood lipid profiles the way more moderate-load training with short rest intervals between sets can. The key to heart-healthy, fat-burning anaerobic training is maintaining a consistent pace and repeating the effort enough times to create an overload on your metabolism. Basically, these workouts will shift your calorie-burning capacity into overdrive.

Speaking of metabolic overloads, now's as good a time as any to examine the impact that strength training has on your metabolism. You've probably heard that adding muscle mass to your body increases your metabolic rate since muscle is metabolically active tissue that needs a constant supply of calories to sustain itself. This is certainly true. It really doesn't tell the whole story, though. Because when you add that to the caloric cost of the workout itself, along with the subsequent elevations in metabolism caused by a workout, you begin to get a real appreciation for why people who lift seriously are often quite lean.

Consider for a second the physiques of bodybuilders, sprinters, and gymnasts. Despite the fact that these individuals do little, if any, aerobic exercise (especially in the case of sprinters), they typically display some of the lowest body fat levels of any athletes. Granted, the high-intensity nature of sprinting has to be factored into that equation, but it only amplifies the impact of anaerobic exercise. It does not, however, change the fact that sprinters also do quite a bit of strength training, as do gymnasts; they just mainly use their own body weight for resistance as opposed to barbells and dumbbells. The point is, here you have three types of athletes for whom strength training comprises the bulk of their daily exercise routine, and yet they're some of the leanest individuals around. This is more than just a coincidence.

While the energy cost of various forms of aerobic exercise has been well documented, you rarely if ever hear anything about the number of calories burned during a strength-training session. It might surprise you to learn that you can burn 5 to 10 calories per minute, depending on whether you work large or small muscles. (The former burn more calories.) Assuming that you did a 40-minute workout consisting of predominantly large-muscle-group exercises like squats, bench presses, deadlifts, and rows, that's a whopping 400-calorie energy expenditure! Not bad for just pumping a little iron. In fact, it's enough to make the folks toiling away on the treadmills pretty jealous, for a number of reasons.

FAT BURNING OF "EPOC" PROPORTIONS

THE FAT BURNING DOESN'T STOP JUST BECAUSE YOUR WORKOUT IS OVER

Not only is it possible for you to burn a significant number of calories during your weight workout, but thanks to a little something known as EPOC (exercise post-oxygen consumption), your metabolism can stay elevated for several hours after you've finished training. Participants in a 1993 study saw significant increases in their resting metabolism for as long as 15 hours after they finished doing resistance exercise. The same usually isn't true of the type of moderate-intensity aerobic exercise most guys mindlessly do for 30 minutes while watching *SportsCenter*. In fact, another study even showed that oxygen consumption returned to resting levels just 40 minutes after subjects performed a full 40 minutes of stationary cycling at 70 percent of their maximal aerobic capacity, or VO_2 max.

Why such a disparity? Well, to be fair, the resistance training study in question did use an extremely grueling 90-minute, high-volume program that's probably well beyond what most people have the time or inclination to do. Using a more realistic, lower-volume protocol, researchers still noticed significant, albeit slightly lower, elevations in metabolic rate as much as several hours later. Some of this may have to do with the fact that weight training causes microtrauma (microscopic damage to muscle fibers) that needs to be repaired during the recovery process. This could certainly account for the increase in metabolic rate, although elevations in heart rate, breathing rate, and the levels of certain hormones may also come into play.

Whatever the cause, it appears that the EPOC generated as a result of strength training is greater than that from aerobic exercise. One study that compared the EPOC of four different forms of training produced some rather interesting results. Researchers compared subjects who performed 40 minutes each of cycling (at 80 percent of maximal heart rate), circuit weight training (4 sets of 15 reps at 50 percent of the individuals' 1-rep max, or the maximum amount of weight they can lift for one repetition), and heavy resistance training (3 sets of 3 to 8 reps at 80 to 90 percent of the individuals' one-rep max). While all forms of exercise increased metabolic rate immediately after the workout, only the two forms of weight training produced increases that were still significant 30 minutes later.

Now, the actual caloric cost of EPOC usually tends to be rather small. So small, in fact, that many experts believe its importance is often overstated, especially in relation to the energy cost of the actual workout itself. After all, even in the study where metabolism stayed elevated for 15 hours, the actual caloric expenditure added up to only about 150 extra calories burned. Over time, however, even this modest calorie expenditure can have a significant impact on body composition. If you burn an additional 100 or so calories three times per week, over the course of a year that's an extra 15,600 calories. Since there are roughly 3,500 calories in 1 pound of fat, you're talking about a little more than an extra 4-pound fat loss on top of the caloric costs of the workouts themselves.

I know what you're thinking: "Who says those extra calories necessarily come from fat?" According to a 1992 study, the more carbs you burn during a workout, the more fat you burn when you've finished exercising. And seeing as how strength training relies predominantly on stored carbohydrates for fuel, your body will be tapping into those fat stores to try to replenish some of the energy you used up. How cool is that? I don't know about you, but if I've got the opportunity to keep my metabolism stoked and give up a few extra pounds of flab in the process, I'm gonna take it! Especially if it involves lifting weights—because the benefits don't end there.

YA GOTTA HAVE HEART

CARDIOVASCULAR BENEFITS OF ANAEROBIC EXERCISE

Even though this is a chapter on fat loss, I'd be remiss if I didn't mention the effect that anaerobic exercise has on your cardiovascular system. I mean, it's nice to look all lean and chiseled, but it's equally nice to not keel over from a heart attack while chasing down your bus in the morning.

Whether you realize it or not, there are numerous cardiovascular benefits to be had from lifting weights and high-intensity interval training such as sprints. Granted, these activities won't do much to improve your ability to consume and utilize oxygen, as aerobic exercise can. But they will improve your cardiovascular function in a number of different ways.

First off, during periods of intensive muscular effort, your heart has to contract more forcefully to pump blood where it's needed. Whether you're doing a bench press or a 40-yard dash, all of that pushing and straining is creating increased resistance against your artery walls, effectively minimizing the space your blood has to travel through. This is different than during aerobic activity, where the muscle contractions are usually less intense and bloodflow isn't impeded to anywhere near the same degree. So just like any of your other muscles, your heart becomes stronger when you do strength training or high-intensity intervals. This is important because there are lots of times when it's handy to have a heart that can endure increased strain.

Take shoveling snow, for instance. Every winter you hear about a few poor souls who have heart attacks while shoveling wet, heavy snow. True, many of them were probably fairly inactive to begin with, and the intense effort just proved to be too overwhelming. But do you think that people who are "aerobically" fit are better off? Okay, perhaps their superior ability to consume and utilize oxygen may help them recover more quickly once they're done, but if they do mainly long-duration, low-intensity activity like, say, jogging, they might be just as susceptible. Shoveling wet snow is intense, anaerobic exercise during which your heart has to overcome the same kind of increased strain it encounters during a strength-training session. No amount of steady-state aerobic training is going to prepare you for that.

Still need more proof that anaerobic training promotes good heart health? As I alluded to earlier, studies have shown that high-intensity strength training can have a favorable impact on both resting blood pressure and cholesterol levels. A 1999 study found that strength training caused significant reductions in blood pressure in people ages 65 to 73 who exhibited "high-normal" resting blood pressures prior to participation in the study. Although the research on blood lipid profiles has been less conclusive, there seems to be enough evidence to support the fact that, at the very least, strength training helps raise the levels of HDL, or "good," cholesterol.

Then there's the landmark Paffenbarger study that followed the health of 6,300 longshoremen for 22 years and found that the longshoremen with the most active jobs had 50 percent fewer heart attacks compared to those with less active jobs. Interestingly, the pro-aerobic crowd jumped all over this study, feeling that it legitimized their stance that regular exercise lowered the risk for cardiovascular disease. I say "interestingly" because the bulk of a longshoreman's day is spent in *anaerobic* metabolism: lifting heavy loads and often holding his breath while doing so. If that isn't the antithesis of aerobic exercise, I don't know what is. If nothing else, this study should help hammer home the point that there is tremendous cardiovascular benefit to be had from doing repeated bursts of high-intensity exercise and that, when added up over time, these can be just as beneficial to long-term health as more aerobic forms of exercise.

The bottom line is an exercise doesn't have to be aerobic to be good for your heart. Yes, there are certain benefits to be had from working aerobically in your so-called target heart rate zone. Things like an improved ability to consume and utilize oxygen and a lower resting heart rate immediately come to mind. That said, there are also numerous advantages to going anaerobic and working above the comfort level of steady-state aerobic metabolism. While I do feel that there's a place for both forms of training in the overall scheme of things, from a time-efficiency standpoint, I think anaerobic exercise is pretty tough to beat.

JOIN THE HIIT PARADE

DISCOVERING THE NUMEROUS BENEFITS OF INTERVAL TRAINING

Looking for a time-efficient yet brutally effective way for getting cardio workouts without spending all day in the gym, people of all ages and fitness levels have recently begun to adopt a style of training called high-intensity interval training, or HIIT. By delivering all of the benefits of traditional aerobic exercise in a fraction of the time, HIIT has become increasingly popular with athletes, bodybuilders, and even regular Joes. Due to its relative brevity (the average workout takes 12 to 15 minutes), HIIT doesn't hinder your ability to recover from your strength workouts the way high volumes of aerobic work often can.

Although there are a variety of ways you can do it, with HIIT you typically warm up for a brief period (3 to 5 minutes) before ramping up the intensity for a short time frame (usually anywhere from 10 to 120 seconds) to a level that you wouldn't be able to maintain for your entire workout if you did it continuously. You then bring things down a notch and partially recover for a brief period (the length of which is determined by the length of your work interval as well as by your individual goals) before once again cranking it back up to the higher intensity level. Then it's just a matter of repeating this process for the desired number of repetitions.

Say for example that you're doing HIIT on an exercise bike. After a brief warmup to get your blood flowing, you might quickly jack up the intensity for about 30 seconds to the point where your thighs started burning and you were huffing and puffing. You would then lower the intensity (for an equal, or in most cases, greater time interval) to the point where you were still working but at least gave yourself the chance to partially recover. Then, once the recovery interval was over, you'd take things back up again.

The great thing about HIIT is that at the end of the workout you find that you've been able to amass much more time working at the higher intensity level than you otherwise could have. Not only that, but since you kept on working even during your recovery periods, you wind up with a much greater caloric expenditure and more potent cardiovascular stimulus than you get from more steady-paced aerobic work. That's because you're basically combining the benefits of both aerobic and anaerobic training in one efficient workout. The high-intensity intervals take you out of your little aerobic "comfort zone" and send your metabolism into overdrive. And the lower intensities allow you to recover while still pumping large volumes of blood through your heart and circulatory system, improving your ability to transport oxygen and nutrients through your bloodstream.

I so prefer HIIT over traditional aerobic exercise that it's the only type I recommend for my clients. I find it to be more effective and efficient in just about every way imaginable. It's also a pretty darn fun way to train. Let's face it, it's a lot more interesting to do a bunch of sprints interspersed with periods of jogging than it is to zone out for a half hour on a stationary bike while you peruse the latest stock quotes. Add some strength training into the mix and now you're talking about a veritable fat-burning inferno! I'm not just speculating here; I've used this training approach to get fat off people of all ages and fitness levels. In fact, it works so well that when sheer fat loss is the goal, I never prescribe traditional steady-state aerobic exercise.

Now before you go playing the beginner card on me, keep in mind that intensity is a relative thing. Nobody's asking you to work at a level you're not capable of. You will, however, be required to push yourself a little during the work intervals. That's why I like using the Borg

Rating of Perceived Exertion (RPE) scale so much (see "Perception Is Reality" on the opposite page). It's a subjective way of gauging intensity that's a step up from the simplistic 1-to-10 scale you used back in Chapter 7. You simply equate a given level of intensity with a number on the scale. Something that feels easy might be a 9 or 10, as opposed to something more difficult, which might be a 14 or 15. The beauty of the scale is that rather than attempting to meet some arbitrary level of intensity, *you* determine how hard to work based on your subjective perception of the effort you're putting forth.

Because this regimen is self-regulated, beginners can easily do it without feeling like they're working over their heads. One of the biggest keys to getting beginners to stick to an exercise program is to keep things manageable. Well, it doesn't get any more manageable than deciding for yourself how hard you need to be working. If you start to get too winded or get one of those nasty little cramps in your side, you know you may have pushed yourself a little too far. Remember, though, that having a skewed perception of the scale works two ways. Don't try to pretend something feels like a 6 or 7 when your heart is pounding out of your chest and you're sweating like Michael Jackson in front of a grand jury.

Misplaced heroics and acting like a weenie notwithstanding, the RPE scale is probably your best way to go for gauging interval intensity. Heart rate doesn't work because besides being too unreliable, it's tough to get a true gauge of how hard your heart is actually working when you're constantly raising and lowering your intensity level every minute or so. About the only way you can keep tabs on it is with one of those fancy heart rate monitors. Maybe it's just me, but that seems like an awful lot of expense just to try to monitor something as variable as heart rate. Besides, in the overall scheme of things it's nowhere near as important as most people make it out to be.

And please, spare me this nonsense about needing to monitor your heart rate to stay in your "fat-burning zone," typically identified as anywhere between 50 and 70 percent of your maximal heart rate. As I mentioned earlier, athletes like sprinters and gymnasts regularly work at intensities well above this for extremely short time frames, and they don't seem to have any trouble keeping off body fat. Athletes like these are so lean largely because the anaerobic forms of exercise they regularly engage in enable them to get that way.

Even if you'll never compete for a medal or hear the roar of an adoring crowd, you can garner tremendous benefit from training the way most athletes do. You name the sport—football, hockey, basketball, soccer, tennis, whatever—most involve quick bursts of intensive effort interspersed with brief, active recovery intervals. So whether you actively participate in any of these sports or just want to look the part, the workouts in this phase are specifically designed to meet all of your needs. They'll improve your cardiovascular function, lower your risk for heart disease, and burn fat at an amazing rate. Best of all, they're fun to do. Sure, they're a little tougher than zoning out on a stationary bike or ambling down a country road, but the results will be well worth it.

Tell you what: If you're attached to doing some low-intensity aerobic training just to cover all your cardiovascular bases, go right ahead. As long as it's something you enjoy, I've got nothing against your going out for a leisurely bike ride or long run every now and then. You could even go ahead and make one or two of your weekly cardio workouts of the low-intensity variety, with the others being HIIT. Just know that from an efficiency standpoint, interval training is pretty tough to beat, regardless of what your goals might be.

PERCEPTION IS REALITY

The Borg Rating of Perceived Exertion (RPE) scale is a way of subjectively monitoring exercise intensity that enables you to gauge your effort by equating it to heart rate. The scale ranges from 6 to 20 because adding a zero to the end of each number would give you the approximate heart rate span that most people would fall under (assuming that resting heart rate is near 60 beats per minute and 200 beats per minute represents maximum heart rate) in going from rest to strenuous exercise. You simply assign the appropriate number to the level of intensity you feel you're working at.

About the only way you can screw up your RPE is if you wuss out and say something feels like a 16 when it's more like a 6. Aside from that, the scale is pretty foolproof.

I like it because it allows me to prescribe interval workouts for a wide variety of people. Let's say I give you a workout where I want the work interval to be in the 15-to-17 range and the recovery interval to be 11 or 12. When using the RPE scale, people of completely different fitness levels can all do the same workout but gauge it to their own specifications. One person might be running at 6 mph for his work interval and the other at 5 mph. Yet they both perceive the effort to be in that 15-to-17 range.

Level of Intensity	RPE
6	20 percent effort: very, very light (rest)
7	30 percent effort
8	40 percent effort
9	50 percent effort: very light (gentle walking)
10	55 percent effort
11	60 percent effort: fairly light
12	65 percent effort
13	70 percent effort: moderately hard (steady pace)
14	75 percent effort
15	80 percent effort: hard
16	85 percent effort
17	90 percent effort: very hard
18	95 percent effort
19	100 percent effort: very, very hard
20	Exhaustion

THE ABC'S OF FAT LOSS

THE BEGINNER'S GUIDE TO INTERVAL TRAINING

I've arranged the interval workouts in this chapter into three main groups according to their intensity and which energy systems they train. The first group features what I like to call the Quick HIITers. These babies are short and sweet but, boy, do they pack a wallop. These brief yet super-intense work intervals are designed to target the more powerful of your two anaerobic energy systems, the alactic, or ATP-PC, energy system. Don't sweat the high-tech name; all it means is that these workouts produce little if any of the lactic acid that causes the nasty little burning sensation you get in your muscles when you're working intensely. And the letters just refer to the stored chemical energy that's used to power your efforts. You call on this energy system for nearly all-out bursts lasting no longer than 10 seconds. Quick HIITers are best suited to younger individuals who've trained in the not-too-distant past. No matter how thoroughly you warm up, wind sprints and jumping rope at a blistering pace don't mix well with a deconditioned, middle-age body. That being the case, let's reserve these workouts for former jocks and seasonal exercisers under the age of 35, initially at least. If that's not you, you can always give them a go later on down the road once your fitness level has improved.

Next up are the Thrash and Burn workouts. With slightly longer work intervals, these are bound to get your attention. As you may have gathered from the name, some lactic acid accumulation is pretty much inevitable here. It won't last too long, though, as this energy system is used only to power efforts lasting from about 30 to 120 seconds. Since you're only a beginner, I've elected to keep the work intervals to a maximum of 45 seconds. Trust me, you'll thank me for it later. Because the intervals are somewhat longer, you can't work as intensely, making these a better choice for newbies of all ages, as well as ex-jocks and seasonal lifters over age 35.

Last but not least are the Rare Air workouts. I call them "rare" because, although they target your aerobic energy system, few people do aerobics like this. Since the aerobic system starts to take over once an activity extends past the 2-minute mark, I figured we'd dance right around that number with intervals just intense enough to allow you to reach that time frame. And when I say "reach," I mean just barely reach. By the time that clock hits 2 minutes, you should be breathing pretty darn heavy and all too happy to drop the intensity a bit. Don't get too comfortable, though, because after an equal 2-minute recovery interval, you'll ramp it right back up. This workout works well for just about everyone, as it's significantly easier than any of the others. Even though it's technically more aerobic than the other two workout groups, so long as you stick to the prescribed RPE levels, you should still find it pretty challenging.

The thing I like best about all of these workouts is the tremendous amount of diversity they allow. You can stick to one specific type that you may like or mix and match them according to your mood. Despite my recommendations, you're free to try any workout you like, regardless of your current fitness level. It's also worth mentioning that any of these workouts can be done with just about any type of equipment, though I will offer you the benefit of my experience as to which modalities are most effective for each type of workout. For instance, it's pretty difficult to do the Quick HIITers with a treadmill, since constantly changing the speed and grade would likely eat into some of your interval time. In the end, the decision about which modality to select lies with you. Just make sure your ego doesn't start writing checks that your body can't cash.

However you choose to go about these workouts, I can guarantee you'll rarely, if ever, get bored. You'll be too busy just trying to catch your breath for that. Plus, since you can use all different kinds of equipment and your RPE levels will change as you become more fit, it'll take a long time before your body adapts to them and renders them ineffective.

Quick HITTers (Alactic, or ATP-PC, System)

Types of beginners: ex-jocks and seasonals under age 35

Recommended forms of exercise: sprints, jumping rope, and cycling

Workout #1

Work interval: 8 to 10 seconds at RPE of 18 or 19

Recovery interval: 30 seconds at RPE of 8 or 9

Work-to-rest ratio: 1:3

Number of intervals: 15

Workout #2

Work interval: 15 seconds at RPE of 17 or 18

Recovery interval: 45 seconds at RPE of 9 or 10

Work-to-rest ratio: 3:1

Number of intervals: 15 to 20

Due to the relatively high intensity of these intervals, extending the recovery interval slightly (i.e., an extra 10 to 15 seconds) as you go along is acceptable. So if you feel like you're not recovered enough to give the next work interval your full effort, feel free to add some time between work intervals. Then, simply strive to stick to the prescribed recovery intervals as your conditioning level improves.

Thrash and Burn (Lactic Acid System)

Types of beginners: newbies of all ages, as well as ex-jocks and seasonals over age 35

Recommended forms of exercise: rowing, stairclimbing, cycling, and swimming

Workout #1

Work interval: 30 seconds at RPE of 17 or 18

Recovery interval: 60 seconds at RPE of 11 or 12

Work-to-rest ratio: 2:1

Number of intervals: 10 to 12

Workout #2

Work interval: 45 seconds at RPE of 16 or 17

Recovery interval: 90 seconds at RPE of 11 or 12

Work-to-rest ratio: 2:1

Number of intervals: 6 to 8

At first the lactic acid buildup caused by these workouts might require you to extend the recovery intervals slightly (i.e., 10 to 20 seconds). That's fine. Just look to keep to the prescribed recovery intervals as your conditioning level improves.

Rare Air (Aerobic System)

Types of beginners: all beginners

Recommended forms of exercise: running (middle distance), hiking, and cycling

Work interval: 2 minutes at RPE of 15 or 16

Recovery interval: 2 minutes at RPE of 12 or 13

Work-to-rest ratio: 1:1

Number of intervals: 5 to 6

Unlike with the other two groups of workouts, I'd like you to stick to the prescribed recovery intervals right from the outset. When working your aerobic system, you don't need to ensure near-complete recovery. This explains why the recovery interval is a higher intensity than in the previous two workout groups. If you tried this with the other workouts, you'd never make it.

SHORT CIRCUIT

THE FAT-BURNING POWER OF CIRCUIT TRAINING

If I had to pick one type of training for beginners interested in losing fat, it would be circuit training. Circuit training is the practice of going through several strength-training exercises at a rapid pace with the goal of increasing both the caloric cost and cardiovascular demands of the workout. Typically this involves using light weights (between 40 and 55 percent of your 1-repetition max) and higher reps as you alternate between upper- and lower-body exercises, with minimal rest between sets. It's an excellent, time-efficient way to train because besides combining some of the benefits of strength training and aerobic exercise, it doesn't expose you to heavy loads before you're ready for them. Yet despite all of these benefits, it's far from perfect.

If you look hard enough, pretty much any form of training will show a few warts, and circuit training is certainly no exception. For starters, it can be darn near impossible to do in a crowded gym. Having designed effective training programs for magazine articles and books, I've received my fair share of complaints from readers about the impracticality of carrying out these workouts in commercial health clubs. I've also heard from home exercisers who've been inconvenienced by constantly changing the amount of weights on the bar between upper- and lower-body exercises. One of the biggest gripes I've heard is that when you take time to change the weight between sets, your heart rate falls, effectively minimizing any potential aerobic benefits. True enough, although it should be mentioned that circuit training has been shown to bring about only minimal improvements in aerobic capacity even when done at a continuous pace. Many also argue that the training loads are too light to bring about significant improvements in strength. Another fair point, though working with relatively light loads does improve muscular endurance.

Despite these criticisms, I still think the traditional form of circuit training, where you alternate between upper- and lower-body exercises, is a fantastic training option for beginners. Known as Peripheral Heart Action (PHA) training, this shunts large volumes of blood from one end of your body to the other, with your large-muscle groups effectively working as peripheral hearts (hence the name) and improving both circulation and overall conditioning. Perhaps the best feature of this type of training is the relatively low amount of lactic acid it generates, making it easier for beginners to stick with it without succumbing to fatigue.

Here are two examples of PHA routines. Remember, to achieve the desired effect, you need to keep the loads light and the reps fairly high (10 to 15 per set). Also, keep your rest intervals between sets as short as possible (15 to 20 seconds max). All you need is enough time to get to the next station and set up your weight, then off you go. Once you've finished all of the exercises, rest for a minute or do a couple minutes of jogging or cycling before going through the circuit once again. Do either of these workouts two to three times per week for 4 to 6 weeks, and you'll be amazed at how much different you look and feel.

PHA Workout #1

Barbell squat or leg press
Cable row
Incline reverse crunch
Lying leg curl
Barbell bench press

PHA Workout #2

Chinup or lat pulldown
Barbell deadlift
Rotational situp
Neutral-grip dumbbell shoulder press
Dumbbell lunge

IT TAKES TWO

PAIRING EXERCISES FOR ADDED INTENSITY

What if you do train in a crowded gym that makes it impossible to secure this many pieces of equipment in a row? Or perhaps you're a home exerciser who finds it difficult to set up the weight for that many consecutive exercises without breaking the flow of your workout. Fear not—I've come up with a series of mini-circuits designed to provide you with the benefits of PHA without all the aggravation. With these, you select two exercises that each work different areas of your body (i.e., upper body and lower body; or lower body and core) and continuously alternate between these until you perform the desired number of sets. You then move on to another pair of exercises and perform them in the same manner. Simply follow the same set and rest interval guidelines as for the previous PHA workouts (10 to 15 reps per exercise with 15 to 20 seconds of rest between sets).

Mini-Circuit Workout #1

Barbell bench press and dumbbell split squat: 3 sets each

Incline reverse crunch and lying leg curl: 3 sets each

Cable row and dumbbell calf raise: 3 sets each

Mini-Circuit Workout #2

Lat pulldown and barbell squat: 3 sets each

Neutral-grip dumbbell shoulder press and rotational situp: 3 sets each

Dumbbell incline bench press and Romanian deadlift: 3 sets each

To intensify the fat burning, you may want to throw in little 1-to-2-minute stints of intense cardio exercise after completing each exercise pairing. This is another way to increase the energy demands and subsequent afterburn of the workouts. So you might elect to throw in 60 to 90 seconds on the rowing machine after your first pairing and then a brief interval on the stationary bike after the second. Just be sure to keep your RPE level manageable (13 to 16) since you're never really getting a chance to recover.

The great thing about PHA training, regardless of how you choose to do it, is that it's great for beginners of all types. The lighter loads and higher reps make it perfect for introducing you to strength training while simultaneously bolstering tendon and ligament strength to help prevent injury. Best of all, PHA enables you to get a tremendous amount of work done in a relatively short time frame without being too drained. This is without question one of the best ways to promote adherence to an exercise program.

POWER SURGE

TAKING CIRCUIT TRAINING TO THE NEXT LEVEL

In addition to the more traditional forms of circuit training, there's also another, more aggressive way to get a good cardio workout with the feel of iron in your hands. Unlike PHA training, it doesn't have a specific name assigned to it. I'm fond of calling it the Power Surge, because it achieves similar results in a much more dynamic way. The biggest difference between the Power Surge and PHA training is the amount of weight being lifted. The Power Surge involves grouping two or more large-muscle-group exercises, like squats and bench presses, at much higher percentages of your 1-rep max (65 to 80 percent) for far fewer reps (5 to 8 per set).

Besides being a better strength stimulus, training this way can also have a pretty significant effect on your metabolism. How's that, you ask? Well, in addition to the short rest intervals between sets, working with heavy loads such as these creates a greater energy demand than you might imagine. As the amount of weight being lifted increases, your mechanical efficiency actually decreases. Because heavier loads require more balance and coordination, more of those little stabilizing muscles need to kick in and help out. The more muscle mass being activated, the greater the energy demands of the exercise. And, as you now well know, the more calories you burn during your workout, the more calories you burn *after* your workout.

Note that I don't advocate this type of training for beginners, at least not initially. I just figured I'd present it as an option for later on down the road, when your conditioning level has improved and you're looking for something to kick your fat burning into a higher gear. If you decide to try it, just be sure to always stress form over weight and to select exercises that you know you can perform correctly. I'd also advise throwing in moderate-intensity periods of cardio work to serve as an active rest between strength-training exercises. Although relatively heavy loads like the ones in question don't produce much lactic acid, the heavy nervous system demand could prove too much for some people.

Perform Power Surge workouts two or three times a week, leaving at least 1 day in between workouts to allow for recovery. Do each exercise for a total of 2 or 3 sets of 5 to 8 repetitions each. You can also do additional core exercises on off days or immediately following your workout.

Power Surge Workout #1

Barbell squat

Barbell bench press

Barbell deadlift

Chinup

90 to 120 seconds on rower (RPE: 12 to 14)

Power Surge Workout #2

Prone dumbbell row

Dumbbell lunge

Dumbbell shoulder press

Lying leg curl

90 to 120 seconds on stairclimber (RPE: 12 to 15)

SEGMENTED SURGE

A STRATEGY FOR CROWD CONTROL

If you train in a crowded gym or have difficulty changing weights quickly enough to maintain a consistent pace, you can break up the Power Surge workouts just as you did with the mini-circuits on the previous page (meaning that you'll do 1 to 2 minutes of cardio after each exercise). This will enable you to keep your cardio stints in between lifts slightly more intense, because you won't expend as much energy performing two consecutive lifts as you would performing four. Perform all exercises to the same set, rep, and loading parameters as in the original Power Surge workouts: 2 or 3 sets of 5 to 8 reps each, at 65 to 80 percent of your 1-rep max. Such workouts might look something like this:

Segmented Surge Workout #1

Barbell squat and barbell bench press

90 to 120 seconds on rower (RPE: 14 to 16)

Barbell deadlift and chinup

90 to 120 seconds on stationary bike (RPE: 14 to 16)

Segmented Surge Workout #2

Prone dumbbell row with elbows out and dumbbell lunge

90 to 120 seconds on stairclimber (RPE: 14 to 16)

Neutral-grip dumbbell shoulder press and lying leg curl

90 to 120 seconds on elliptical trainer (RPE: 14 to 16)

AB-STINENCE?

WHY YOU DON'T NEED DIRECT ABDOMINAL WORK TO HELP YOU LOSE THAT GUT

Go ahead, say it: You've looked over all these workouts, and you can't believe how little abdominal work they contain. Aside from a couple of sets of reverse crunches and some situps, there seems to be an omission of direct

FAT CHANCE

Five common fat fallacies

1. It's possible to spot-reduce. My apologies to those of you who think that broomstick twists will whittle down your waist or that squats will reduce the size of your butt, but it just doesn't work that way. When you lose fat, you do it from all over your body, not just those areas you wish to see it banished from the most.

2. Water weight stays off. If you're tempted to wear a rubber reducing suit when you exercise or perhaps do squats and pushups in the sauna, I'm begging you not to. As entertaining as you would be for the rest of us, you'd end up hurting yourself. You might feel a lot lighter once you finish, but that's only because you would have dehydrated yourself. As soon as you had a couple of glasses of water, you'd be right back where you started.

3. Low-intensity cardio exercise burns more fat than higher-intensity exercise. This one's actually got some truth to it. When you exercise at a lower percentage of your VO_2 max (the maximal rate at which your body can consume and utilize oxygen)—say, at about 40 to 50 percent—you do burn a greater percentage of calories from stored body fat than you do when working at higher intensities (such as 75 to 90 percent of VO_2 max). However, it's also true that working at higher intensity burns more total calories, so, if your workout duration is similar to that of a low-intensity session, you actually end up burning more fat calories as well. Say, for instance, you do 30 minutes on the treadmill at the lower intensity and burn 200 calories. Approximately 60 percent, or 120, of those calories will come from stored body fat. Now, let's say the next day you do 20 minutes of higher-intensity HIIT and burn 400 calories. Only 40 percent of those calories will come from fat. However, 40 percent of 400 equals 160 calories—40 more than during the low-intensity session. Not bad for working out 10 minutes less than you did the day before.

4. If you stop working out, your muscles turn into fat. Right, and Britney Spears and her husband are going to live happily ever after. C'mon, folks, this is complete bunk. Muscles do two things: They get bigger (hypertrophy) and smaller (atrophy). That's it! They don't miraculously turn to fat if you stop exercising. If you ask me, this is just an old wives' tale concocted by people looking for an excuse not to start going to the gym.

5. You don't start burning fat until 20 minutes into your workout. Tell that to a sprinter the next time you see one whizzing down the track without an ounce of visible body fat on him. Your body burns a mixture of fats and carbohydrates all the time. Granted, it tends to switch over more to fat as exercise duration increases, but to think you use no fat between the onset of exercise and the 20-minute mark is simply erroneous.

abdominal exercises. Must be some sort of oversight, right? Nope. I did it for a reason. Most of the exercises in this phase involve your core quite heavily. Don't believe me? Give one of those Power Surge workouts a whirl and tell me that the next day you don't feel like you got kicked in the gut by a mule. So you see, there's really no need for too many specific abdominal exercises. Besides, it's not like doing them is going to burn any additional fat from around your waist (see "Fat Chance" on the previous page).

Call me crazy, but in my never-ending quest to change people's perceptions about physical fitness, I saw this as an opportunity to drive home the point that direct abdominal training simply isn't necessary if fat loss is your goal. You might still want to throw in a few exercises to keep your core strong—feel free to do so by choosing some of the numerous exercises provided in this book. Just don't think they're going to amplify the results of these fat-burning workouts. That just isn't possible. There's not a single ab exercise that's going to burn fat more effectively than the workouts contained in this chapter.

I know it's a hard pill to swallow, especially since so many of us have been brought up on the belief that getting down on the floor and doing various forms of situps and crunches is the key to having a flat stomach. Like any other muscle group, your abs get pumped when you work them. When they engorge with blood and press tightly against your skin, you feel like your abs have gotten tighter and firmer. This is a temporary sensation that has no impact whatsoever on the size of your waistline. It might sound weird, but things like squatting, lunging, and interval cardio will help you shed way more belly flab than crunches ever will.

BARBELL SQUAT

Hold a barbell with an overhand grip so that it rests comfortably on your upper back (not on your neck). Set your feet shoulder-width apart, knees slightly bent, back straight, eyes focused straight ahead.

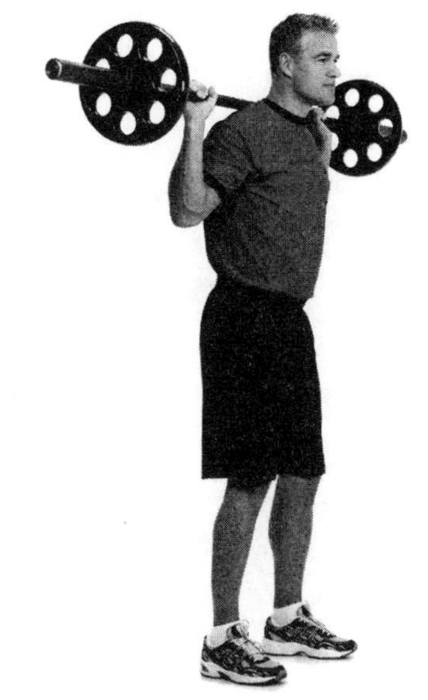

A

Next, slowly lower your body as if you were sitting back into a chair, keeping your back in its natural alignment and lower legs nearly perpendicular to the floor. When your upper thighs are parallel to the floor, pause, and then return to the starting position.

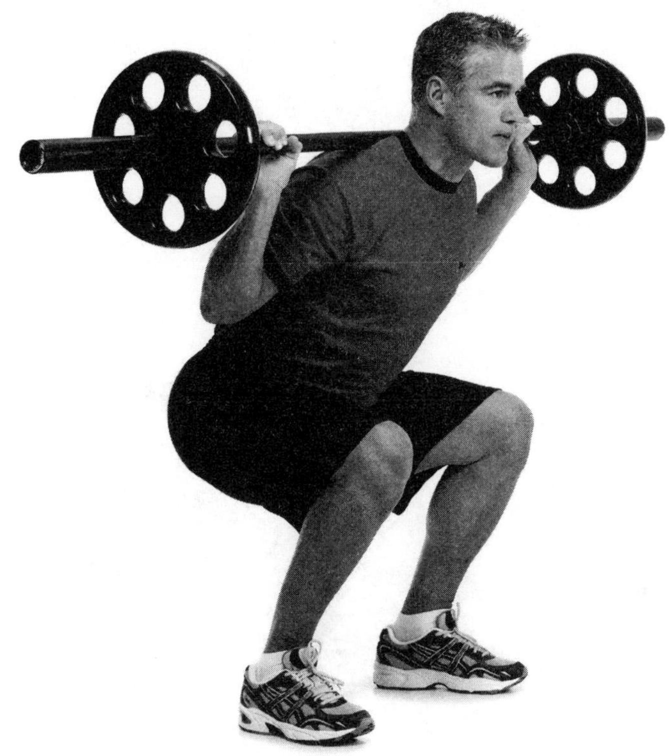

B

DUMBBELL SPLIT SQUAT

Grab a pair of dumbbells and hold them at your sides. Stand in a staggered stance with one foot 2½ to 3 feet in front of the other.

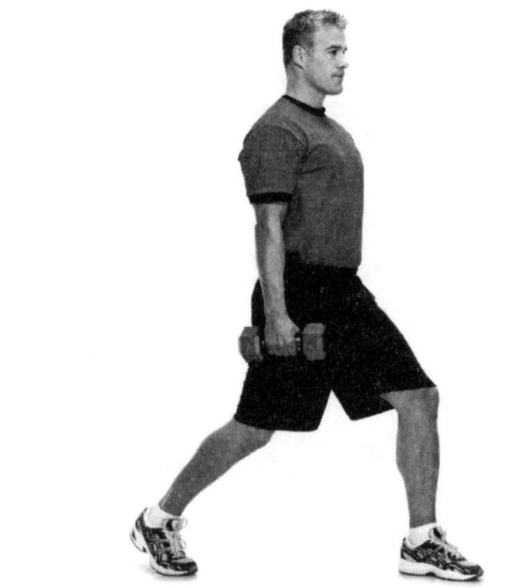

Lower your body until your front knee is bent 90 degrees and your rear knee nearly touches the floor. Your front lower leg should be perpendicular to the floor and your torso should remain upright. Push yourself back up to the starting position as quickly as you can. Finish all of your repetitions, then repeat the exercise with your opposite foot in front.

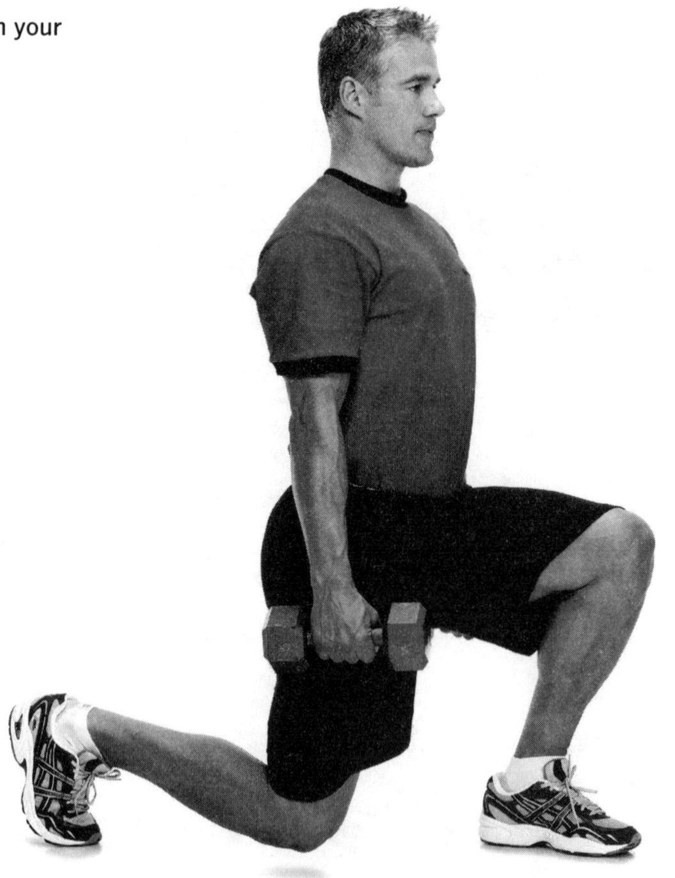

B

DUMBBELL CALF RAISE

Grab a dumbbell in your right hand and stand on a step or a block. Put your left hand on something for balance—a wall or weight stack, for instance. Cross your right foot behind your left ankle and balance yourself on the ball of your left foot, with your heel hanging off the step. Lower your left heel as far as you can.

Pause, and then lift it as high as you can. Finish the set with your left leg and then repeat with your right (while holding the dumbbell in your left hand).

Note: This exercise can also be done using a calf raise machine if you train in a gym.

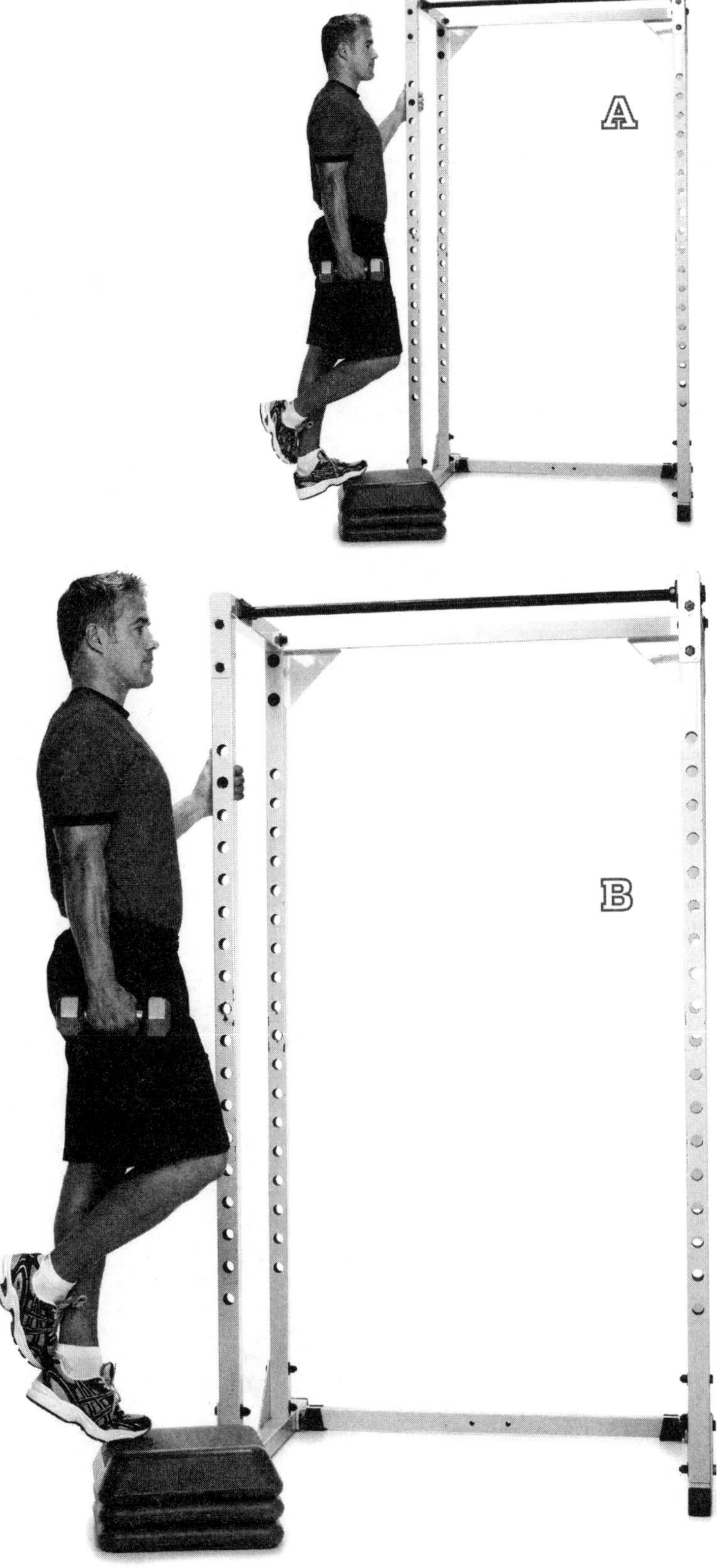

LEG PRESS

Position yourself in a 45-degree plate-loaded leg press sled with your feet about shoulder-width apart and your lower back pressed into the pad.

Begin by unlocking the sled and slowly lowering the weight down toward your chest. Once your thighs are parallel to the force plate, pause for a second and push back up to the starting position.

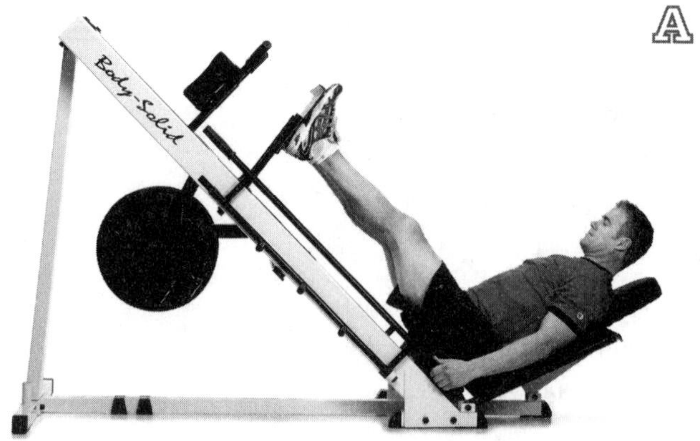

A

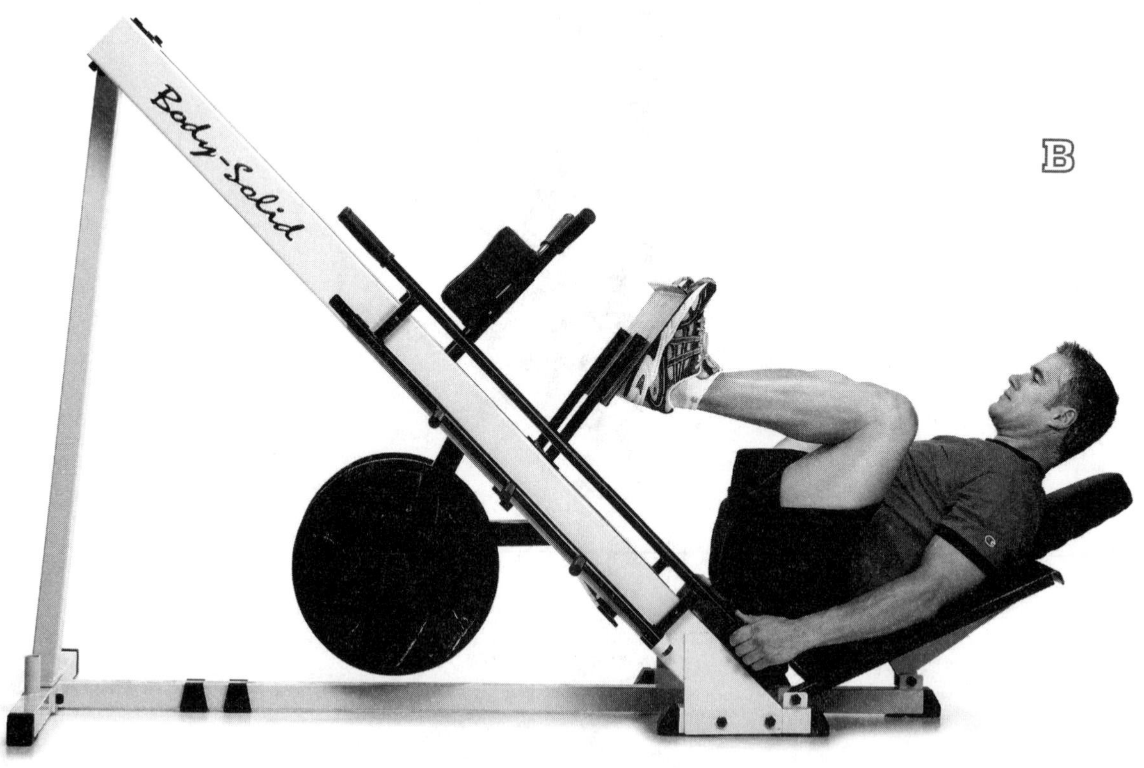

B

CABLE ROW

Sit in front of a cable station with your feet up against the support plate and grabbing the bar with a pronated (palms facing away from you) grip.

Keep your torso right over your hips and pinch your shoulder blades together as you pull the bar in toward the base of your sternum (breastbone). Be sure to keep your elbows flared out, away from your body. Pause for a second and return the weight to the starting position.

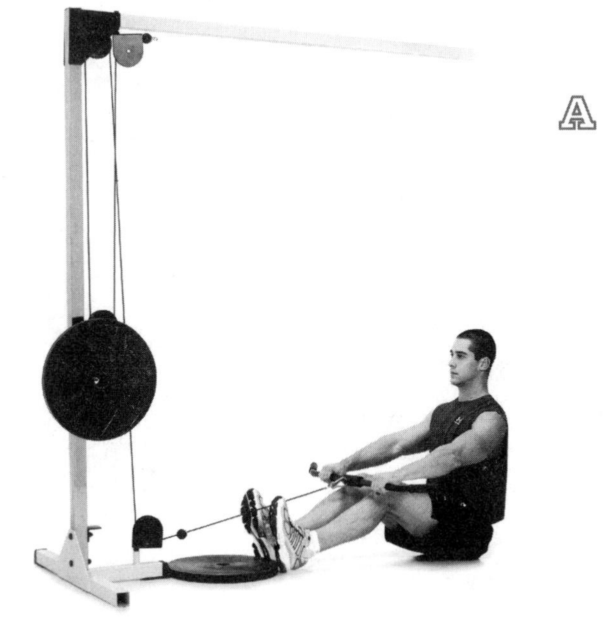

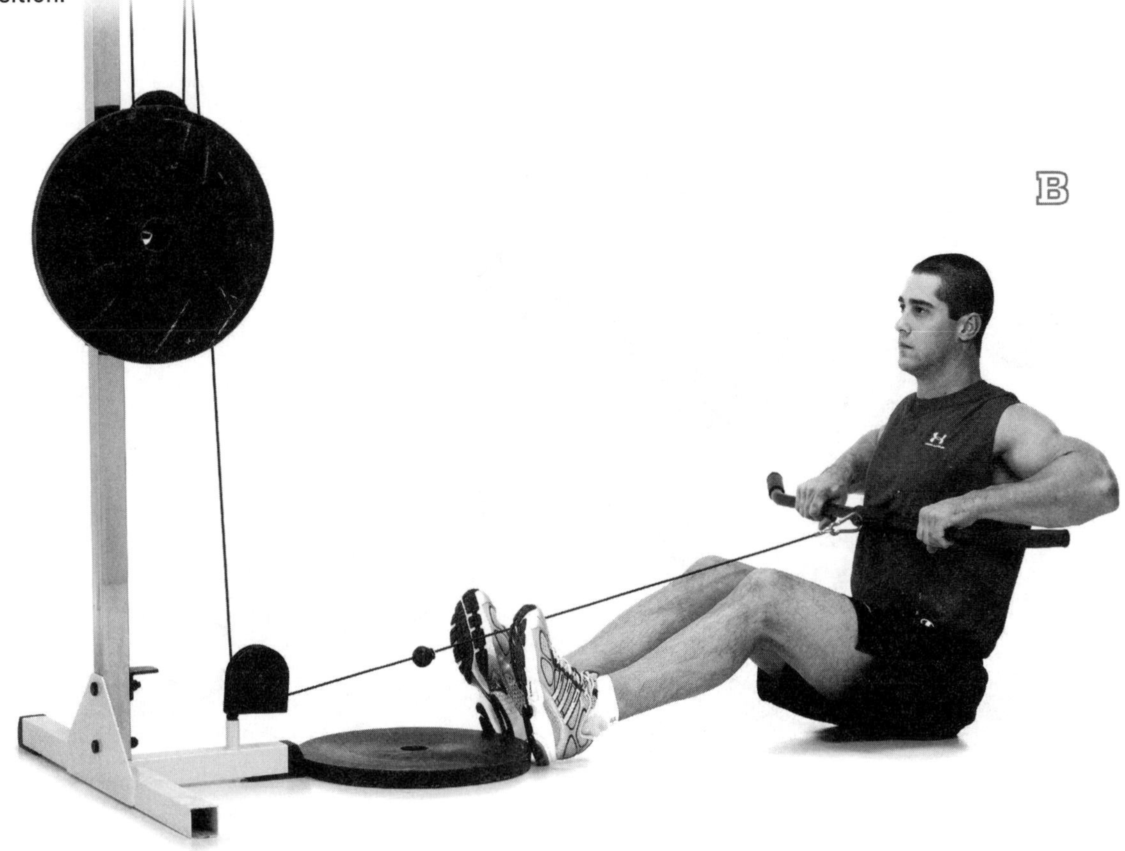

INCLINE REVERSE CRUNCH

Lie on a slant board with your hips lower than your head. Grab the bar behind your head for support. Bend your hips and knees 90 degrees.

Pull your hips upward and crunch them inward, as if you were emptying a bucket of water that's resting on your pelvis. Keep your hips and knees at 90-degree angles throughout the exercise. Pause and then slowly lower your hips to the starting position.

A

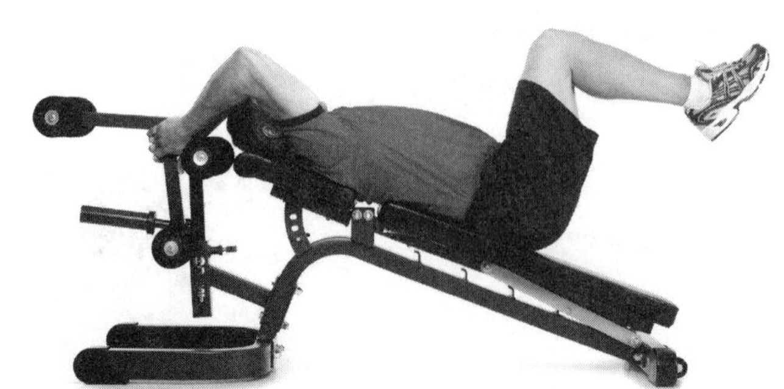

B

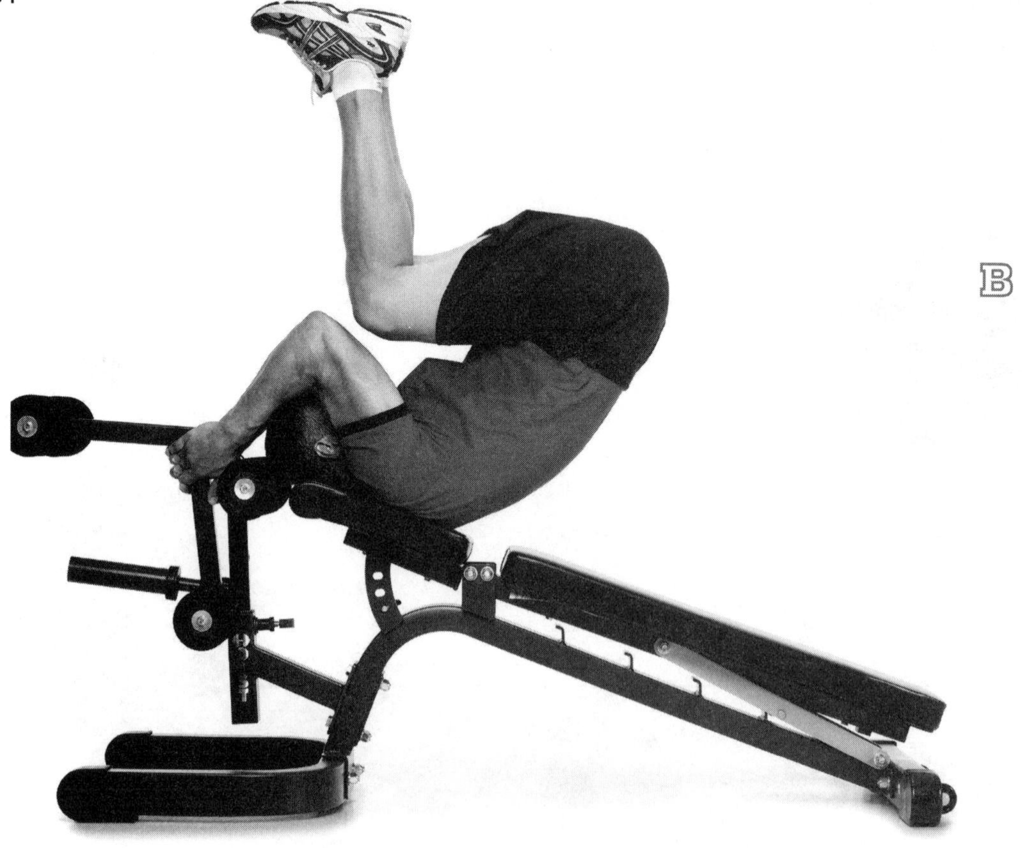

INCLINE DUMBBELL BENCH PRESS

Grab a pair of dumbbells and lie faceup on a bench set to a low incline (15 to 30 degrees). Lift the dumbbells so they're over your chin and hold them with your palms turned out (thumbs facing each other).

Slowly lower the weights to your upper chest, pause, and then push them back up over your chin.

A

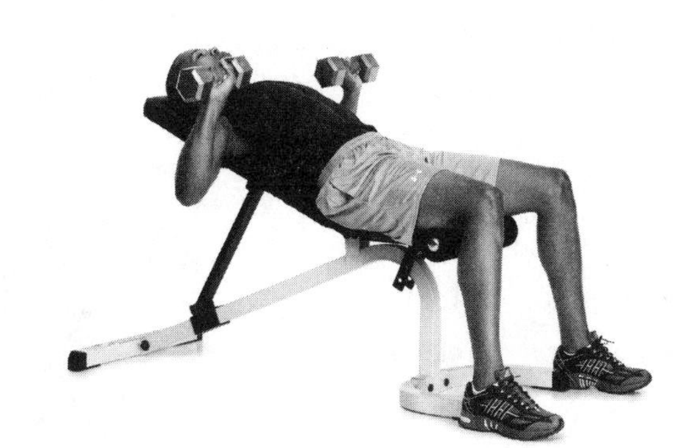

B

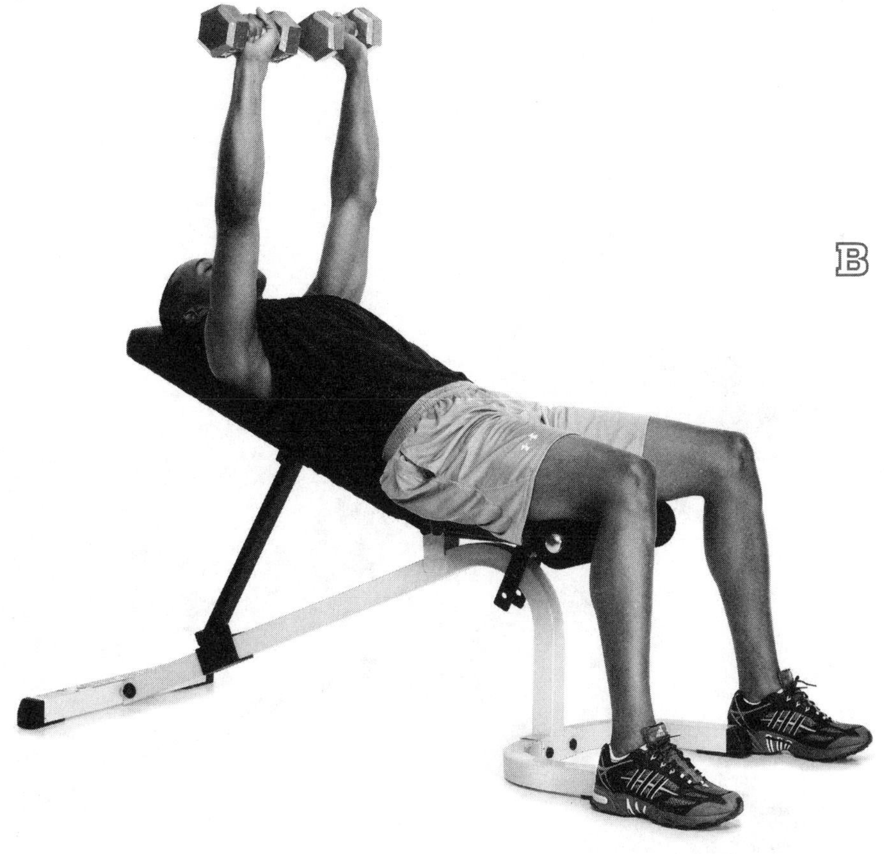

LYING LEG CURL

Lie in the leg-curl machine with the pads against your lower legs, above your heels and below your calf muscles.

Without raising your body off the pad, bend your legs at the knees and pull the weight toward you as far as you can. Pause and then slowly return to the starting position.

A

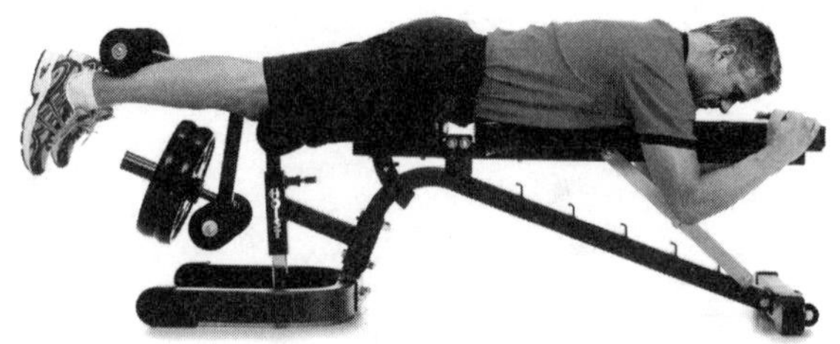

B

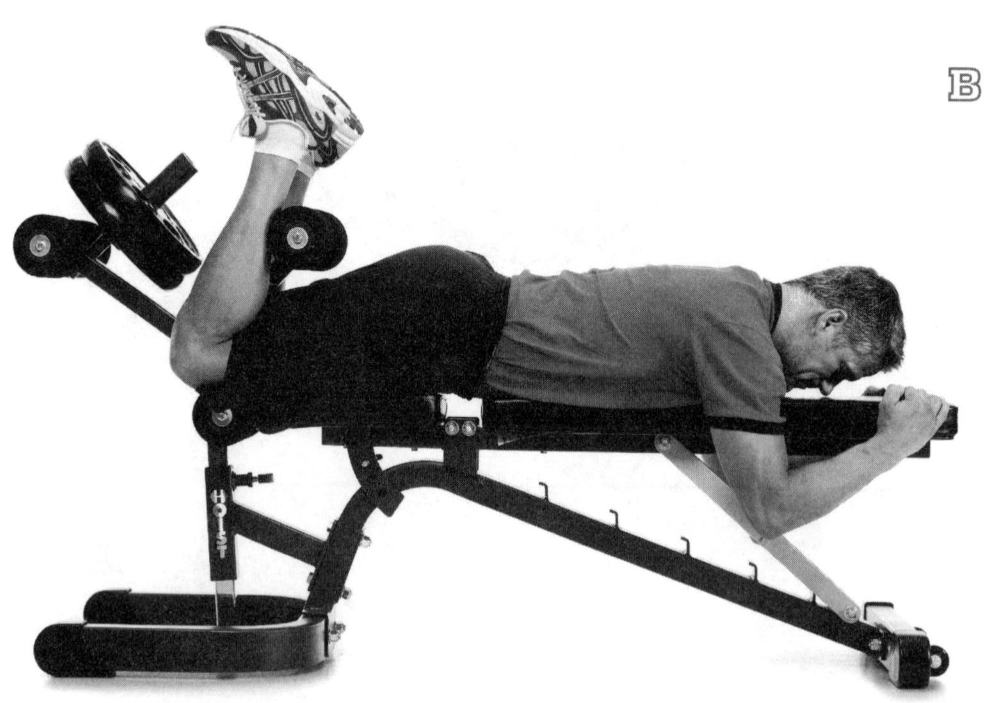

BARBELL BENCH PRESS

Grab the bar with your hands just wider than shoulder width. Lift the bar off the uprights and hold it over your chest.

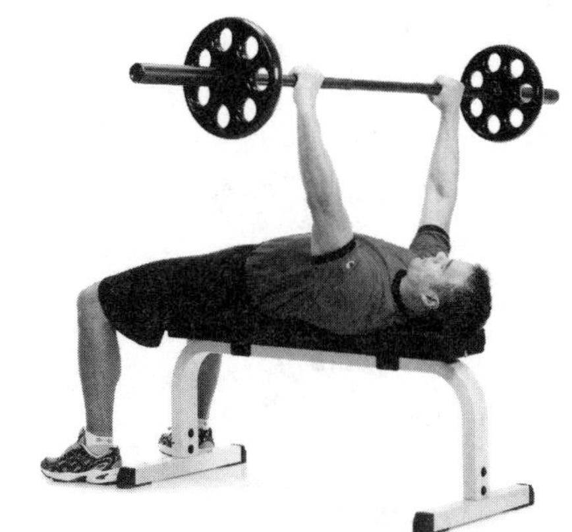

Next, lower the bar to your chest, pause, and then push it back to the starting position.

Note: You can make this exercise easier on your shoulders by using a closer grip and keeping your elbows in closer to your body.

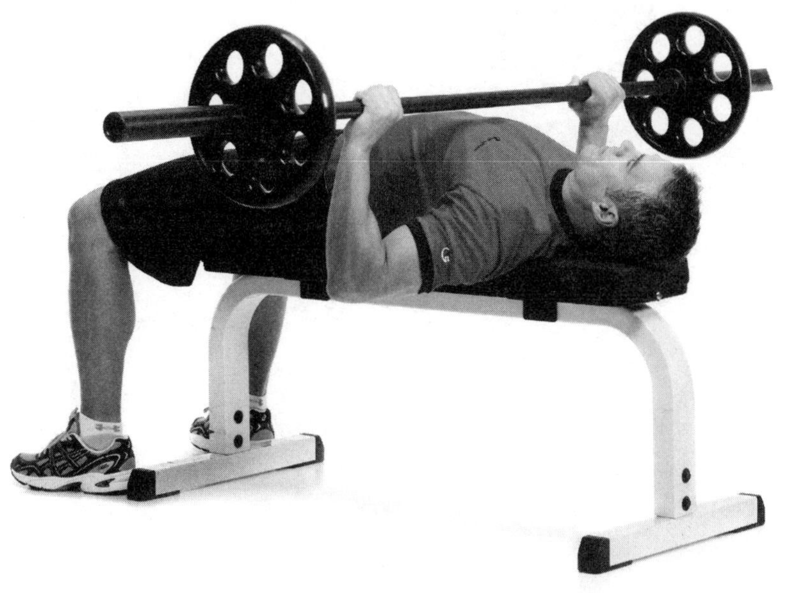

B

CHINUP

Grab the chinup bar with a shoulder-width, underhand grip, as you bend your knees and cross your ankles behind you to hang from it.

Keeping your chest out, pull yourself up until your chin clears the bar. Pause there for a second and then slowly return to the starting position.

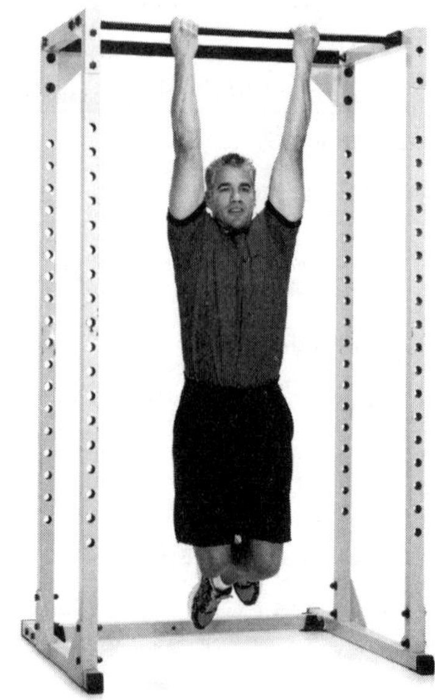

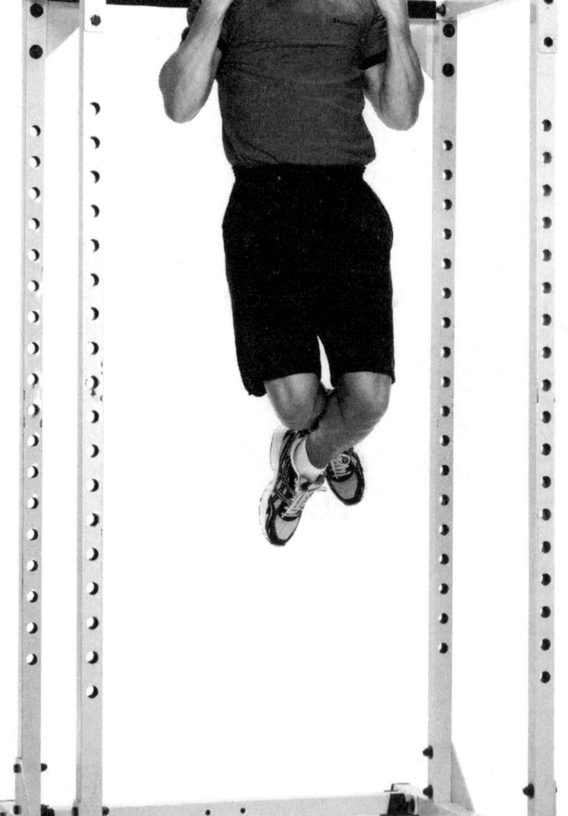

B

LAT PULLDOWN

Grab the bar of a lat pulldown machine (or a straight bar on the high pulley of a cable station) with a shoulder-width, overhand grip.

Moving only your arms, pull the bar down to your chest by squeezing your shoulder blades together. Hold for a second and then bring the bar back to the starting position.

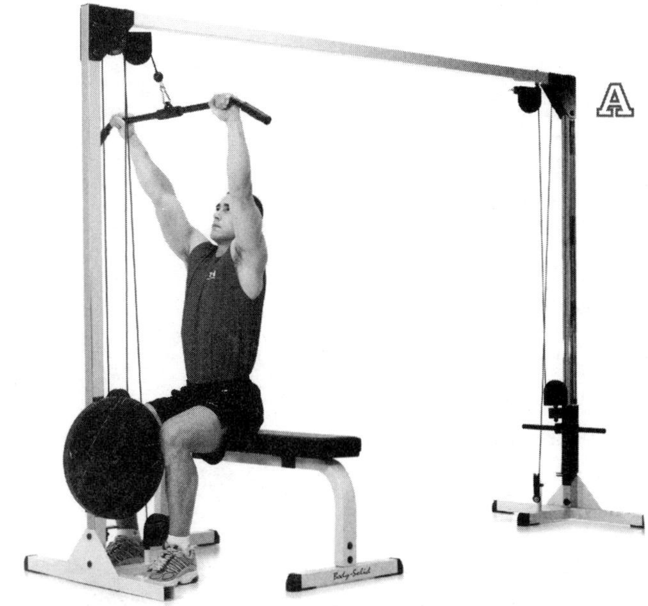

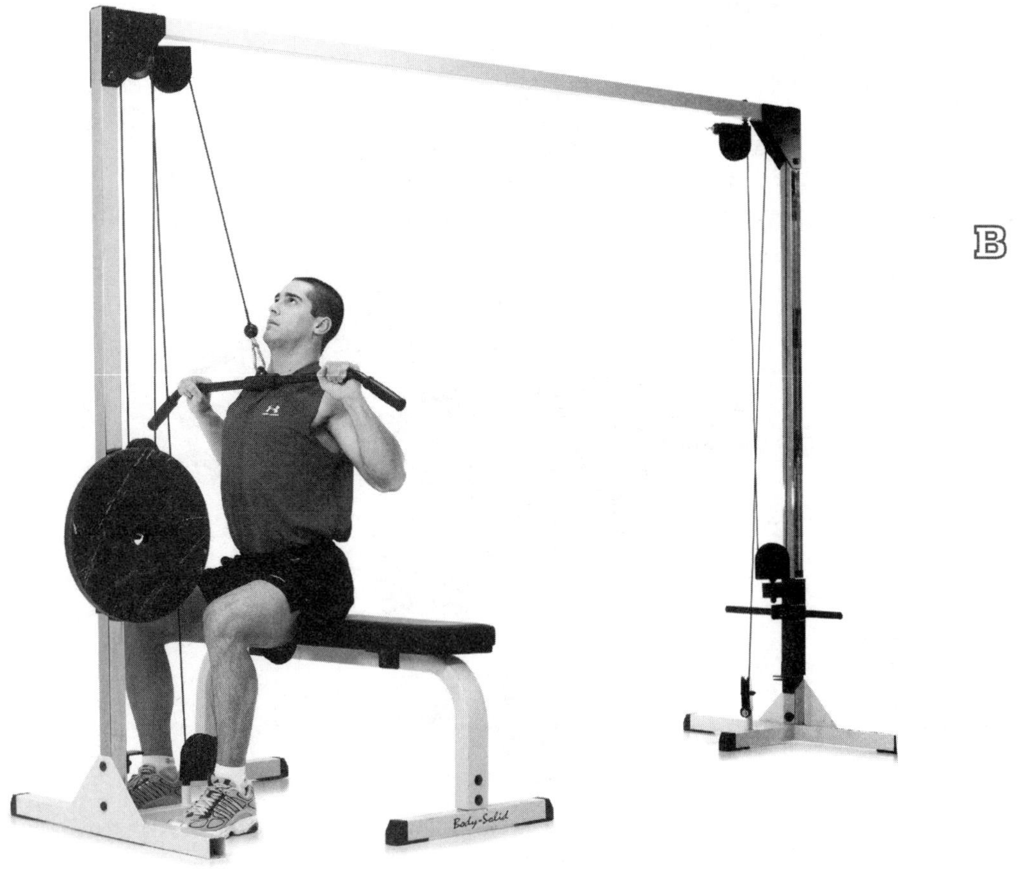

BARBELL DEADLIFT

Set a barbell on the floor and stand facing it. Squat down and grab it overhand, your hands just outside your legs.

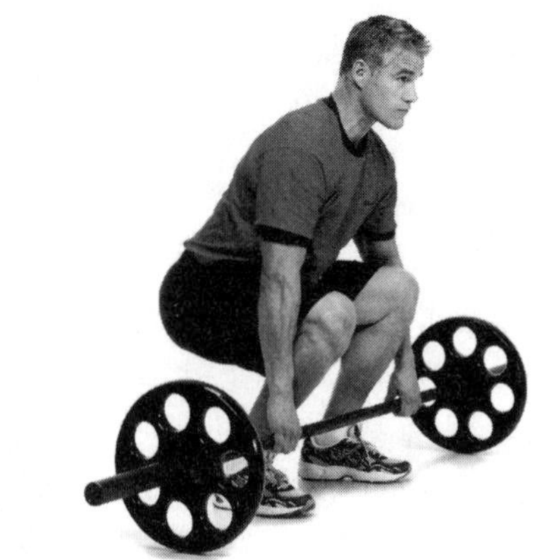

With your back flat and head up, stand up with the barbell, pulling your shoulder blades back. Then slowly lower the bar to the starting position.

Note: Those of you who have lower-back issues may want to either start from the top position (by taking the bar off the supports in a squat rack) or not go as low. Or do the exercises with dumbbells held at your sides, which allows you to maintain a more upright posture and reduced lower-back strain.

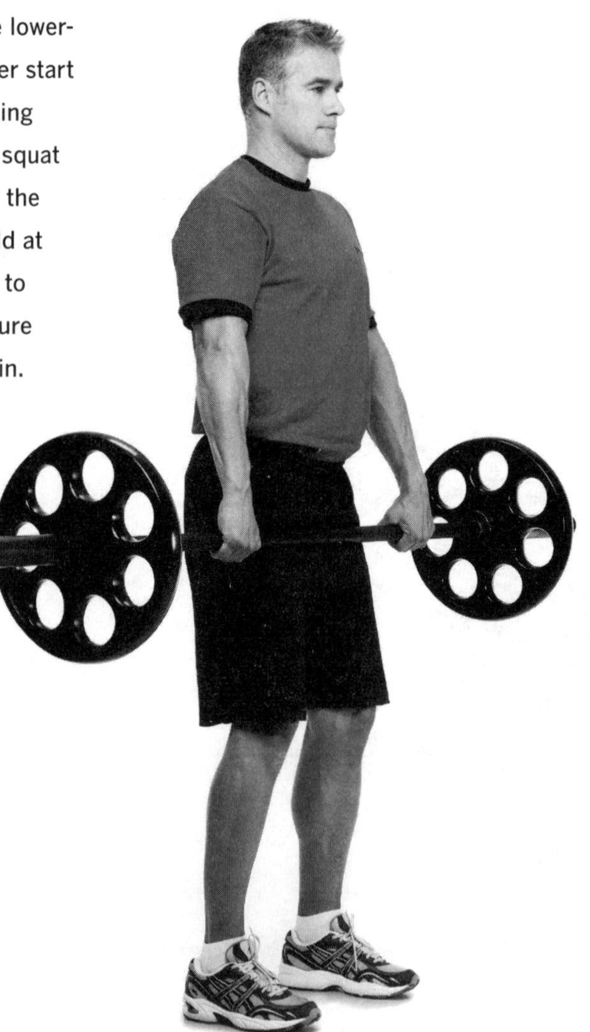

B

ROMANIAN DEADLIFT

Grab an unloaded barbell (feel free to add weight to it as you get stronger) with an overhand grip that's just beyond shoulder width. Stand holding the bar at arm's length and resting on the fronts of your thighs. Your feet should be shoulder-width apart and your knees slightly bent. Focus your eyes straight ahead.

Slowly bend at the hips as you lower the bar to just below your knees. Don't change the angle of your knees. Keep your head and chest up and your lower back flat or slightly arched. Lift your torso back to the starting position, keeping the bar as close to your body as possible.

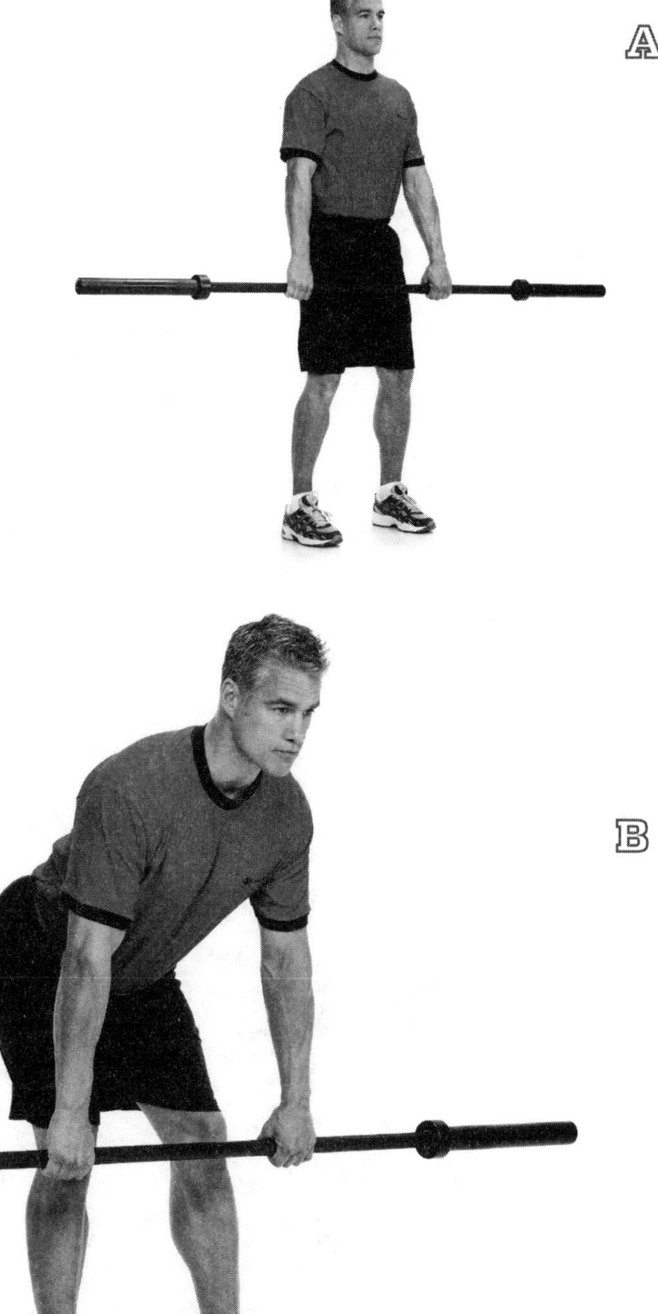

ROTATIONAL SITUP

Lie on the floor with your knees bent and feet flat.

Next, with your hands held at the sides of your head, sit up and rotate as you bring one armpit toward the opposite knee. Lower back down and repeat to the other side.

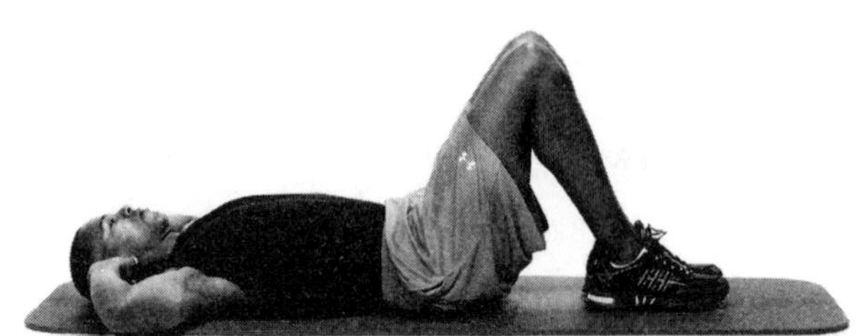

B

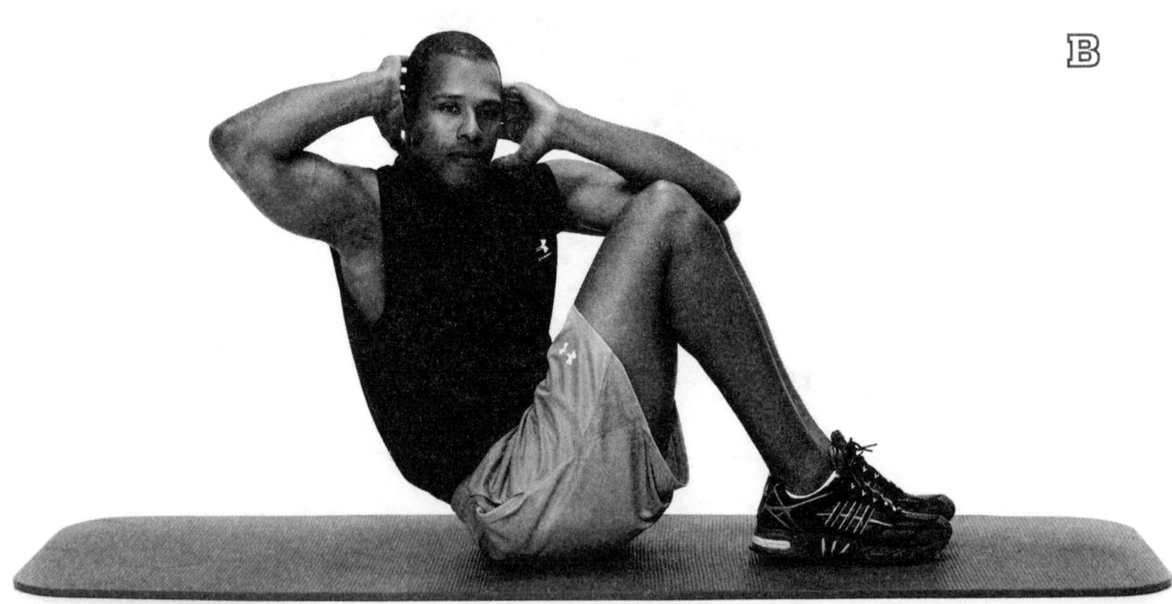

NEUTRAL-GRIP DUMBBELL SHOULDER PRESS

Stand holding a pair of dumbbells just outside your shoulders, with your arms bent and your palms facing each other.

Push the weights straight overhead (like a referee signaling a touchdown). Pause, then lower them to the starting position.

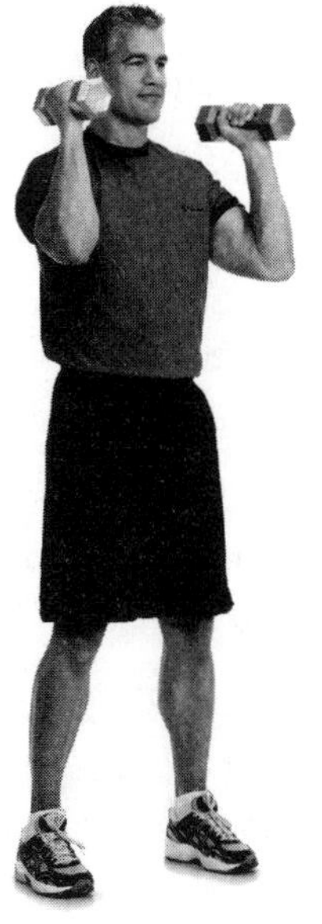

A

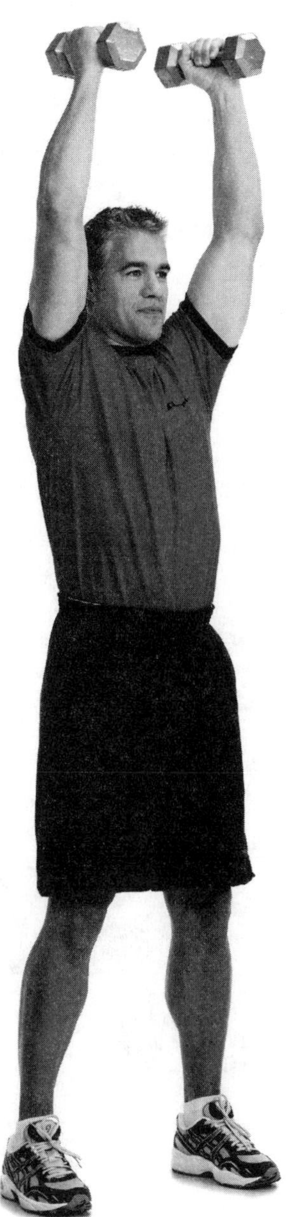

B

DUMBBELL LUNGE

Standing with your feet hip-width apart, grab a pair of dumbbells and hold them at your sides.

Step forward with one leg and lower your body until your front knee is bent 90 degrees and your rear knee nearly touches the floor. Your front lower leg should be perpendicular to the floor and your torso should remain upright. Push yourself back up to the starting position as quickly as you can and repeat with your other leg.

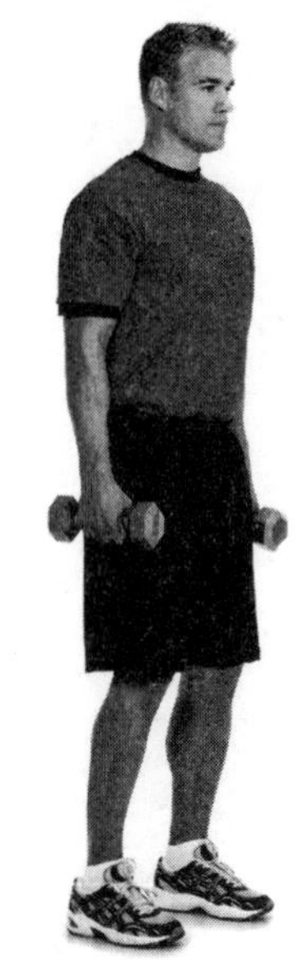

A

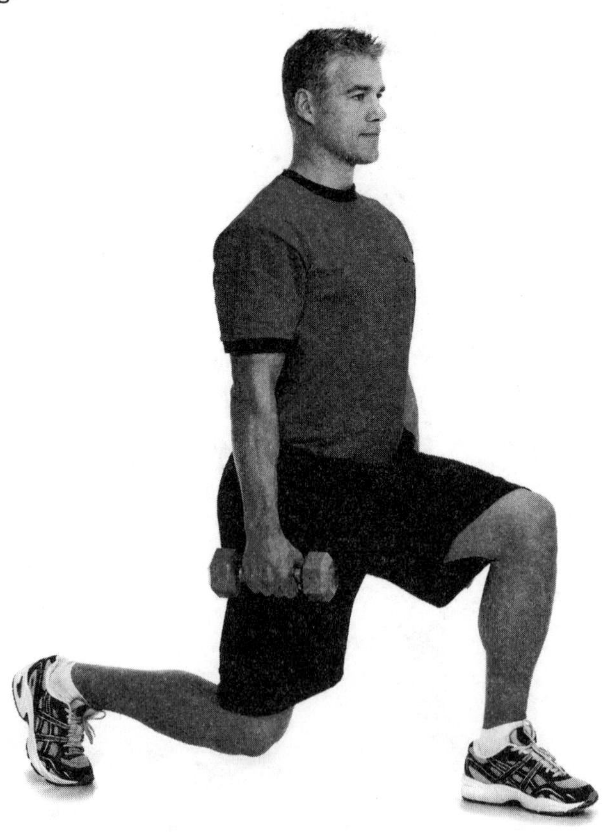

B

PRONE DUMBBELL ROW WITH ELBOWS OUT

Lie facedown on an incline bench set to a 30- to 45-degree angle holding a pair of dumbbells at arm's length with your palms facing behind you.

Lift your upper arms as high as you can by bending your elbows and squeezing your shoulder blades together. Your forearms should be pointing toward the floor throughout the movement. Pause, then slowly lower the weights to the starting position.

A

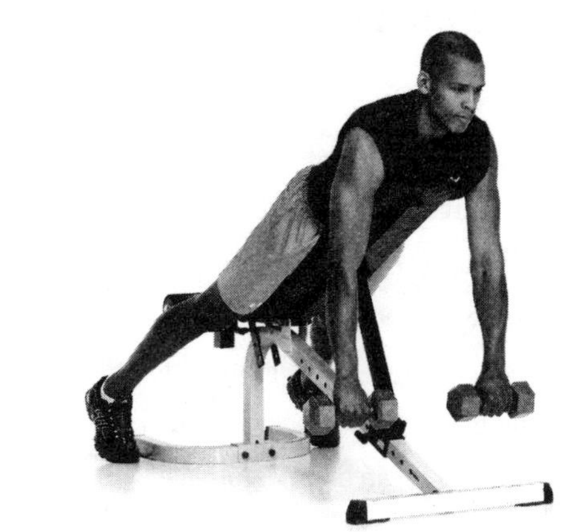

B

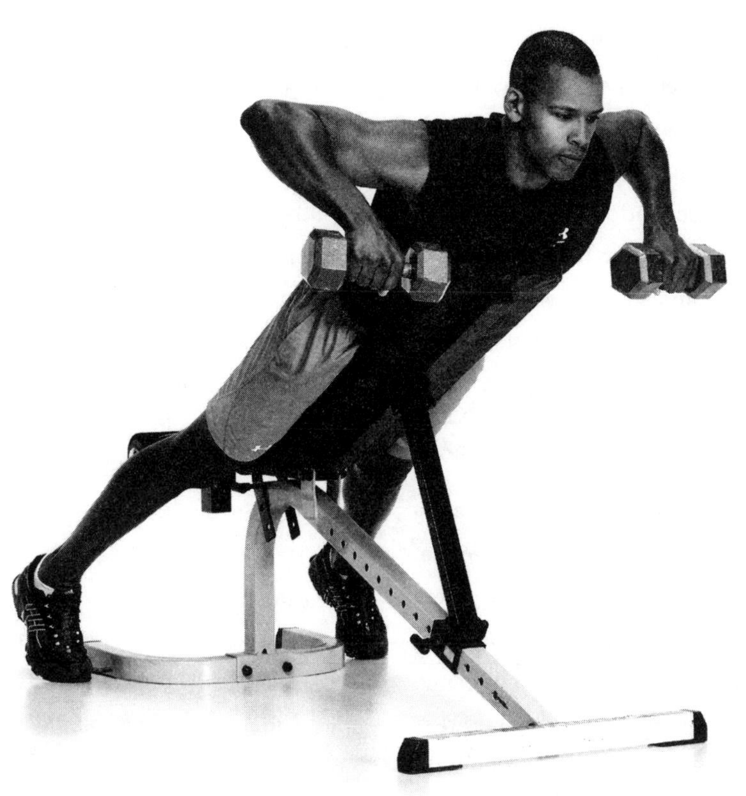

EAT, DRINK, AND BE WARY

NUTRITIONAL STRATEGIES FOR FAT LOSS

Right about now I can picture you sitting there, rubbing your hands together, saying "C'mon, give it to me!" You've patiently read through the rest of this chapter desperately hoping for me to reveal some of the real "secrets" to fat loss once you reached the nutritional section. You're probably expecting to hear a bunch of tips like how eating grapefruit on an empty stomach will help you burn more body fat or why the elimination of evil carbohydrates is the key to finally achieving that elusive six-pack. Well, sorry to disappoint you, but it just doesn't work that way. When it comes to fat loss, there are no secrets or quick-fix solutions. It basically boils down to eating less and exercising more.

Okay, perhaps that is an overly simplistic way of stating it. Burning body fat takes hard work and lots of discipline. If you're really serious about dropping excess poundage, you have to pay close attention to everything you put in your mouth. Not that you have to be so strict that you can never enjoy yourself. But if you think you can eat whatever you want just because you've started working out, you're sadly mistaken.

The good news is there are strategies you can employ to help achieve your goals a little more quickly.

Eat based on your upcoming activities. By eating based on what you'll be doing for the next couple of hours, you'll avoid that tired, sluggish feeling that often accompanies overeating. For instance, if you know that after lunch you'll be sitting down to a bunch of paperwork at your desk, keeping your meal light and fairly low in carbohydrates will allow you to focus better because it won't cause huge fluctuations in your blood sugar levels. After you eat a meal high in carbohydrates (i.e., where carbs comprise 50 to 75 percent of the total caloric content), blood sugar levels typically rise at a rapid rate. (High-glycemic carbs cause a greater rise than do those of the low-glycemic variety.) This causes the hormone insulin to be released into your bloodstream in an attempt to bring your blood sugar levels back down to more stable levels. The greater the rise in blood sugar, the larger the insulin release. And the larger the insulin release, the lower your blood sugar levels will drop. This in turn will leave you feeling tired and make it difficult to concentrate. As if that weren't bad enough, too much insulin circulating through your body also has the nasty little habit of increasing fat storage. So, needless to say, keeping insulin levels in check is pretty important when you're trying to get as lean as possible.

Conversely, if shortly after your meal you'll be engaging in some sport or vigorous exercise, a slightly larger meal that's somewhat rich in carbohydrates might be a better choice. You still want to pay close attention to the types of carbs you'll be consuming, via the glycemic index. But a bigger meal is warranted since you'll shortly be putting the energy to good use.

Keep your metabolism guessing. Just as you figured out, in phase 4, how much of a calorie surplus you needed to consume to build muscle, you'll need to determine how much of a deficit you're willing to endure to burn fat. This needn't be extreme—remember, starvation diets don't work. They rob your body of precious muscle mass and actually cause your metabolism to slow. Depending on what your daily energy needs are, once again figure on a 15 to 20 percent calorie reduction in order to start seeing a reduction in your waistline.

So say your daily energy needs are around 2,300 calories. Eating 300 to 400 calories below that, or 1,900 to 2,000, would start making a nice dent in your body fat percentage before long. It's enough of a caloric restriction to get your attention but not drastic enough to force your body into starvation mode, where you start sacrificing existing muscle tissue to meet your energy needs. Feel free to tweak things as you see fit. If you start losing weight too quickly or don't think you're progressing quickly enough, you could always adjust these amounts up or down a bit.

The one thing you do not want to do is become predictable. The human body is a truly amazing organism, one that adapts rather quickly to demands placed on it. As soon as your body begins to figure out that you're restricting energy intake, it will respond by attempting to slow down your metabolism. That's why you can't let it get used to one set level of food consumption. This entails basically tricking your body into giving up that stored fat by slightly altering your caloric intake from day to day.

Say you want to take in 1,900 calories or so. Rather than simply strive to hit that exact number each day, you're better off dancing around it by eating slightly more or less over the course of several days. So one day you might take in 2,000 calories, the next 1,600, and then 1,800 the day after that. This simple manipulation in your daily energy intake can often be enough to keep your metabolism off balance and keep the fat-burning process going.

Of course, like any other highly evolved organism, your body will eventually figure out what you're doing. Another great trick you can use is to periodically select one day where you eat well above your maintenance numbers as a means of forcing your metabolism to speed up. So after several days of staying near the 1,900-calorie level, once every 5 to 7 days take in 2,400 or so. It's a highly effective strategy that I recommend, if for no other reason than to help you keep your sanity during what could be a prolonged period of calorie restriction. Knowing that every once in a while you can splurge and take in some extra calories for one day can often be the difference between reaching your goals and throwing up your arms in disgust.

Increase your fiber intake. Besides helping to lower your cholesterol levels and prevent heart disease and cancer, increasing your intake of dietary fiber can also be an effective way to decrease body fat. Both soluble fiber (which dissolves in water) and insoluble fiber (which does not) help fight fat, in different ways. Soluble fiber is known to help reduce cholesterol levels and even plays a role in helping regulate blood sugar levels. Insoluble fiber, aka roughage, helps speed the transit times of carbs and fat through the small intestine, leaving less time for them to be absorbed by your body.

While most nutritionists recommend between 25 and 30 grams of fiber per day, most Americans are lucky to average even half of that. In case you're wondering how you can get more fiber into your diet, the "True Grit" list below will provide you with a nice variety of choices. Be careful not to add too much fiber too soon, though. Radical increases in dietary fiber can lead to unpleasant side

TRUE GRIT

Good sources of dietary fiber

Soluble Fiber	*Insoluble Fiber*
Dried fruit	Wheat bran
Oat bran	Whole grains
Rolled oats	Leafy greens
Barley	Bananas
Citrus fruits	Peas
Pinto beans	Pears
Brown rice	Parsnips
Nuts	Flaxseed
Apples	Strawberries

effects like cramping, gas, and bloating. You also need to make sure you increase your fluid intake to help ease fiber's passage through the small intestine.

Become a late-night burner. There's more to burning calories than just engaging in strenuous exercise. This isn't where I make a case for miracle fat-loss supplements. I'm referring to the energy cost of digestion, also known as the thermic effect of food. Whether you're aware of it or not, your body expends energy just breaking down the various foodstuffs you eat. Here's the cool part: The harder the food is to break down, the more calories your body has to expend to properly digest it.

As luck would have it, your body expends more energy breaking down protein than it does either carbohydrates or fat. Since most of us tend to be less active during the evening hours, favoring protein over carbohydrate- or fat-laden foods both for dinner and after-dinner snacking can serve as an effective strategy for fighting fat. It also acts as a sort of insurance policy that you're taking in all the protein you need, in case you came up a little short throughout the course of the day.

As far as how much protein you actually need, opinions tend to differ amongst nutritional experts. Some dietitians still cling to the old recommendation of 0.8 gram per kilogram of body weight (to determine your body weight in kilograms, simply divide your weight by 2.2). In recent years, the new norm for athletes and people who work out on a regular basis has become 1.0 to 1.5 grams per pound of body weight. Personally, I typically recommend about a gram per pound of body weight for most of my clients, with athletes and serious bodybuilders taking in 1.5 to 2 times that amount.

Drink lots of water. Good ol' H_2O does a lot more than just quench your thirst and help fiber pass through your system. I bet you'd be surprised to learn that drinking water is also one of the best tools for getting rid of body fat. In fact, most nutritional experts would go so far as to say that drinking enough water will have a more dramatic impact on your ability to burn fat than any of those overhyped supplements you constantly see being advertised. Yet you rarely if ever hear anything other than vague generalizations about why drinking water is so important. So what say we get into some of the specifics of how water helps you lose fat?

For starters, without enough water your kidneys can't function properly and end up dumping some of their workload onto your liver. What's so bad about that? Well, seeing as how one of your liver's primary functions is to help burn stored body fat, if that organ has to pick up the slack for your kidneys, it can't do its own job at optimal levels. Translation: You end up burning less fat!

But wait, there's more. When you don't drink enough water, your body begins to conserve what it has out of fear that it won't be getting more. The result is that you end up retaining water, which can obscure the visual effect of those muscles you're working so hard to show. So, ironically, one of the best ways to prevent water retention is to *drink more water.* Once your body sees that it's getting all of the fluid it needs, it will begin letting go of some of that stored water weight. You'll immediately feel lighter and have a more visually pleasing physique. Granted, this isn't really a loss of fat, per se. But in my experience, once the numbers on the scale start to go down and muscles start to become more visible, people become inspired to start working even harder.

Then of course there's the whole temperature regulation issue to contend with. Much the way that protein causes your body to work harder to digest it, drinking cold water forces your body to expend more calories to heat it to a temperature at which it can more readily be used. This energy expenditure is minimal (only 100 to 150 calories per day, or 1 pound a month), but over the course of a year, it can add up to a substantial weight loss (12 pounds or so).

A BURNING QUESTION

DOES THIS STUFF REALLY WORK?

If at this point you still need more convincing that there are other, more effective ways to burn fat than endless hours of aerobic exercise and starvation diets, I don't know what else to tell you. I've presented you with sound scientific evidence to support my claims and offered the physiques of some of the world's leanest athletes as a testament to the power that anaerobic exercise has on metabolism. I've even given you some insights into how I've successfully used this type of training with numerous clients over the years. Most important, I've made it clear that you can adopt this type of approach without worrying that you're sacrificing cardiovascular health.

I realize that at times throughout this chapter it may have seemed like vanity was the driving force behind these recommendations. Many in the pro-aerobics crowd have criticized this as being a more narcissistic approach to becoming healthy and fit. It's really a more efficient approach. I'm not saying that you can't burn fat and improve cardiovascular function by doing traditional aerobic exercise. It'll just take you a longer time to do it than if you adopted the strategy detailed in this chapter. And when it comes to burning fat, most people want to see results in the shortest time frame possible.

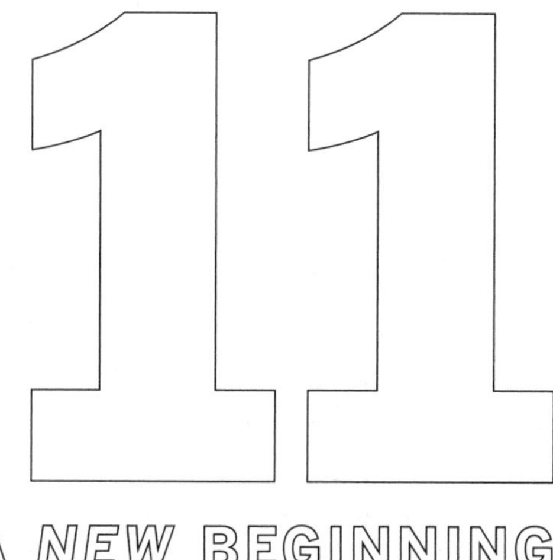

A NEW BEGINNING

TAKE THE NEXT STEP INTO YOUR FITNESS FUTURE

Whew! You finally made it. It's been a long time getting to this point. You've been hit with an awful lot of information over the course of the past couple of hundred pages. So much, in fact, that I almost feel like I owe you some sort of certificate of completion. At the very least, perhaps a T-shirt with the phrase "Who you calling a Beginner?" emblazoned across the chest. Because let's face it, once you've gone through this program in its entirety, you'll be pretty far removed from beginner status. You'll understand and appreciate the importance of things like assessing your physical abilities prior to starting a program and adequately preparing your body before jumping into intensive training. Best of all, you'll know that a properly periodized program is the key to making continued progress.

The big question now is: What comes next? Remember, at best you're looking at enough programs to last you about a year. Assuming that you're not going to stop there, you are going to need some alternative sources of information. As thorough as the contents of this book may be, they don't evolve with you past a certain point. I suppose you could go back and repeat certain phases that you may have liked more than others. It's just that the second time around, your body will likely adapt to them much more quickly, rendering them less effective than they were the first time through.

Some of you could also go back and try some of the programs you may not have had the confidence or ability to attempt on the first go-round. Things like the all-free-weight fat-burning workout or the weighted flexibility routine or maybe even one of the muscle-building or strength workouts you felt were a bit beyond your reach at the time. And there are certainly enough cardio routines strewn throughout the pages of this book to keep you busy for a while. Like I said, though, if you're lucky, that'll just about take you through your first full year of training. Obviously, to make fitness a lifelong commitment, you're going to need a little bit more of a long-term solution that that.

Perhaps I'm jumping the gun a bit here. After all, I am pretty much assuming that you're going to just seamlessly breeze through every phase, knowing exactly what path to take based on the criteria I've presented along the way. Sure, I suppose it could happen. Chances are, though, you're going to run into a little snag or two somewhere down the line. So rather than just assume that you're going to know how to piece all of this information together, perhaps it would help if I showed you how two types of beginners with completely different needs went about constructing their programs. At the very least, this will give you an opportunity to see what the various phases look like laid out in order.

A MAN WITH A PLAN

PUTTING IT ALL TOGETHER FOR MAXIMUM RESULTS

Scenario #1

Status: Newbie, age 27

Training goals: Lose 20 pounds and drop about 3 inches off waist (obtain the vaunted six-pack), while adding a couple of inches to the chest, shoulders, back, arms, and thighs

Available equipment: Full-service gym membership

Available training time: 3 days per week/1 hour per session

Phase 1: Self-Assessment

Postural: Moderate forward head, kyphosis, and lordosis (due to having a desk job). Some scapular winging as well.

Flexibility: Scored poorly on the overhead squat (knees pinching/feet collapsing inward somewhat) and had very limited rotational ability

Strength: Don't even ask. Zero chinups and one-legged squats.

Endurance: Could perform only 2 neutral-spine pushups at the specified tempo

Core: Again, fairly weak across the board. Failed the slow situp and barely made it past 75 degrees on the leg-lowering test.

Cardio: Because he runs sporadically, he didn't test quite as poorly here, but there's still plenty of room for improvement.

Phase 2: Corrective (4 weeks)

Based on the results of his assessment, I've picked out the appropriate exercises and stretches he needs to do to fix everything that's wrong. I'll list them first, then show you how he arranged them into a workout.

Exercises

Prone dumbbell row with elbows out

Reverse fly

Swiss ball hip extension

Cable hip abduction

Prone front raise

Side-lying external rotation

Negative chinup

Negative situp

Unilateral dumbbell touch

Plank

Pelvic tilt

Medicine ball wall rotation

Static Stretches (to be done both at the end of workouts and on off days from lifting)

Pec wall stretch

Internal rotator broomstick stretch

Hip flexor stretch

Butterfly adductor stretch

Hamstring doorway stretch

Pike calf stretch

Seated rotational stretch

Wall chin tuck

Dynamic Stretches (to be done as a warmup prior to lifting)

Spiderman

Reverse gate swing

Medicine ball wraparound

Reverse lunge with rotation

The following schedule would work well in keeping with his 3-day-per-week time commitment: two total-body workouts done on a rotating schedule, i.e., week 1 would be A/B/A and week 2 would be B/A/B. The workouts would be arranged as follows:

Workout A

Prone dumbbell row with elbows out: 2 sets × 6 to 10 reps

Swiss ball hip extension: 2 sets × 6 to 10 reps

Prone front raise: 2 sets × 8 to 10 reps

Unilateral dumbbell touch: 2 sets × 6 to 8 reps (each side)

Side-lying external rotation: 2 sets × 10 reps (each side)

Negative situp: 2 sets × 8 to 10 reps

Pelvic tilt: 2 sets × 10 to 12 reps

Plank: 2 sets × 20 to 30 seconds

Medicine ball wall rotation: 2 sets × 5 or 6 reps (each side)

Workout B

Negative chinup: 2 sets × 6 reps

Reverse fly: 2 sets × 8 to 10 reps

Cable hip abduction: 2 sets × 8 to 10 reps

Prone front raise: 2 sets × 6 to 10 reps

Negative situp: 2 sets × 8 to 10 reps

Pelvic tilt: 2 sets × 10 to 12 reps

Plank: 2 sets × 20 to 30 seconds

Medicine ball wall rotation: 2 sets × 5 or 6 reps (each side)

Notice that the exercises are divided up into two different total-body workouts (with the exception of the core exercises, which will be done every time he trains) so he won't feel overwhelmed by doing too many exercises in each workout. I'd also like you to pay particular attention to the set and rep recommendations. Since the aim is to correct imbalances and retrain muscles to work the way they're supposed to, largely through repetition, the repetitions often start at 8 and go as high as 12 per set for some exercises. For other, much more difficult exercises (negative chinups, for example), 6 reps per set will be plenty. The higher reps for certain exercises are not about burning fat but about bolstering tendon and ligament strength while building a good overall conditioning base. This young newbie will undoubtedly notice that they'll also allow him to get a good sweat going so he'll feel like he's doing some real work during this phase.

Speaking of working up a sweat, because the cardio portion of the workouts will be light and relatively unstructured, he could opt to include it either prior to strength work, as a warmup, or immediately after he's finished training. It really doesn't make much of a difference since the intensity will be fairly low. All we're trying to do here is get him used to some form of continuous, low-intensity exercise to increase bloodflow and improve circulation to his working muscles. We'll save the more intensive cardio work for later phases.

Phase 3: Basic Training (4 weeks)

In this phase, he goes from fixing weak links to upping the intensity slightly to prepare his body for the next two phases. He's also going to switch from a 3-day-per-week plan to a 4-day, adding one extra brief cardio workout. This will allow him to get in two strength/core workouts and two cardio/flexibility workouts per week. The emphasis on daily stretching will continue; he'll do a little extra following his cardio workouts. The plan shakes out as follows, with a slash (/) between two exercises indicating that that pairing is to be performed as a superset.

Strength/Core: 2× per week

Dumbbell squat, hammer curl, and press/lat pulldown: 2 or 3 sets × 6 to 10 reps of each

Alternating lunge: 2 or 3 sets × 6 to 10 reps (each leg)

Dumbbell bench press/one-arm row with elbow out: 2 or 3 sets × 6 to 10 reps of each

Unanchored situp: 2 sets × 10 to 12 reps

Russian twist: 2 sets × 5 or 6 reps (each side)

Lateral crunch: 2 sets × 8 to 10 reps (each side)

Superman: 2 sets × 10 to 12 reps

Because he'll be using heavier weights during this phase, I'm prescribing slightly longer rest intervals between sets (60 seconds) to help facilitate recovery. He'll also have the option of doing an extra set on all of the large-muscle-group exercises if he feels he can handle the increased training demand. There are also a few new and more challenging exercises sprinkled into the workouts.

The cardio/flexibility part of his program will be relatively short and sweet. He'll shoot for two brief, yet intense interval workouts lasting no longer than 20 minutes total, including warmup and cooldown. The best modes of exercise for these cardio workouts include running, stairclimbing, rope-jumping, and rowing.

Work interval: 15 seconds

Recovery interval: 45 seconds

Number of intervals: 12 to 15

Intensity of work intervals: 8.5 to 9.5

Recovery intervals: 5 to 6.5

As far as stretching goes, he'll perform the appropriate mobility sequences from Chapter 7 (Workout A on page 130) prior to his lifting workouts and static stretching after both strength-training and cardio work.

Phase 4: Muscle Building (4 weeks)

Here our subject makes a pronounced effort to start adding some muscle mass. Assuming he also makes the appropriate nutritional modifications outlined in Chapter 8, the following workouts should prove very effective toward reaching that goal.

Perform these workouts on a rotating schedule each week: A/B/A one week, B/A/B the next. All of the exercises have been arranged into supersets and require longer rest intervals than those used in the previous phase: 90 seconds.

Workout A

Squat/incline dumbbell bench press: 2 or 3 sets × 6 to 10 reps

Lying leg curl/one-arm row: 2 to 3 sets × 8 to 10 reps

Calf raise/cable external rotation: 2 or 3 sets × 10 to 12 reps

Lateral bridge/Swiss ball crunch: 2 or 3 sets × 5 or 6 reps

Workout B

Chinup or lat pulldown/deadlift: 2 to 3 sets × 6 to 10 reps

Standing barbell shoulder press/dumbbell lunge: 2 or 3 sets × 8 to 10 reps

Upright row/reverse fly: 2 or 3 sets × 8 to 10 reps

Back extension/Incline reverse crunch: 2 or 3 sets × 10 to 12 reps

Considering this phase's goal of building muscle mass, the cardio recommendation here is that each off day he should do one workout of a sufficient intensity to maintain cardiovascular fitness. However, because the workout is of such a short duration, he could opt to add in an additional workout following strength training one other time during the week if he so chooses.

The Pyramid (12 minutes)

Works best with: Bike sprints, rowing machine, VersaClimber, and Upper Body Ergometer (UBE)

Work intervals: Follow a pyramid scheme of 15 seconds/30 seconds/45 seconds/60 seconds/45 seconds/30 seconds/15 seconds

Recovery intervals: 30 seconds/60 seconds/90 seconds/120 seconds/90 seconds/60 seconds/30 seconds

RPE levels: 8 to 9 for the work intervals and 6 to 7 for the recovery intervals

Phase 5: Strength (4 weeks)

Since our newbie is a bit on the younger side, he'll be doing the more aggressive of the two strength workouts. He must still take care to stress form over weight. The higher-rep range for the reverse fly and prone external rotation is due to the postural components of those exercises and the fact that they isolate muscles and therefore make heavy loading difficult.

Workout A

Squat or leg press: 4 sets of 4 to 6 reps

Barbell push press or incline dumbbell bench press: 4 sets of 4 to 6 reps

Prone dumbbell row with elbows out: 4 sets of 4 to 6 reps

Split squat: 4 sets of 4 to 6 reps

Reverse fly: 3 sets of 8 to 10 reps

Workout B

Turkish get-up: 4 sets of 4 to 6 reps (each side)

Reverse pushup (supinated grip): 4 sets of 4 to 6 reps

Overhead squat: 4 sets of 4 to 6 reps

T-pushup: 4 sets of 4 to 6 reps (each side)

Lower-body rotation: 3 sets of 8 to 10 reps

Workout C

Chinup or lat pulldown: 4 sets of 4 to 6 reps

Clean pull or dumbbell deadlift and shrug: 4 sets of 4 to 6 reps

Barbell bench press: 4 sets of 4 to 6 reps

Swiss ball leg curl or lying leg curl: 4 sets of 4 to 6 reps

Prone external rotation: 2 or 3 sets × 10 to 12 reps

Here he can opt for a 2- or 3-day cardio approach since the extra energy output likely won't negatively impact strength development. The following should work well.

Work interval: 3 minutes

Recovery: 3 minutes

Number of intervals: 4 to 5

Work interval intensity: 7 to 8

Recovery interval intensity: 5.5 to 6.5

Works best with: Running (moderate pace), hiking, stairclimbing, and bike riding

Phase 6: Fat Loss (4 Weeks)

Time to shed that unwanted flab with some circuit training. Seeing as how our newbie trains in a commercial gym, I'd advise that he go with the more concentrated version of the PHA protocol. Given the brevity of these workouts, he could opt to include some brief interval training and extra core work of his choosing, either after his workouts or on off days if he has the time.

Mini-Circuit Workout #1

Do 10 to 12 reps of each exercise and rest 30 to 60 seconds between supersets.

Barbell bench press and split squat: 3 sets each

90 to 120 seconds on rower

Incline reverse crunch and lying leg curl: 3 sets each

90 to 120 seconds on VersaClimber

Cable row and dumbbell calf raise: 3 sets each

90 to 120 seconds on stationary bike

Mini-Circuit Workout #2

Lat pulldown and squat: 3 sets each

90 to 120 seconds on rower

Neutral-grip dumbbell shoulder press and situp: 3 sets each

90 to 120 seconds on VersaClimber

Dumbbell incline bench press and Romanian deadlift: 3 sets each

90 to 120 seconds on stationary bike

Scenario #2

Status: Ex-jock, age 55

Training goals: Increase strength and flexibility, improve cardiovascular fitness, and redistribute weight by losing about 2 inches from waist and adding a few inches to upper body and thighs for hiking and swimming

Available training equipment: Works out at home and has a set of PowerBlocks, a barbell, some free weights, a bench, and a Swiss ball

Available training time: 2 days per week/45 minutes per session

Phase 1: Self-Assessment

Postural: Severe forward head and kyphosis

Flexibility: Low score on modified sit and reach test and poor overhead squat (arms drifted way forward, back rounded), not to mention that the lower he got, the more his feet turned out (externally rotated)

Muscular strength: Not totally pathetic—3 chinups, almost did 1 full one-leg squat (stopped due to excessive back rounding)

Muscular endurance: Able to do 5 neutral-spine pushups

Core: Made it to about 15 degrees from the floor on leg-lowering test and passed slow-situp test

Cardio: Due to lots of swimming and hiking, scored well on Queens College step test. Would, however, still like to improve cardiovascular fitness.

Phase 2: Corrective (4 to 6 weeks)

As you'll notice from the results of his assessment, this guy doesn't have as many weaknesses as the first subject. Because of this and the fact that he can commit to only two workouts per week, I elected to have him do all of his exercises each time he trains. I just flipped the order from one workout to the next to keep things interesting for him. I included several good core drills (bird dog, plank, and Russian twist) that are worthwhile for most guys regardless of whether they scored poorly on related self-assessment tests. Here are the stretches and exercises he'll be doing.

Exercises

Cable row

Reverse fly

Side-lying external rotation

Unilateral Romanian deadlift

Swiss ball hip extension

Bird dog

Plank

Russian twist

Static Stretches

Wall chin tuck

Pec wall stretch

Internal rotator broomstick stretch

Lat stretch
Hamstring doorway stretch
Pike calf stretch
Glutes and piriformis stretch

Dynamic Stretches
Frankenstein
Gate swing
Medicine ball woodchopper
Hip walk

And here's what the exercises look like arranged into workouts:

Workout A
Prone dumbbell row: 2 sets × 10 to 12 reps
Reverse fly: 2 sets × 10 to 15 reps
Side-lying external rotation: 2 sets × 10 to 15 reps
Unilateral Romanian deadlift: 2 sets × 8 to 10 reps (each side)
Swiss ball hip extension: 2 sets × 10 to 12 reps
Superman: 2 sets × 10 to 15 reps
Plank: 2 sets × 20 to 30 seconds
Russian twist: 2 sets × 6 to 8 reps (each side)

Workout B
Russian twist: 2 sets × 8 reps (each side)
Plank: 2 sets × 20 to 30 seconds
Superman: 2 sets × 8 reps
Swiss ball hip extension: 2 sets × 8 reps
Unilateral Romanian deadlift: 2 sets × 6 reps (each side)
Side-lying external rotation: 2 sets × 10 to 15 reps
Reverse fly: 2 sets × 10 reps
Prone dumbbell row: 2 sets of 10 to 12 reps

In case you're wondering about the complete omission of direct chest work for this guy, as well as for the newbie, realize that each of them had an issue with kyphotic posture. Including pec work at this point would only exacerbate the problem. After 4 weeks of intensive stretching and upper-back strengthening, both guys will likely be able to add in some chest work in the next phase.

Given the fact that this guy is already in decent cardiovascular shape, he'll adopt an unstructured approach to his cardio workouts during this corrective phase, doing them either before or after his weight workout, or if he has the time, on off days from training. He'll also follow the same warmup and stretching guidelines as our first subject.

Phase 3: Basic Training (4 weeks)

Here, again, he'll perform the same workout two times per week, this time keeping the order of the exercises constant.

Strength/Core: 2× per week
Dumbbell squat: 2 sets × 8 to 10 reps
Dumbbell bench press: 2 sets × 8 to 10 reps
Reverse lunge: 2 sets × 8 to 10 reps (each leg)
One-arm row with elbow out: 2 sets × 8 to 10 reps
Unanchored situp: 2 sets × 8 to 10 reps
Neutral-grip dumbbell shoulder press: 2 sets × 8 to 10 reps
Bicycle: 2 sets × 8 to 10 reps (each side)
Oblique jackknife: 2 sets × 8 to 10 reps (each side)
Swiss ball back extension: 2 sets × 8 to 10 reps

For his first structured form of cardio, twice a week he'll go with an interval workout slightly less intense and longer in duration than the subject in our first example. His flexibility focus will be on dynamic warmups (either of the two on page 130) prior to workouts and static stretching once he's finished training.

Work interval: 30 seconds

Recovery interval: 60 seconds

Number of intervals: 14 to 16

Work interval intensity: 7.5 to 8

Recovery interval intensity: 6 to 7

Phase 4: Muscle Building (4 to 6 weeks)

This former BMOC will do two intense total-body workouts each week that prioritize lower-body lifts in order to capitalize on the hormonal release triggered by using larger muscle groups.

Workout A

Barbell squat: 2 sets × 8 to 10 reps

Swiss ball leg curl: 2 sets × 6 to 8 reps

Barbell bench press: 2 sets × 8 to 10 reps

Prone dumbbell row with elbows out: 2 sets × 8 to 10 reps

Dumbbell calf raise: 2 sets × 8 to 10 reps

Cable external rotation: 2 sets × 10 to 12 reps

Incline reverse crunch: 2 sets × 8 to 10 reps

Dumbbell woodchopper: 2 sets × 10 to 12 reps (5 to 6 per side)

Workout B

Barbell deadlift or dumbbell deadlift: 2 sets × 8 to 10 reps (each leg)

Lunge: 2 sets × 8 to 10 reps (each leg)

Chinup or lat pulldown: 2 sets × max reps (if more than 5)

Standing barbell shoulder press: 2 sets × 8 to 10 reps

One-arm row with elbow out: 2 sets × 8 to 10 reps

Back extension: 2 sets × 10 to 12 reps

Lateral bridge: 2 sets × 8 to 10 reps (4 to 5 per side)

Swiss ball crunch: 2 sets × 8 to 10 reps

For his cardio, he'll do the Yo-Yo, a workout that works well with a variety of cardio drills including skipping rope, sprints, rowing machines, and stairclimbing.

Work intervals: 15 seconds and 45 seconds (6 to 8 rounds)

Recovery intervals: 30 seconds and 90 seconds (6 to 8 rounds)

RPE levels: 8.5 to 9 for the work intervals; 6.5 to 7 for the recovery intervals

During this phase he'll also continue with both dynamic and static stretching before and after his workouts, respectively.

Phase 5: Strength (4 to 6 weeks)

This is the first phase where I'd ask him to work out a third day per week. If that weren't possible, I'd simply have him alternate between the two workouts.

Workout A (Monday & Friday)

Turkish get-up: 4 sets × 4 to 6 reps (each leg)

Reverse pushup (supinated grip): 4 sets × 4 to 6 reps

Elevated one-leg squat: 4 sets × 4 to 6 reps (each leg)

Overhead squat: 4 sets × 4 to 6 reps

Lower-body rotation: 3 sets × 8 to 10 reps

Workout B (Wednesday)

Barbell deadlift (or dumbbell deadlift): 4 sets × 4 to 6 reps

Barbell push press (or incline dumbbell bench press): 4 sets × 4 to 6 reps

Split squat: 4 sets × 4 to 6 reps (each leg)

One-arm row: 4 sets × 4 to 6 reps (each leg)

Prone external rotation: 2 to 3 sets × 10 to 12 reps

For cardio, we're still going with intervals here, just not at the same intensity used in previous phases. The following protocol can be applied to any number of cardio activities, including cycling, stairclimbing, running, and rowing.

Work interval: 3 minutes

Recovery interval: 3 minutes

Number of intervals: 4 or 5

Work interval intensity: 7 or 8

Recovery interval intensity: 5.5 to 6.5

Phase 6: Fat Loss (4 weeks)

Since he trains at home alone, full PHA circuits are on the menu here. To avoid hassles with changing the weights between sets, I've indicated whether the exercises should be done with either a barbell or dumbbells. This should help keep the flow of the workouts running smoothly. These workouts are different than the PHA circuits provided in Chapter 10, to give our subject (and you, too) the opportunity for more variety. Perform each exercise for 10 to 12 reps with a 60- to 90-second rest interval between circuits.

PHA Workout #1
Squat (barbell) or split squat (dumbbells)
Prone row (dumbbells)
Incline reverse crunch (bodyweight)
Swiss ball leg curl (bodyweight)
Bench press (barbell)

PHA Workout #2
Chinup or reverse pushup (bodyweight)
Deadlift (barbell)
Rotational situp (bodyweight)
Shoulder press (dumbbell)
Lunge (dumbbell)

He's actually got a couple of options for cardio. He could choose to add 1 to 2 minutes of intense cardio activity (RPE of 13 to 16) at the end of each circuit. Or he could opt to include an interval workout of his choice when he's through lifting. Static flexibility exercises should, as always, be done at the end of his workouts and on off days from lifting.

THE NEXT STEP

At this point our subjects—and you, of course—will have gone through between 20 and 24 weeks of training, or roughly 5 to 6 months. In going forward, you have the following options to choose from.

1. **Attempt to create your own workout routine.** Honestly, though, you're probably not experienced enough for this yet.
2. **Go back and try some of the programs in this book that you haven't done yet.** There are probably enough to take you through at least another couple of months. Take the young newbie in this chapter's first scenario, for example. Now that he's built up his body to withstand more intensive forms of training, he can take a more aggressive approach to burning off any leftover flab he might have. He could always try 3 to 4 weeks of the all-free-weight fat-loss workout from Chapter 8, perhaps followed by a month of mixing and matching various lifting programs and cardio workouts just to spice things up a bit. The ex-jock in scenario #2 has even more options at his disposal. Because his age initially relegated him to many of the easier routines in each phase, he could always run through them again, this time selecting some of the more challenging workouts. Or he could opt to try things like the free-weight fat-burning workout, "Weighty Issues," on page 155. And, as with our first subject, there are certainly more than enough cardio workouts for him to choose from.

Despite these alternatives, in the end this book can take you only so far. Once you've completed the majority of the programs in it, you're going to need to consider the final option. . . .

3. **Follow some pre-made routine from a magazine, book, or Web site.** This is certainly an option; after all, you are far better equipped to do so now than you were several months ago. However, I doubt you'd see the same kind of results you've experienced using the more individualized approach. So if you're going to use such a routine, make sure it's from a quality information source. To that end, I've compiled a list of some other places you can turn to for the very latest, cutting-edge dietary and training information.

- ***Scrawny to Brawny.*** This book and the companion Web site, www.scrawnytobrawny.com, are comprehensive guides to natural muscle building courtesy of yours truly and my co-author, John Berardi. Though they are targeted mainly toward skinny guys who have a hard time gaining muscle, they also have a lot of application for guys of all shapes and sizes who are interested in getting bigger. They're especially valuable for teens due to their strong anti-steroid message. You'll find training routines, diets, and even muscle-building recipes. Not to mention the Web site's online forum where John and I personally respond to any questions you might have.
- ***The Men's Health Home Workout Bible:*** This is a book that I co-authored with noted fitness writer Lou Schuler. If you train at home, this one is simply a must-have. Aside from detailed pictures and descriptions of more than 400 exercises you can do in your own home, it also includes beginner, intermediate, and advanced workout routines that you can do regardless of what type of setup you have. Plus, it includes complete workout logs to help track your progress.
- **JohnBerardi.com:** There's that name again. There's a reason for that, though: John is one of the best and most highly sought-after nutritional specialists in the world. Also an accomplished strength and conditioning coach in his own right, John currently consults with top professional athletes throughout the United States and Canada. What I like best is that, despite his elite status, his site includes tons of useful information for people of all ages and fitness levels. Whether you want to learn about the power of antioxidants, food allergies, what to put in your post-workout shake, or the latest findings in the field of nutritional research, you'll find it all at John's site.
- **Jpfitness.com (forums):** Celebrated personal trainer John Paul Francouer hosts an amazing message board on his Web site. You can enter into discussions on a staggering array of topics including how to improve functional strength, the best age for kids to start training, the impact that the timing and composition of your meals have on your workouts, and on and on. Not to mention the fact that highly regarded experts including Francouer himself typically field your questions.
- **ExRx.net:** A great site where you can find either pictures or video clips of just about any exercise or stretch you can possibly think of. Deserves to be bookmarked by anyone who's serious about fitness.

IT'S ALL UP TO YOU NOW

I've done just about all I can to get you started on what will hopefully become a lifelong commitment to staying healthy and fit. You no longer have to feel awkward or unsure when you walk into a gym or fear that you won't know what to do if you exercise at home. As long as you surround yourself with the proper equipment, you can rest assured that you now have the knowledge you need to reach your goals, regardless of what those might be. In fact, I'd even go so far as to say that you know just as much—if not more—about keeping fit than most of the people who frequent gyms. And that includes most of the trainers!

Knowledge alone, however, will take you only so far. You have to be able to implement it for it to have any real value. That takes lots of hard work and dedication, which is something that no book, regardless how comprehensive, can provide. So in the end, it really comes down to a question of how badly you want it. For years now, you've talked about wanting to become more fit, but you have always been able to fall back on the excuse that you didn't know how to get started. Well, now you have a definitive plan of action for doing just that—one that, if followed correctly, can produce results the likes of which you never even thought possible. I've done my part; the rest is up to you.

YOUR MUSCLES, FRONT VIEW

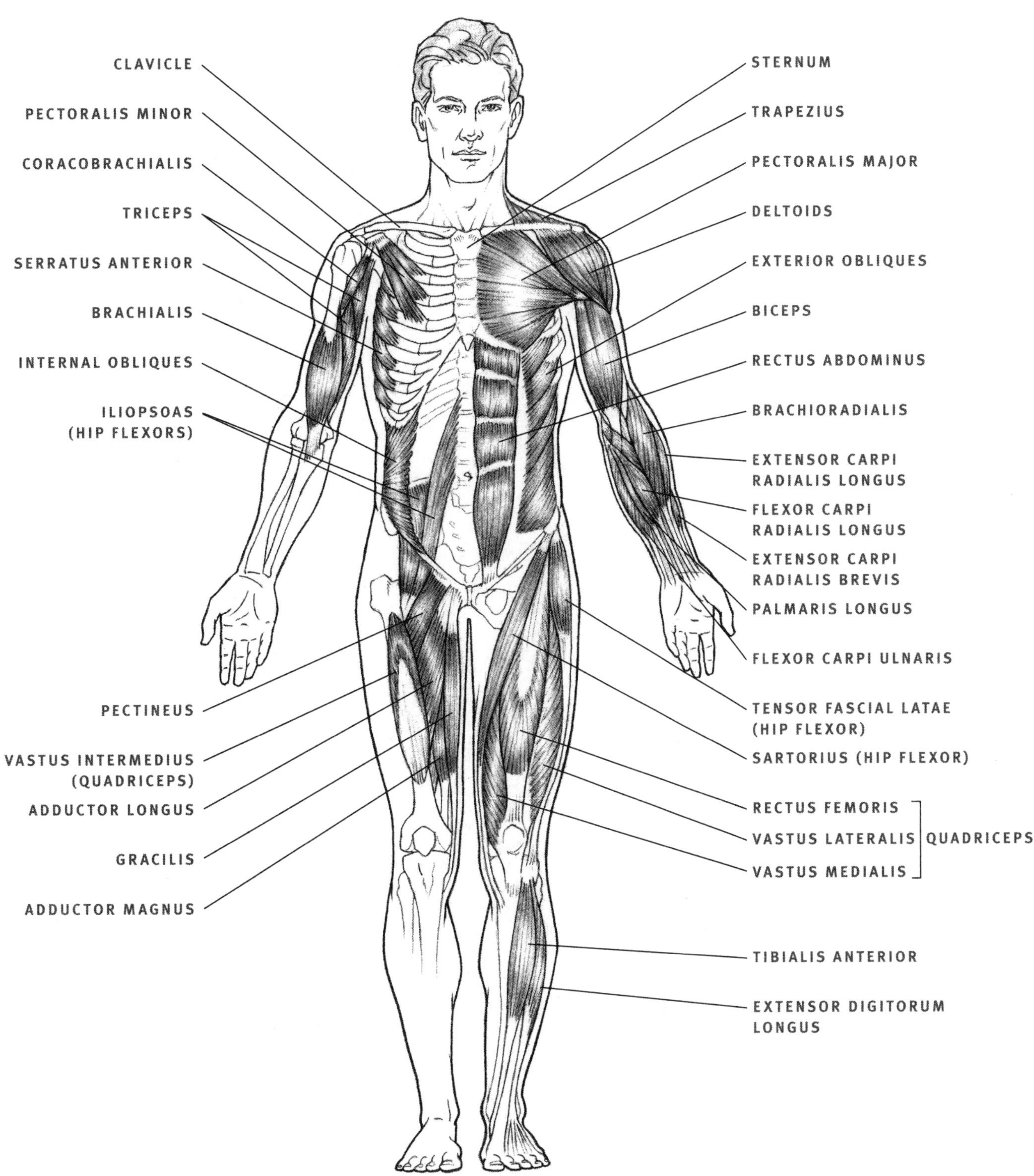
CLAVICLE
PECTORALIS MINOR
CORACOBRACHIALIS
TRICEPS
SERRATUS ANTERIOR
BRACHIALIS
INTERNAL OBLIQUES
ILIOPSOAS
(HIP FLEXORS)
PECTINEUS
VASTUS INTERMEDIUS
(QUADRICEPS)
ADDUCTOR LONGUS
GRACILIS
ADDUCTOR MAGNUS
STERNUM
TRAPEZIUS
PECTORALIS MAJOR
DELTOIDS
EXTERIOR OBLIQUES
BICEPS
RECTUS ABDOMINUS
BRACHIORADIALIS
EXTENSOR CARPI
RADIALIS LONGUS
FLEXOR CARPI
RADIALIS LONGUS
EXTENSOR CARPI
RADIALIS BREVIS
PALMARIS LONGUS
FLEXOR CARPI ULNARIS
TENSOR FASCIAL LATAE
(HIP FLEXOR)
SARTORIUS (HIP FLEXOR)
RECTUS FEMORIS
VASTUS LATERALIS
VASTUS MEDIALIS
QUADRICEPS
TIBIALIS ANTERIOR
EXTENSOR DIGITORUM
LONGUS

YOUR MUSCLES, BACK VIEW

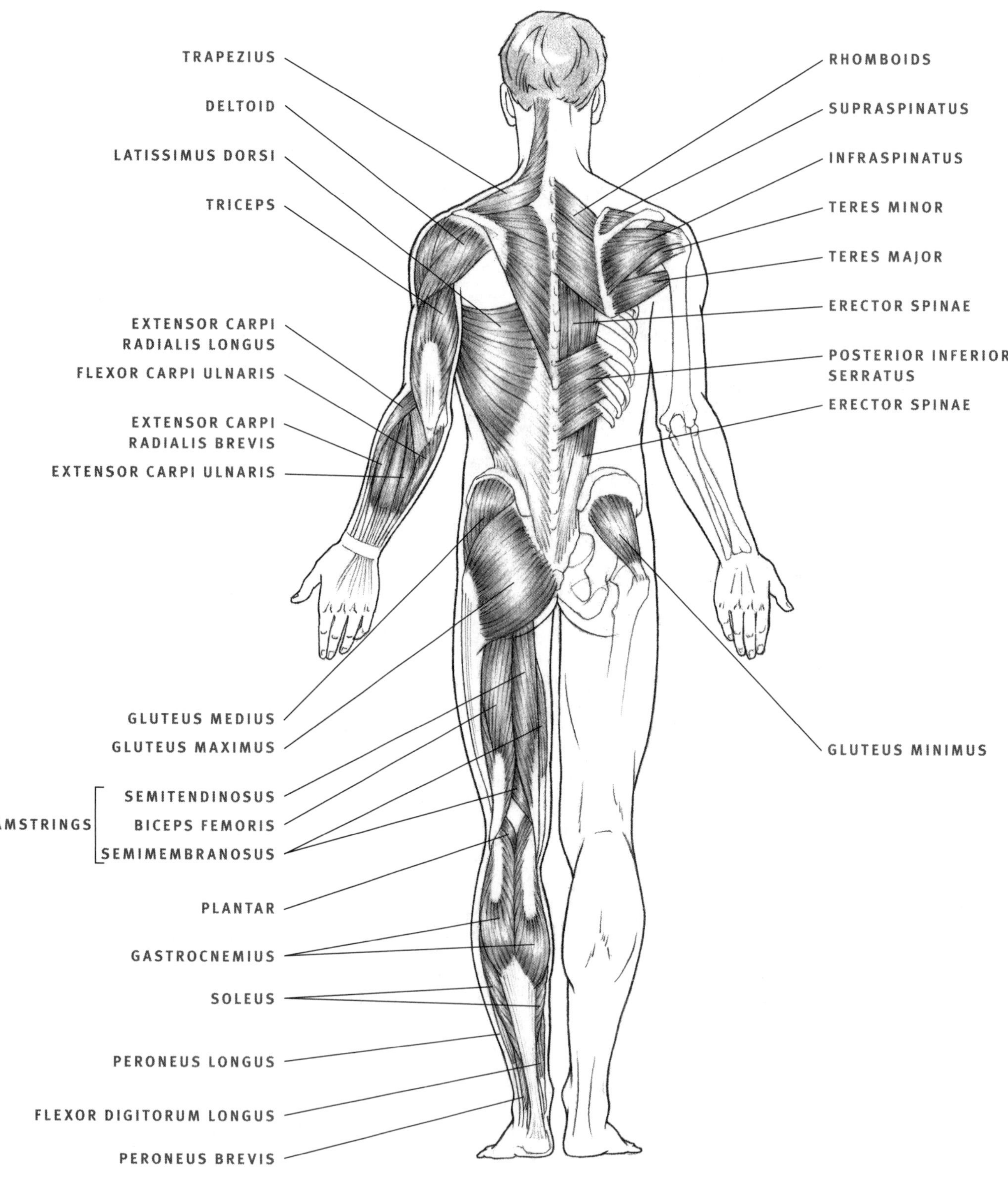

TRAPEZIUS
DELTOID
LATISSIMUS DORSI
TRICEPS
EXTENSOR CARPI RADIALIS LONGUS
FLEXOR CARPI ULNARIS
EXTENSOR CARPI RADIALIS BREVIS
EXTENSOR CARPI ULNARIS
GLUTEUS MEDIUS
GLUTEUS MAXIMUS
HAMSTRINGS
SEMITENDINOSUS
BICEPS FEMORIS
SEMIMEMBRANOSUS
PLANTAR
GASTROCNEMIUS
SOLEUS
PERONEUS LONGUS
FLEXOR DIGITORUM LONGUS
PERONEUS BREVIS
RHOMBOIDS
SUPRASPINATUS
INFRASPINATUS
TERES MINOR
TERES MAJOR
ERECTOR SPINAE
POSTERIOR INFERIOR SERRATUS
ERECTOR SPINAE
GLUTEUS MINIMUS

GLOSSARY

Abduction: Movement of a limb away from the middle of the body, such as bringing an arm from a hanging-down position to shoulder height.

Adduction: Movement of a limb toward the middle of the body, such as bringing an arm from an extended position at the shoulder down to the side.

Aerobic exercise: Exercise with oxygen; any activity in which the body is able to supply adequate oxygen to the working muscles for a period of time. Running, cross-country skiing, and cycling are examples of aerobic activities.

Agonist: Muscle directly engaged in contraction that is primarily responsible for movement of a body part; i.e., when performing a curl with the arm, the biceps is the agonist.

Anaerobic exercise: Exercise without oxygen; any activity in which the oxygen demands of the muscles are so high that they rely upon an internal metabolic process for oxygen, resulting in lactic acid buildup. Short bursts of "all-out" activities such as sprinting or weight lifting are examples of anaerobic exercise.

Antagonist: Muscle that counteracts the agonist, lengthening when the agonist muscle contracts; i.e., the triceps are the antagonist of the biceps.

Antioxidants: Vitamins A, C, and E, along with various minerals, which protect the body from free radicals, unstable cells that are naturally created in the body and also are caused by factors such as smoking and radiation. Free radicals may cause cell damage that leads to disease.

Barbell: An iron weight used for exercise, consisting of a rigid handle 5 to 7 feet long, with detachable metal discs, or plates, at each end.

Basal metabolic rate (BMR): The rate at which the body burns calories while awake but at rest (usually measured in calories per day).

Bioimpedance: The resistance of a path through the body (typically measured between the feet and/or hands), most often used to estimate body fat percentages because fat conducts electricity more poorly than muscle.

Body fat percentage: The amount of fat in your body, generally expressed as a percentage. While some body fat is necessary for temperature regulation and the conduction of nerve impulses, a high percentage has been proven to be hazardous to health.

Bulking up: Gaining body weight by adding muscle, body fat, or both.

Carbohydrate: Digestible food components such as starches and sugars that are composed of carbon, hydrogen, and oxygen but not nitrogen. Carbohydrates are the main constituent of most vegetables and fruits, provide four calories per gram, and are present only in small quantities in animal products.

Cardiovascular training: Physical conditioning that strengthens the heart and blood vessels, resulting in a greater level of conditioning in terms of the body's increased ability to utilize fuel more effectively.

Catabolism: The breakdown of lean muscle mass, normally as a result of injury, immobilization, and poor nutrition.

Central nervous system (CNS): The brain and spinal cord.

Cholesterol: A lipid (fat) with both good and bad implications within the human body. Good cholesterol, known as high-density lipoprotein (HDL), is required for the production of many steroid hormones. Bad cholesterol, called low-density lipoprotein (LDL), is associated with heart disease and stroke.

Circuit training: Going quickly from one exercise station to another and doing a prescribed number of exercises or length of time on each station, the goal of which is to provide your body with a good cardiovascular and strength workout in minimal time.

Collar: Any kind of sleeve that may be slipped over the end of a weight bar and then tightened to hold weight plates securely on the bar, preventing the plates from slipping off, shifting position, or rattling during the exercise.

Compound movement: An exercise that targets more than one muscle or muscle group simultaneously; usually the movement involves flexing or extending at least two joints. Lat pulldowns, squats, and bench presses are all compound movements; curls, leg extensions, and flies are not.

Concentric muscle contraction: A contraction where a muscle shortens to perform work. Curling a barbell to your shoulders is an example of a concentric contraction.

Creatine: Naturally occurring in muscle tissue, creatine functions as a secondary reservoir for short-term energy to be drawn upon when ATP (adenosine triphosphate) stores—the energy storage molecule that drives muscular contraction—are depleted. Supplemental creatine monohydrate added to the diet will increase the concentration of creatine phosphate within muscle tissue, which may improve one's ability to perform brief, high-intensity exercise.

Crunch: A type of abdominal exercise that works your abs through a relatively small range of motion while simultaneously reducing lower-back strain.

Deadlift: One of the "big three" lifts (the other two being the squat and bench press) where the weight is lifted off the floor to approximately waist height.

Dehydration: Excessive loss of body fluid, sometimes caused by excessive perspiration (exercising intensely in the heat), urination (from consuming too many caffeinated beverages), or illness. Dehydration can also exist at more moderate levels due to inadequate fluid intake over a prolonged period.

Delayed onset muscle soreness (DOMS): Discomfort that is often felt 24 to 72 hours after intense or unfamiliar exercise. Part of the body rebuilding process, it is thought to be caused by microtears within muscles.

Dietary fat: Often referred to as *lipids* or *triglycerides*, this macronutrient contains nine calories per gram and serves a variety of functions in the body.

Dumbbell: Weight consisting of a rigid handle about 14 inches long with either fixed weights or detachable metal discs (plates) at each end.

Eccentric muscle contraction: A contraction where a muscle lengthens to perform work. Lowering the bar to your chest during a bench press is an example of an eccentric contraction.

Electrolytes: These particles capable of conducting electricity in a solution are used in many bodily activities. Potassium, sodium, and chloride are all forms of electrolytes.

Endurance: The ability of a muscle to produce force continually over a period of time.

Essential fatty acids (EFAs): Oils that are required by the body but obtainable only from food sources. EFAs include flaxseed oil and safflower oil.

Extension: Movement of a body part (i.e., hand, neck, trunk, etc.) from a bent to a straight position.

Fast twitch: Refers to muscle fibers that fire quickly and are utilized in anaerobic activities such as sprinting and power lifting.

Fiber: An indigestible component of food that is chemically classified as a carbohydrate (and may be included in the total carbohydrate content listed on food labels) and found primarily in unprocessed vegetables, nuts, grains, and fruits. Fiber does not provide calories but offers significant health benefits including the prevention of diseases such as diabetes, heart disease, and cancer.

Flexibility: Range of motion (ROM) in a joint or group of joints.

Glycemic index (GI): A system of measuring the extent to which various foods raise the blood sugar level. The benchmark is white bread, which has a GI of 100. The higher the score, the greater the rise in blood sugar.

Glycogen: The principle form of carbohydrate energy (glucose) stored within the muscles and liver.

Growth hormone: An anabolic hormone naturally released by the pituitary gland. It promotes muscle growth and the breakdown of body fat for energy; unfortunately, its levels are greatly reduced after the age of 20.

High-density lipoprotein (HDL): A blood substance that picks up cholesterol and helps remove it from the body; often referred to as "good cholesterol."

Hypertension: High blood pressure.

Hypertrophy: Increase in the size of muscle fibers.

Isometric muscle contraction: A contraction where a muscle maintains a constant length and joints do not move as it performs work. An isometric exercise is usually performed against a wall or other immovable object.

Lactic acid: A substance caused by anaerobic training; its buildup prevents continuation of exercise.

Ligament: Strong, fibrous band of tissue connecting two or more bones or pieces of cartilage, or supporting a muscle, fascia, or organ.

Low-density lipoprotein (LDL): A core of cholesterol surrounded by protein, often referred to as "bad cholesterol."

Lumbar: Lower region of the spine, vertebrae L1 to L5. Used for bending and extending the body forward and back, with the aid of the abdominal and erector spinae muscles.

Max: Maximum effort for 1 repetition of an exercise.

Muscle: Tissue consisting of fibers organized into bands or bundles that contract to cause bodily movement. Muscle fibers run in the same direction as the action they perform.

Muscle tone: Condition in which muscle is in a constant yet slight state of contraction and appears firm.

Peripheral Heart Action (PHA): A system of training in which you go from one exercise to another with little or no rest, preferably alternating upper-body and lower-body exercises. Designed for cardiovascular training and to develop muscle mass.

Prime mover: A muscle or group of muscles whose contraction produces the movement in an exercise.

Prone, pronation, pronated: Facedown or palm down.

Pumped: Slang meaning the muscles have been made large by increasing blood supply to them through exercise.

Repetition: One complete movement of an exercise.

Resistance training: Training with weights or other sources of resistance above and beyond the movement itself.

Rest interval: Pause between sets of an exercise, which allows muscles to recover partially before beginning the next set.

Rotator cuff: Four muscles (supraspinatus, infraspinatus, teres minor, and subscapularis) that run from the shoulder blade to the upper arm, or humerus, and together stabilize the shoulder joint.

Set: Fixed number of repetitions. For example, 10 repetitions may comprise 1 set.

Slow twitch: Muscle fibers that contract slowly, are resistant to fatigue, and are utilized in endurance activities such as long-distance running, cycling, or swimming.

Spinal erectors, erector spinae: Paired muscles on either side of the spine in the lower back, whose function is to straighten the spine.

Spot: Assist called upon by someone performing an exercise.

Spotter: Person who watches a person closely to see if any help is needed during a specific exercise.

Stabilizer: Muscle that assists in the performance of an exercise by steadying the joint or limb being moved without increasing the force being applied.

Static stretch: A stretch that is held in the stretched position for several seconds, without movement.

Sticking point: The most difficult part of a movement or exercise. Typically it is the midpoint during lifts such as bench presses and squats.

Strength: The ability of a muscle to produce maximum force.

Superset: Alternating back and forth between two exercises until the prescribed number of sets is completed.

Synergist: Muscle that assists in the performance of an exercise by adding to the force required to execute the movement.

Tendon: A band or cord of strong, fibrous tissue that connects muscle to bone.

Testosterone: Principal male hormone that accelerates tissue growth and stimulates bloodflow.

VO_2 max: The maximum amount of oxygen a person can utilize per minute of work. Often recorded as an evaluation of cardiovascular efficiency.

Warmup: Light, gradual exercise performed to get the body ready for more intense physical activity; it is often a slower version of the activity to follow: i.e., a light jog before a run.

INDEX

Boldface page references indicate photographs. Underscored references indicate boxed text

D

I

J

K

L

M

N

O

P

T

U

V

W